ASIAN STUDIES ASSOCIATION OF AUSTRALIA
Southeast Asia Publications Series

NO. 14
DEATH AND DISEASE IN SOUTHEAST ASIA

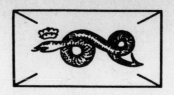

ASIAN STUDIES ASSOCIATION OF AUSTRALIA
Southeast Asia Publications Series

1 John Ingleson,
   Road to Exile: The Indonesian Nationalist Movement, 1927–1934

2 Heather Sutherland,
   The Making of a Bureaucratic Elite: The Colonial Transformation of the Javanese Priyayi

3 J. C. Jackson & Martin Rudner (eds.),
   Issues in Malaysian Development

4 Anthony Reid & David Marr (eds.),
   Perceptions of the Past in Southeast Asia

5 Alfons van der Kraan,
   Lombok: Conquest, Colonization and Underdevelopment, 1870–1940

6 Wang Gungwu,
   Community and Nation: Essays on Southeast Asia and the Chinese

7 Alfred W. McCoy & Ed. C. de Jesus (eds.),
   Philippine Social History: Global Trade & Local Transformations

8 Charles A. Coppel,
   Indonesian Chinese in Crisis

9 R. E. Elson,
   Javanese Peasants and the Colonial Sugar Industry

10 Benjamin A. Batson,
   The End of the Absolute Monarchy in Siam

11 Patrick Guinness,
   Harmony and Hierarchy in a Javanese Kampung

12 John Ingleson,
   In Search of Justice: Workers and Unions in Colonial Java, 1908–1926

13 Richard Robison,
   Indonesia: The Rise of Capital

14 Norman G. Owen (ed.)
   Death and Disease in Southeast Asia: Explorations in Social, Medical and Demographic History

DEATH AND DISEASE IN SOUTHEAST ASIA

Explorations in Social, Medical and
Demographic History

edited by
NORMAN G. OWEN

A publication of the
Asian Studies Association of Australia

SINGAPORE
OXFORD UNIVERSITY PRESS
OXFORD NEW YORK
1987

Oxford University Press
Oxford New York Toronto
Petaling Jaya Singapore Hong Kong Tokyo
Delhi Bombay Calcutta Madras Karachi
Nairobi Dar es Salaam Cape Town
Melbourne Auckland

and associates in
Beirut Berlin Ibadan Nicosia

ISBN 0 19 588853 7

Sole distributors in Australia and New Zealand for the
Asian Studies Association of Australia
George Allen & Unwin Australia

National Library of Australia
C.I.P. Entry

Death and disease in Southeast Asia.

Includes index.
ISBN 0 04 301280 9.

1. Mortality – Asia, Southeastern – History. 2. Epidemics – Asia,
Southeastern – History. 3. Health – Asia, Southeastern – History. I. Owen,
Norman G. II. Asian Studies Association of Australia. (Series: Southeast
Asia publications series; 14).

304.6'4'0959

Typeset in the Philippines by Vera-Reyes, Inc.
Printed in Malaysia by Peter Chong Printers Sdn. Bhd.
Published by Oxford University Press, Pte. Ltd.,
Unit 221, Ubi Avenue 4, Singapore 1440

Contents

Contributors   x

Acknowledgements   xii

I   INTRODUCTION   **1**

1 Toward a History of Health in Southeast Asia
  NORMAN G. OWEN   3

II   THE DEMOGRAPHIC EVIDENCE   **31**

2 Low Population Growth and Its Causes in
  Pre-Colonial Southeast Asia
  ANTHONY REID   33
3 Morbidity and Mortality in Java, 1820–1880:
  Changing Patterns of Disease and Death
  PETER BOOMGAARD   48
4 Morbidity and Mortality in Java, 1880–1940: The
  Evidence of the Colonial Reports
  PETER GARDINER AND MAYLING OEY   70
5 Measuring Mortality in the Nineteenth Century
  Philippines
  NORMAN G. OWEN   91

III CULTURE AND CURING   **115**

6 Bali: Myth, Magic and Morbidity
  BARBARA LOVRIC   117
7 Asiatic Cholera in Siam: Its First Occurrence and
  the 1820 Epidemic
  B. J. TERWIEL   142
8 Vietnamese Attitudes Regarding Illness and Healing
  DAVID G. MARR   162

IV THE BIOLOGY AND POLITICS OF DEATH 187

9 Death and Disease in Nineteenth Century Batavia
SUSAN ABEYASEKERE 189
10 Plague in Java
TERENCE H. HULL 210
11 The Influenza Pandemic of 1918 in Indonesia
COLIN BROWN 235
12 Blame, Responsibility and Remedial Action: Death, Disease and the Infant in Early Twentieth Century Malaya
LENORE MANDERSON 257

Index 283

Figures

4.1 Indices of Reported 'Native Deaths' and Epidemic
Deaths, Java and Madura, 1870–1903   71
4.2 Reported Deaths by Selected Epidemic Diseases,
Java and Madura, 1870–1903   77
5.1 Variation in Vital Rates by District, Bikol Region,
1845–46   100
5.2 Monthly Variation by Zone, Bikol Region,
1845–46   105
8.1 Sino-Vietnamese Conceptions of Man and the
Universe   165
8.2 Taking the Pulses, Vietnam, c. 1940   167
8.3 Medical Practitioner and Assistant Preparing
Ingredients, Vietnam, c. 1900   169
9.1 Population of Batavia, by Ethnic Group,
1815–1900   190
9.2 Ethnic Distribution of the Population of Batavia,
c. 1885   191
10.1 Plague Deaths in Java, 1910–39   211
10.2 House Improvements in Java, 1910–39   212
10.3 Inspection of houses and household effects during
the plague-fight in Java   217
10.4 Plague Deaths and House Improvements in Java,
by District, 1910–39   224
12.1 Infant Welfare Centre, Balik Pulau, Penang,
c. 1933   268
12.2 Chinese Grandmother and Toddler, Singapore,
c. 1910   270

Tables

2.1 Population Growth in Southeast Asia, 17th–18th
Centuries   35
2.2 Population Estimates for Southeast Asia in 1600   36
2.3 Population Estimates for Java, 1652–1880   46
2.4 Population Estimates for Indonesia outside Java,
1800–1930   47
3.1 Calculated Death Rate by Decade, Java, 1820–80   51
3.2 Estimated Excess Mortality, Java, 1820–80   51
3.3 Factors Affecting Malaria in Nineteenth Century
Java   59
4.1 Crude Death Rates in Java (Village Registration),
1915–29   73
5.1 Comparative Crisis Fertility and Mortality by
District, Bikol Region, 1845–46   99
5.2 Crisis Mortality by Month, Sample Parishes, Bikol
Region, 1845–46   103
5.3 Comparative Mortality, Selected Modern Asian
Famines   108
10.1 Plague Deaths in Java, by District, 1910–39   231
10.2 House Improvements Sponsored by the Plague
Service in Java, by District, 1911–39   233
11.1 Index of Flu-Related Mortality Rates, by Regency,
Java and Madura, 1918   238
12.1 Medical Facilities, Straits Settlements and
Federated Malay States, 1936   278

Maps

Map 1   Nineteenth Century Southeast Asia   32
Map 2   Colonial Java   54
Map 3   Bikol Region   98
Map 4   British Malaya   259

Contributors

Susan Abeyasekere is a Senior Lecturer at the Footscray Institute of Technology, Melbourne. She is the author of *One Hand Clapping: Indonesian Nationalists and the Dutch* (1976) and *Jakarta: A History* (forthcoming), and the editor of *From Batavia to Jakarta* (1985).

Peter Boomgaard is currently employed as Editor of the series of historical statistics on Indonesia, *Changing Economy in Indonesia*, at the Koninklijk Instituut voor de Tropen, Amsterdam. His main interests are the demographic and agricultural history of nineteenth century Java.

Colin Brown is a Senior Lecturer in the School of Modern Asian Studies at Griffith University, Brisbane. He is the author of several articles on modern Indonesian history and politics.

Peter Gardiner, formerly a visiting staff member at the Population Studies Center, Gajah Mada University, is now a private consultant in Jakarta. He has written extensively on Indonesian demography and economics, including such topics as vital registration, urbanization and rural credit.

Terence H. Hull is a Senior Research Fellow in Demography at the Australian National University, with a special interest in the Indonesian population. He is the author of a number of articles on the Indonesian Family Planning Programme, mortality trends, and the social and cultural determinants of fertility.

Barbara Lovric is currently completing a doctoral dissertation on Balinese rituals and medical traditions at the University of Sydney.

Lenore Manderson is a Senior Lecturer in the School of Sociology, the University of New South Wales. She is currently on secondment to the Department of Pacific and Southeast Asian History, Australian National University, where she is writing a book on health care and medical services in colonial Malaya. Her research interests have focused on Malaysia and on gender and health, and her earlier books are *Overpopulation in Java: Problems and Reactions* (1974) and *Women, Politics and Change* (1980). She is also editor of *Women's Work and Women's Roles* (1983).

David Marr is a Senior Fellow in Southeast Asian History at the Australian National University. His publications include *Vietnamese Anti-colonialism, 1885–1925* (1971) and *Vietnamese Tradition on Trial, 1920–1945* (1981).

Mayling Oey is a Research Associate at the Institute of Social and Economic Research, Faculty of Economics, University of Indonesia. She has published extensively on migration, fertility, and development in Indonesia.

Norman G. Owen has just taken up an appointment in the Department of History, University of Hong Kong, having been Senior Research Fellow in Pacific and Southeast Asian History, Australian National University, during the writing and editing of this volume. He is the author of *Prosperity Without Progress: Manila Hemp and Material Life in the Colonial Philippines* (1984), and editor/co-author of *Compadre Colonialism* (1972) and *The Philippine Economy and the United States* (1983).

Anthony Reid is Senior Fellow in Southeast Asian History at the Australian National University. His books include *The Contest for North Sumatra* (1969), *The Indonesian National Revolution* (1974) and *The Blood of the People: Revolution and the End of Traditional Rule in Northern Sumatra* (1979). He has recently edited *Slavery, Bondage and Dependency in Southeast Asia* (1983).

Barend Jan Terwiel is a Senior Lecturer in the Asian History Centre, Australian National University. He is the author of *Monks and Magic* (1975; 2nd edn 1979), *The Tai of Assam* (2 vols., 1980–81) and *A History of Modern Thailand 1767–1942* (1983). He has also edited *Seven Probes in Rural South East Asia* (1979), *Buddhism and Society in Thailand* (1984) and *Development Issues in Thailand* (1984).

Acknowledgements

THE idea for the conference that led to this book was planted long before I first set foot in Australia. Glenn A. May, Anthony Reid and David Marr of the Department of Pacific & Southeast Asian History, Research School of Pacific Studies, Australian National University, were the progenitors and prime movers of this event. Ably assisted by Jennifer Holmgren, Dr May was the principal organizer of the conference and should receive major credit for its success. The Research School of Pacific Studies provided funding and facilities. Participants came from all over Australia and around the world; besides those whose papers are included here we should like to express our gratitude to all who gave papers, chaired panels or served as discussants — J. C. Caldwell, Ian Catanach, Donald Denoon, Frank Fenner, James Fox, Paul Hinderling, Valerie Hull, Reynaldo C. Ileto, John Ingleson, Ann Kumar, Anton Lucas, Peter McDonald, Virginia Matheson, Doug Miles, William O'Malley, James Rush, Lado Ruzicka, Susan Serjeantson, F. B. Smith and the late Neville Stanley — as well as to others who attended and contributed their ideas so generously.

When the time came to prepare the papers for publication, the editorship fell to me by default, though I continued to benefit from consultations with Drs Reid, Marr, May and Jennifer Brewster. Dr Reid also co-ordinated the project while I was overseas and Dr Brewster, with the keyboard help of Dorothy McIntosh, Julie Gordon and Karen Haines, assembled the manuscript in a form fit for publishers to read. Robert Elson supplied excellent, if unofficial, editorial advice, particularly on matters Javanese. Suzie Jeffcoat and Keith Mitchell of the Cartography Section, Department of Human Geography, Research School of Pacific Studies, provided the maps and graphs. Finally, the Wellcome Trust awarded a most welcome grant toward the expenses of typesetting this volume, enabling us to present these essays to a wider public.

I INTRODUCTION

It is very naive to claim to understand men without knowing what sort of health they enjoyed.

MARC BLOCH
Feudal Society

1 Toward a History of Health in Southeast Asia

NORMAN G. OWEN

OVER the past few years historians of Southeast Asia have begun to discuss with each other the revolutionary findings of the 'new social history' in Europe and to wonder whether its questions and approaches might be systematically applied to the Southeast Asian past. Among many topics worthy of exploration—including urban history, popular mentalities, family and sexual relations, costume, entertainments, and both social and geographic mobility—perhaps the most fundamental are those that focus on the human body itself, in sickness and health.[1] The brute facts of 'birth, copulation and death' (in T. S. Eliot's phrase) manifest themselves in different ways at different places and times. Moreover, they are essentially egalitarian, which is of great importance to the continuing effort to write a non-elite history of Southeast Asia. Regardless of rank, wealth or ethnicity, everyone is entitled to just one birth and one death—even if in Southeast Asia, as elsewhere, rich and powerful men do get more than their share of copulation. To understand the history of these elements in the Southeast Asian past is to gain an important insight into the world that Southeast Asians inhabited and to which they responded.

In 1982, members of the Department of Pacific and Southeast Asian History of the Australian National University began to make plans for an exploratory conference on this topic, which had never been systematically approached from a historical perspective. They decided to focus on morbidity and mortality (rather than on nuptiality and fertility) in the hope that the dramatic nature of death, particularly by epidemic disease or other disaster, would make it relatively well documented. This conference, on 'Disease, Drugs and Death: Their History in Modern Southeast Asia,' was held at the Australian National University, 6–8 May 1983; no participant emerged unenlightened by the proceedings. The essays selected for this volume represent not just the ideas we

3

individually brought to the conference, but the revisions—often quite extensive—that the comments of our colleagues forced or inspired us to make.[2]

The topic itself seemed relatively straightforward at first. Death and disease are real; they appear to have a more 'objective' quality than the elusive *mentalité* of an eighteenth century Javanese aristocrat or a twentieth century Filipino peasant, and thus should be less susceptible to distortion by subjective interpretations or preconceptions. Human physiology can be studied without regard to varying human value systems; micro-organisms do their deadly or debilitating work independent of the culture of those they infest.

In practice it is not so simple. There are significant interactions between states of mind and states of body (psychosomatic afflictions are more common and complex than once believed) and there are culturally prescribed behaviours that directly affect human hospitality to various micro-organisms. More fundamentally, our knowledge of the physical past is itself transmitted through culture, whether Southeast Asian or colonial. It is hard enough, micro-biologists tell us, to identify a disease today, when the organisms involved may be isolated and placed under powerful microscopes. How much more difficult it is to know the nature of the 'great sicknesses' mentioned in Balinese legends, Thai chronicles, or the histories written by Spanish friars in the Philippines! When informed or reminded that the diseases themselves are also mutable,[3] so that the sources might be describing a syndrome that no longer even exists, historians may easily despair of ever learning 'what really happened', even in the most simple physical terms.

Each chronicler also makes decisions as to what is, and is not, recorded, and these decisions in turn are based on assumptions we can only partially decipher. What did it mean to be ill? How were illnesses perceived—as assaults by evil spirits, as evidence of physical or spiritual disharmony, as spiritual entities, as attacks by physical pathogens?[4] What made a particular disease worth mentioning at all—the number of victims, the distinctiveness or disruptiveness of its symptoms (leprosy, smallpox and cholera are almost always better documented than tuberculosis or indeterminate 'fevers'), the rapidity of its onslaught, its symbolic significance? It might be thought that at least counting the living and the dead would be a straightforward proposition, but we frequently discover that infants and marginal members of society (foreigners, slaves, hill tribes) are apparently underrepresented, implying cultural distinctions as to the relative importance of various types of human lives.[5]

The history of death and disease can be distorted not only by the cultures of those who left the records but by our own preconceptions about the Southeast Asian past. We may assume, for example, that the passing observations of travellers confirm what we already envisage as a linear sequence from regional 'underpopulation' in the nineteenth century to 'overpopulation' at present. We may extrapolate simple Western-based models of 'demographic transition' theory to assert that high mortality must have accompanied high fertility in pre-modern Southeast Asia. As beneficiaries of 'scientific' medicine today we may accept too readily colonial claims about its efficacy in the past. And those of us who are Westerners have always to contend with our secret belief that the jungle is *not* neutral, but full of nameless horrors and 'tropical' diseases that make the region far less safe than the salubrious temperate zones where our own civilization flourishes. Part of our task in studying death and disease in Southeast Asia must be to try to exorcise our own mythologies about the subject.

Yet if the difficulties in attempting such a study are great, so are its prospective rewards. Investigating the history of death and disease is not only valid—and fascinating—in its own right, but it can lead into many other areas of social history. Family size and structure depend not only on the demographic probabilities of survival of parents, spouses and children, but on popular perceptions of mortality; we need to explore whether Southeast Asians responded to the likelihood of early death by producing all the children they could or, as some sources suggest, by artificially restricting family size to improve their standard of living, and thus the odds of their survival as a family.[6] Mortality and morbidity also have important implications for the question of state power, which in the Southeast Asian past was typically based on control of labour and thus ultimately on the size and health of the population available for service. Even such institutions as slavery may have been affected, as they were in nineteenth century Africa, where epidemic losses increased the demand for slaves.[7]

Above all, the study of death and disease forces us to confront a world in which the vulnerability of human life was visible in a way unfamiliar to those of us living in the West today. Did the Southeast Asian past, characterized by high infant mortality, short life expectancy and the ever-present threat of irresistible epidemics,

resemble our own past, the plague-ridden Europe so vividly portrayed by Barbara Tuchman in *A Distant Mirror*? Was the dramatic recent diminution of mortality similarly prompted or
reinforced by improved nutrition, new medical and agricultural
technologies, and a more secular outlook on life in general? Or
was Southeast Asia as distinctive in the biological as in the cultural
sphere? Is there, in short, a uniquely Southeast Asian history of
health?

The essays that follow represent a wide range of methodologies
applied to an even wider range of historical questions, posed by
anthropologists, political scientists, sociologists and demographers
as well as historians.[8] The very diversity of the essays suggests the
excitement and potential frustration inherent in opening up a new
field; none of us yet knows which approaches will prove to be most
rewarding in future scholarly investigations. Yet there are patterns
in this seeming randomness, suggesting the extent to which the
field has been—and may continue for some time to be—shaped
not only by our questions but by the availability of sources.

One obvious tendency has been to emphasize crises, such as
cholera or influenza epidemics, at the expense of 'background'
mortality, the everyday deaths that carried away the majority of
Southeast Asians. Our knowledge of these episodes, extraordinary
by definition, reflects the bias of sources that, like ancient chronicles and contemporary news broadcasts, devote far more attention to periodic disasters than to the daily tragedy of lives cut
short. Tuberculosis, for example, tends not to be dramatic (until
art transfigures it), yet it killed far more Filipinos over the past two
centuries than all the cholera epidemics put together. In the
National Archives of the Philippines, however, there are many
boxes filled with documents on cholera; one would have to look
long and hard to locate a single file devoted to tuberculosis. Dutch
records would undoubtedly reveal a similar imbalance between,
for example, plague and infantile diarrhoea.

The disproportion in emphasis between the spectacular and the
ordinary is even greater when morbidity is taken into account.
Most Southeast Asians of the past, like their descendants today,
would have suffered from myriads of debilitating diseases, yet we
cannot with assurance measure this invalidity for even a single
historical period. Much of this everyday ill health, moreover,
would have been due to malnutrition and parasitic infestation,
whereas most of the demographic catastrophes (except for out-

right famine) are attributable to infectious diseases. The imbalance of attention may, if we are not careful, lead to a skewed vision of the real threats to the well-being of Southeast Asians in the past. Nor can this difficulty be surmounted simply by being aware of it; where local studies of morbidity or estimates of nutritional levels (often crudely defined as volume of grain consumption per capita) do exist they are not normally comparable, so we cannot readily assess change over time. We remain almost in the dark as to one of the most important elements in the history of Southeast Asian health.

The asymmetric availability of sources has also led the majority of historians to examine questions of health at a national or regional level. Recently demographers, while continuing to analyse such large units, have also demonstrated the value of a 'micro-approach' in understanding some of the subtler dynamics of change in behaviour and attitudes.[9] Such studies are impossible, however, where data on mortality and descriptions of health and healing practices are available only for higher levels of aggregation, as is normally the case with Southeast Asian historical records. Only in the Philippines, where numerous parish registers of baptisms, weddings and burials have survived, are we likely to be able to examine in detail such potentially significant factors as the average age at marriage or the correlation of crisis mortality with social class.[10]

The nature of the available evidence also underlies an apparent gulf between attempts to specify or quantify diseases 'objectively' and efforts to understand what they meant to those who suffered from them. Colonial documents, the most numerous and accessible historical sources for the modern period, often record the symptoms (or even the scientific names) of diseases and provide estimates of the number of deaths, but they rarely tell us anything about how Southeast Asians perceived their own mortality. What we know about these perceptions, on the other hand, has been painstakingly pieced together from passing references in indigenous texts (often obscure and hard to date), fragments of descriptions of behaviour buried in journalistic or official accounts of crises, the observations of early ethnographers, and judicious backward extrapolation from more recent medical anthropology. Under the circumstances it is not surprising that detailed analyses of demographic growth or mortality crises may say little about indigenous responses to such changes, or, conversely, that studies of local attitudes towards sickness and healing may be difficult to correlate with specific developments in the 'objective' history of disease.

Despite all these limitations, I believe that these essays collectively show that some fundamental questions about the history of health in Southeast Asia can be answered, though we have not yet arrived at any consensus, even on matters of basic methodology or interpretation of major trends. Terwiel and Lovric have very different attitudes toward the use of obscure references to disease in early texts; Reid, Boomgaard, and Gardiner/Oey provide alternative explanations for the phenomenon of nineteenth century population growth (and my version differs slightly from all of theirs).[11] All the contributors would also, like good Southeast Asian specialists everywhere, insist upon stipulating the significance of diversity: before we begin, we must acknowledge not only changes over time and differences between areas governed by differing colonial regimes, but the likelihood of variation among uplands, lowlands, swamps, frontiers, cities and plantation or mining enclaves.

Nevertheless, if the field is to develop, we may have to overlook (temporarily) all these variations and contradictions and begin to speculate on the general shape that a history of Southeast Asian health might take. What follows is my own sense of the field as we now know it; no other contributor would formulate it in quite the same way. Every proposition is, of course, subject to refutation; each, I hope, also contains agendas for future research.

Demography and Death

In trying to reconstruct the *longue durée* in Southeast Asian health, we begin with only the vaguest of demographic principles and a historiographic near-vacuum. The principle is that of approximation to demographic equilibrium. Given the population estimates that we have for the sixteenth to nineteenth centuries and the power of geometric growth (as illustrated by compound interest tables), it is virtually impossible that there should have been a sustained and substantial birth surplus throughout the region prior to the eighteenth century.[12] But that principle tells us little more. Such an equilibrium might have been maintained through either moderate or high rates of fertility and mortality; these rates may have been either relatively stable or characterized by episodic rises and falls, perhaps with decades of slow net growth dramatically reversed by spasms of catastrophic death.[13]

Our evidence for the state of Southeast Asian health prior to the sixteenth century is sparse indeed. We discover in inscriptions and chronicles obscure references to unidentified epidemic diseases; we encounter what purport to be numbers of soldiers or vassals or taxpayers, numbers which might enable us to infer some absolute or relative size of population; we begin to comprehend the cosmologies through which death and disease, like other phenomena, were interpreted. Beyond that, however, all is speculation.

The Portuguese conquest of Melaka in 1511 marks not only the establishment of a permanent European presence in the region but a historiographic, if not a historic, landmark in the story of Southeast Asian health. There is no clear evidence that Westerners had any great epidemiological impact, such as that which they had on the more 'naive' populations of Australia, the Americas, the Pacific and tropical Africa, but they do seem to have been more interested in recording numbers, sizes, shapes and descriptions than Southeast Asians ever were. The result is that our knowledge of the physical features of the region and its people takes a quantum leap upward after their arrival. When combined with indigenous sources, these descriptions and accounts enable us to speculate somewhat more intelligently as to the nature of the demographic equilibrium that still prevailed throughout the region as a whole.[14]

Two to three centuries after the arrival of the Europeans, a critically important and apparently anomalous development occurred in Southeast Asia: the beginnings of sustained and rapid population growth. In the Philippines it may have begun in the eighteenth century—the nominal annual growth rate from 1735 to 1800 was nearly 1.0%, although the data are none too reliable—but is most evident in the early and mid-nineteenth century, when it reached the extraordinary level of 1.8% before falling to 1.1% between 1870 and 1903, when the Philippines was afflicted by a remarkable number of mortality crises.[15] In Java, too, there is some evidence for accelerating eighteenth century growth after the peace of 1755,[16] but again the trend is much clearer in the nineteenth century. Even after adjusting the early population estimates, which gave a nominal annual rate of growth of 2.2%, the lowest calculations based on the evidence are on the order of 1.4% up to 1850 and 1.75% thereafter, averaging 1.6%

over the course of the century.[17] For the rest of Southeast Asia the evidence is much shakier, but many estimates are consonant with high rates of natural increase (1–2% per annum) in the nineteenth century.[18]

It is possible that this growth is in part simply a statistical artifact, explicable as the extension of central (record-keeping) control over an ever-growing percentage of a static population, but the evidence is too detailed to be simply explained away by this means. If the growth is not, then, illusory it presents us with two anomalies. First, it violates conventional demographic theory, in which 'transition' is generally assumed to begin first in Europe, and there only as a result of distinct (though not yet agreed-upon) socio-cultural developments connected with 'modernization'. Sustained growth of this sort is indeed the exception in human history; we can find no firm evidence anywhere for national rates of natural increase above 1.0% over a period of fifty years or more prior to the mid-eighteenth century.[19]

The second anomaly is that the start of demographic growth in Southeast Asia does not coincide neatly with the most obvious historical developments that might be invoked to explain it. It apparently began hundreds of years after Europeans first arrived in the region, yet before the intensive exploitation and 'modernization' that we associate with high colonialism: the 'cultivation system' in Java (introduced in 1830), steamships, railroads, and most of the advances in tropical medicine. The colonial connection cannot be dismissed out of hand, however. The Philippines and Java, where early population growth is better documented than anywhere else in the region, were also more thoroughly controlled by colonialism; they are well documented, in fact, precisely because they were relatively well controlled. And the colonial era was certainly a time of dramatic socio-economic changes throughout the region, whether deliberately introduced by colonialists or inadvertently precipitated by them. The *pax imperica* (and its counterpart in the extension of Bangkok's control over the outlying regions of Siam), the enforced production of agricultural surpluses, the creation of more efficient physical and bureaucratic mechanisms for famine relief, and some of the pioneering efforts at direct medical intervention, such as smallpox vaccination, may have reduced mortality. On the other hand, the nasty colonial wars that preceded and accompanied the *pax imperica*, the heavy labour demand of colonial corvée and capitalist plantations, and the stronger connection of Southeast Asia with global markets and thus with trade-following pandemics like cholera might have increased it.

Indirect effects are even more obscure. It has been suggested that the demand for labour in nineteenth century Java increased the demand for children and thus fostered population growth through reduction in infant and child mortality (by reallocation of the domestic food supply) or through abandonment of traditional contraceptive and abortion practices.[20] The transition from shifting to sedentary agriculture appears to be associated with an increase in fertility, though it is not clear whether this is a result of a lightening of the female work load or of some other factor.[21] As cities are typically centres of high mortality, and as trade tends to spread epidemics, there may well have been demographic changes associated with the decline of traditional Southeast Asian cities and the rise of new colonial port-capitals.[22] The extensive migration to frontier areas (particularly the mainland deltas and the outer islands of Indonesia and the Philippines) that occurred over the last two centuries in Southeast Asia[23] could have resulted either in better nutrition, through extension of the area under cultivation, or in greater exposure to disease—or both. It is easy to get so mired in general hypotheses about the effects of colonialism on indigenous health as to lose sight of the need to specify and try to document the actual mechanisms of demographic change.

In attempting to account for population growth we cannot exclude the possibility of a rise in fertility as well as, or instead of, a decline in mortality.[24] In Southeast Asia a hypothetical increase in birth rates from moderate levels (35–40 per thousand?) to the higher levels recorded around 1900 (up to 50 per thousand)[25] might in fact account for most of the recorded population growth. Yet we have at present no clear evidence for such a rise or for any of the intervening variables which might account for it: lower age at marriage,[26] reduced incidence of celibacy and unmarried widowhood (the latter important in any society in which high mortality makes many widows), shorter lactation periods,[27] or alteration of customary sexual patterns within marriage (e.g., length of postpartum abstinence, age at terminal abstinence). We know that Southeast Asian women were familiar with indigenous methods of contraception and abortion—one recent study notes that at least thirty-seven abortifacients are known in the central Philippine city of Cebu[28]—but to assume that population growth is

essentially explained by the abandonment of these techniques
entails three unproven propositions: that they were actually efficacious, that they were once practised on a demographically significant scale, and that they were for some reason forsaken in the
eighteenth or nineteenth century.[29]

Much of the difference between the sustained growth that began
in the eighteenth or early nineteenth century and the relative
demographic equilibrium prevailing earlier may therefore be attributable to a net decline in mortality, despite the recurrent crises
which continued to characterize the region in the nineteenth and
early twentieth century. Cholera was apparently the newest and
most terrifying scourge, but smallpox, influenza and unspecified
'fevers' (malaria, typhoid?) also exacted a terrible toll, as did
famines, wars and rebellions. These spectacular manifestations of
death and disease must be kept in perspective, however. The data
are poor and the definitions imprecise, but it appears that in Java
such crises accounted for only about 10% of total mortality between 1820 and 1880, rising to about 14% at the end of the century
before falling again after 1900.[30] In the Philippines, the late-
nineteenth century rise was sharper, with crises responsible for as
many as a quarter of all deaths between 1876 and 1905. But even
this calculation means that at least three of four Filipinos died
'ordinary' deaths, mostly from endemic infectious diseases such as
tuberculosis, dysentery and infantile diarrhoea.[31]

The fact that in the nineteenth century 'background' mortality
was so much greater than crisis mortality does not mean that the
latter was demographically or culturally inconsequential. It is
possible that in earlier periods crisis mortality had been even
higher than it was in the better-documented epidemics, famines
and wars after 1800.[32] Within the last hundred years variations in
crisis frequency and severity have affected net growth significantly;
the doubling of Philippine growth rates between 1876–1905 and
1905–39 can largely be accounted for by the virtual disappearance
of major epidemics (except influenza in 1918) during the latter
period.[33] In psychological and cultural terms the terrible swiftness
and ubiquity of epidemics often give them an impact disproportionate to their demographic effects. Just as wars and revolutions often provide the historian with a deeper understanding of
political systems at peace, so episodes of crisis mortality may shed
light on ordinary years and on the endemic afflictions from which
most Southeast Asians actually died.[34]

At present, however, we have little direct evidence for a decline in either crisis or background mortality, so any attempted explanation offers at most hypotheses for further examination. In view of the apparent chronological coincidence with the beginnings of sustained growth both in Europe and in parts of India and Latin America,[35] it is tempting to think in terms of general, rather than local, explanations. Yet any truly global explanation would have to confront the fact that during the nineteenth century population grew slowly (at rates of under 0.5% per annum) in China, Japan and most of India, and may actually have declined in Africa. We also have to account for the apparent decline of diseases extraordinarily diverse in terms of agents, vectors, hosts, and patterns of pathogenicity.[36] Thus a single 'explanation' seems less likely than some complex multi-causal equation.[37]

It is now widely acknowledged that direct medical intervention had little impact in Europe until the decline of mortality was well established, so the virtual absence of such measures in nineteenth century Southeast Asia poses no analytical problem.[38] Of the changes in attitudes and behaviour which may have led to alterations in patterns of European health—a higher value placed on the lives of children, increased concern for public and private hygiene, a more secular and managerial approach to disease and famine control—we can only say that we have no real evidence yet of contemporary parallels in Southeast Asia.[39]

The exploitative nature of colonialism in Southeast Asia makes it at first sight improbable that nutrition improved during the eighteenth and nineteenth centuries, leading (as in Europe) to increased resistance to infectious diseases, but the possibility cannot be dismissed out of hand. If the *pax imperica* had a demographic effect, it is likely to have been more significant in this area than in reducing the number of violent deaths or even in limiting the spread of infection by marching armies or seaborne raiders. The endemic petty and frequent large-scale warfare that characterized traditional Southeast Asia must have been extremely disruptive to agriculture, both through physical destruction of crops, draught animals, fields and irrigation systems and through loss of field labour.[40] At the same time, Southeast Asia was adopting some of the same American food crops that were critical in Europe's 'second agricultural revolution', particularly maize and root crops such as sweet potatoes and cassava. Further research may help us estimate how much they contributed to Southeast

Asian nutrition, particularly to the alleviation of severe hunger caused by the failure of rice crops.[41]

Finally, it is also possible that the putative decline in mortality was due to some alteration in the delicate balance between microorganisms and human hosts which produces disease. William McNeill hypothesizes a general 'homogenization of civilized infectious diseases' after 1700, with epidemics declining into endemicity as the principal microparasites and the peoples of Eurasia and the Americas adapted to each other.[42] We cannot even exclude the possibility of some as-yet-undiscovered global decline in the virulence of various micro-organisms (perhaps connected with climatological change, which is well documented for temperate zones, though not yet for the tropics),[43] uncongenial as such exogenous explanations appear to be for some anthropocentric scholars.[44]

When we move forward into the twentieth century we are on much more secure ground. The major theme, familiar to most of us from medical and imperial history, is that of progress, associated with the institutional triumph of 'scientific' medicine. The frequency and virulence of epidemics diminishes. Some classic pestilences, such as smallpox, eventually disappear entirely. Basic improvements in water supply and sewage disposal, though far short of adequate, greatly reduce the incidence of cholera and typhoid fever. Background mortality, particularly that of infants, also falls, perhaps as a result of improved sanitation or some other factor. Death has hardly been conquered, but it does not conquer Southeast Asians quite so quickly or easily as before.[45]

There can be no doubt as to the trend, though colonial medicine was often not nearly as efficacious as it pretended to be. It rarely helped as much as it might have (underfunding was chronic), frequently did no good at all, and all too often did actual, if unintended, harm. Nevertheless, the facts are clear: people lived longer. In this situation the task of historians is more straightforward than in the chaos and ambiguities of earlier periods. We already know 'what happened'; our job is simply to ascertain which diseases declined, when (how much of the decline, for example, occurred before World War II?), where (urban or rural, lowlands or uplands?), how (sanitation and medicine or economic and environmental changes?), and among whom (infants or adults, males or females, peasants or landlords?).

The triumph of scientific medicine in Southeast Asia was apparently not paralleled, however, by comparable advances in nutrition and thus in human resistance to disease. There is even some evidence pointing to actual declines in per capita food consumption during the late colonial period, although Ian Brown has recently shown that these data are far from reliable.[46] The net effect of capitalist colonialism was not to enrich most Southeast Asians but to stabilize their real income at a level just high enough to permit survival, reproduction and a modicum of productive labour.[47] In part this resulted from the conscious efforts of officials, merchants and planters, who devoted much ingenuity to calculating just how little the 'natives' would have to be paid or fed to keep them working productively and peacefully. The system they devised was characterized by a delicate equilibrium between a market economy that forced the poorest right to the brink and a combination of agricultural specialization, improved transportation, and local famine relief that normally kept most of them from toppling over.

The colonial will to exploit was counterbalanced by the will of Southeast Asians to survive, whether through preventing (by implicit or explicit threat of violence) officials and landlords from pushing them below the subsistence level or through expanding domestic production of such secondary staples as maize and root crops, used everywhere to stave off starvation. Thus the Great Depression, though it undoubtedly caused physical as well as psychic suffering, did not produce a demographic catastrophe. (The great famine of 1944–45 in Vietnam substantiates this perversely, by indicating what could happen when the system lost its precarious equilibrium.) There was hunger, but little starvation; there was sickness, but no great swelling in the ranks of death.[48]

The paradox of the twentieth century, then, is that the reduction of morbidity apparently did not keep pace with the remarkable decline in mortality.[49] The former is always, because of difficulties of diagnosis and record-keeping, much more difficult to study than the latter, but it cannot be omitted from our analysis. The facts are simple: most Southeast Asians are poor, most Southeast Asians are malnourished, and many of the diseases which still afflict Southeast Asians, such as tuberculosis, helminthic diseases (schistosomiasis, etc.) and infantile diarrhoea, are associated with or exacerbated by poverty and malnutrition. Direct medical intervention has by no means reached the limits of its possibilities, but much of the impetus required to reduce morbidity to the level of the more developed countries must now come from a genuine rise in the standard of living, from political economy rather than from medicine.[50]

Disease, Society and Culture

When we turn our attention from the physical to the cultural, from the disease regime in Southeast Asia to the range of responses to it, we confront problems of a different dimension. Here we have evidence going back to the earliest traces of human habitation in Southeast Asia (often burial sites) and coming up to the present. For some of the most fundamental questions, however, we still have no answers.[51] We may be able to tease from the texts various indigenous concepts of the after-life (heaven or hell, reincarnation or nothingness?) or a comparative ethnography of mourning customs, but we lack the self-revelatory documents that might tell us how ordinary Southeast Asians actually felt about the fact of death. Cholera epidemics, apparently new to the region in the nineteenth century, seem to have produced great fear,[52] but to what extent were they and other mortality crises perceived as extraordinary? From great scholarly distance we may conclude that periodic crises were part of the demographic 'normality' of the pre-colonial era, but is that how they appeared to those whom they struck? Were they considered routine cosmological catastrophes, like earthquakes, typhoons and volcanic eruptions? If so, was the fear of sudden death pervasive, or was its sharp edge dulled by familiarity? How did Southeast Asians perceive their own expectancy of life—the likelihood that an infant would grow up, the likelihood that parents would survive to see their children marry? Did the ubiquitous menace of disease and death help to reinforce the 'fatalism' so often attributed to Southeast Asians by Western observers?

We are on somewhat firmer ground when we discuss traditional Southeast Asian approaches to diagnosis and healing, although we still cannot establish when and how most of these beliefs evolved. Many illnesses were attributed to the actions of supernatural beings, though we do their diversity an injustice by lumping together under this rubric powerful deities, demons, ghosts, dragons, local spirits, and the familiars of unfriendly magicians. Such beings might be placated by prayers and offerings, 'confronted' by *mantra*s, or even frightened away by smoke and loud noises. A surprisingly large number of ritual responses were of a group nature—processions, prayers, chanting, dancing and feasts—suggesting that in death, as in life, the individual was seen as part of a community.[53]

Alongside these personalistic interpretations of disease were more naturalistic etiologies, with illness attributed to violation of natural laws or divine principles of harmony.[54] Cure was then seen as a matter of restoring physical and moral balance through diet and right living. Both interpretations—disease as the consequence of the angry or capricious actions of a supernatural being and disease as metaphysical disharmony—were rooted in larger religious cosmologies; in traditional Southeast Asia, as in most pre-modern societies, religion (broadly conceived) was all-pervasive, and death carried extraordinary spiritual significance.

These religious dimensions of disease did not by any means exclude treatment based on carefully described symptoms and prescribed medication from a rich indigenous pharmacopoeia. External attempts to classify Southeast Asian medical systems rigidly tend to founder on their own distinctions between natural and supernatural, metaphysical and material. There is inherent ambiguity in such concepts as *yin* and *yang*, which can be regarded as spiritual essences or simply as metaphors for physical processes. A more fundamental difficulty is the fact that Southeast Asians frequently distinguish between ultimate or efficient causes (often perceived as supernatural) and the immediate or instrumental agent of misfortune (often recognized as natural). Thus the Manobo of Mindanao believe that spirits (*diwata*s) may carry germs (*kagaw*) of cholera, leprosy, typhoid or smallpox; Cebuano sorcerers are believed to employ natural poisons given extra potency by their own magic.[55]

One recurrent theme in indigenous approaches to healing was, in fact, that of pluralism or syncretism—the antithesis of modern exclusivistic medicine, with its implicit claim to prospective, if not present, omniscience. In selecting from the medical menu available to them the appropriate diagnosis and cure for any ailment, Southeast Asians were generally pragmatic. Different treatments might be employed sequentially, or even concurrently, until one worked: its success then retroactively validated a particular etiology for that case, without by any means denying that the next case could respond to a totally different type of diagnosis and cure. The death of the patient might imply a different etiology, often supernatural.[56] The same medicinal herb might be taken to drive away a demon, to cool a hot distemper, or simply to alleviate immediate pain—distinctions which are critical to any effort to decode Southeast Asian systems of thought, though of little relevance to an analysis of the therapeutic efficacy of the remedy.

In all this, of course, Southeast Asia resembled the pre-modern West; many of the same attitudes survive as well in the modern West, despite our public commitment to 'scientific' medicine.[57] In the nineteenth century it is not at all hard to find parallels between colonial and Southeast Asian responses to disease: fires used to clear the air of 'miasmas' or ghosts; holy water used to cure the sick and protect the whole; public processions driving off the cholera demons in Buddhist Bangkok, Islamic Batavia and Catholic Manila.[58] Certain etiological notions then current in the region, including a formal dichotomy between 'hot' and 'cold' (foods, diseases and temperaments) and a recognition of three to five essential 'elements' or 'humours', demonstrate fascinating convergences among several different cultural traditions. Some of these ideas may have been indigenous, while others were adapted by Southeast Asians from Chinese, Indian (Ayurvedic), Arabic (Unanic) or European medicine, the latter two sharing common roots in classical Greek thought.[59]

Although by the nineteenth century advanced medical thinkers in Europe no longer subscribed to most of these beliefs, the typical colonialist was scarcely an advanced thinker, a fact which permitted a measure of mutual intelligibility in the medical sphere. And as Western medicine was scarcely able to save lives in Europe itself prior to about 1850, and was even less effective in the culturally and epidemiologically alien environment of Southeast Asia, it met and mixed with local traditions on essentially equal terms. Siamese kings questioned Western physicians about cholera remedies (at a time when colonial doctors were touting 'cholera drinks' based on opiates and brandy!); Dutch botanists attempted to classify Javanese medicinal herbs; citizens of Saigon, Manila and Batavia were able to avail themselves of as many different medical traditions as they could afford.

The role of healer seems to have been broadly defined and informally assumed. Apparently there was little professionalization, and no strong institutional distinction among shamans, herbalists, masseurs, midwives and physicians trained in the 'great traditions' of medicine.[60] In strictly biological terms, it is doubtful whether any of these practitioners offered much hope of curing or preventing most serious disease.[61] The best of them inspired enough confidence or provided enough comfort to alleviate suffering or even, at times, to allow the body to heal itself. Where the science of medicine was inadequate, the art of medicine had to suffice.

This harmonious medley of rather ineffective medical traditions was disrupted in the later nineteenth and twentieth centuries by the development and imposition of what might be called 'imperial medicine'.[62] In its initial stages it represented more an affirmation of faith—or hubris—than a policy based on experience. Although smallpox vaccination had achieved some success in Southeast Asia, and European residents of major cities enjoyed better health as a result of improved hygiene in their quarters (if not in the rest of the city), the number of lives actually saved by imperial medicine was relatively insignificant at the time it became official ideology. 'Tropical medicine', which emerged as a formal specialty or subdiscipline at the turn of the century, involved not only promising recent discoveries in microbiology (most of which did not yet lend themselves to therapeutic application) but imperial arrogance. It suggested that diseases such as malaria and cholera, which had often devastated Europe itself, were primarily associated with climate rather than with social conditions; it reversed earlier tendencies toward mutual borrowing, which had implied there was something to be learned from Asian medicine; it tacitly denied the role of poverty and malnutrition in causing disease, thus relieving the colonial government of responsibility; it justified racial segregation ('the first law of hygiene in the tropics'); and it provided a pretext for the extension of state power into the everyday lives of its subjects.[63]

In Southeast Asia, colonialists burned dwellings, destroyed draught animals and desecrated the dead in the name of medicine.[64] They devoted a disproportionate share of the budget, ultimately derived from indigenous labour and taxes, to health measures designed primarily to benefit themselves, with 'hill stations' such as those in Baguio, Bogor (Buitenzorg), Dalat and the Cameron Highlands merely the most conspicuous manifestations of this self-concern.[65] Yet despite—or because of—their arrogance, sometimes they saved lives, more lives than had been saved by any medical system the region had ever known.

What we still need to discover is how Southeast Asians perceived the effects of imperial medicine, how they weighed its bungling insensitivity against its occasional triumphs. Although in recent years anthropologists and demographers have made remarkable advances in understanding current attitudes and behaviours in the area of health and healing,[66] they have barely tapped the historical evidence for Southeast Asia. Too often their writings are synchronic, conveying no sense of change over time beyond a contrast between the present and 'traditional' past that began in the mists of antiquity and lasted until roughly World War II. It remains, therefore, for historians to uncover and analyse those sources (including the reports of early ethnologists) that might illuminate the evolving responses of Southeast Asians to the increasingly intrusive claims of imperial medicine.

Meanwhile, we can speculate as to what those sources might suggest. Belief in, and recourse to, imperial medicine seems to have come from the top down and spread, like other components of imperial ideology, with urbanization and education. Institutionally, imperial medicine was first established in the major cities and, if accessible to Southeast Asians at all, was costlier than traditional remedies. It also represented a direct challenge to indigenous conceptions, a radically different explanation of the nature of the universe. To some intellectuals (generally drawn from the wealthier classes) it became one of the symbols of Western superiority, part of an entire constellation of concepts, values and practices that had to be adopted if their own countries were to be strong and free again. It is not surprising that such Southeast Asians as José Rizal and Tjipto Mangunkusomo joined the international tradition of physicians-turned-radicals that was to include Sun Yat-sen, Salvador Allende and Ernesto 'Che' Guevara.

Though some Southeast Asians accepted the exclusivist pretensions of imperial medicine—Filipino physicians typically translate *arbolaryo* (herbalist) as 'quack'—others, probably the majority, incorporated the new learning within an existing pluralistic repertory. Most were not directly confronted with the intellectual claims of medical science. Instead they formed their attitudes toward it on the basis of observation and performance, often concluding (rightly, on the basis of then-available evidence) that it was a hit-or-miss proposition. Nineteenth century processions, bonfires, 'cholera drinks', and half-hearted quarantine and sanitation programmes cannot have convinced many Southeast Asians of colonial wisdom. Even in the twentieth century the failure of medical authorities to cure cholera in Luzon, to identify the correct plague vectors in Java, or to stave off the influenza pandemic anywhere can scarcely have increased public confidence that they knew what they were doing.[67]

There was, nevertheless, a perceptible change in indigenous attitudes toward health and healing during the twentieth century, though at present we see only glimpses of it. At the most obvious and superficial level there seems to have been a general recognition that certain specific ailments had material causes and thus were appropriately treated by imperial medicine, although others, particularly those for which there was a customary diagnosis of supernatural causation, remained in the domain of traditional medicine.[68] The demand for injections grew rapidly in the twentieth century, presumably because experience had proved them effective against certain diseases.[69] Given the general Southeast Asian bent toward syncretism, it is not surprising that ideas were also blended, with the concepts and vocabulary of medical science often being incorporated into indigenous etiology and cures.

What we do not yet know is the part played by alterations of patterns and perceptions of death and disease within the larger transformation of Southeast Asian *mentalités*. There were under late colonialism (and the concurrent efforts to modernize Siam) an extraordinary number of innovations in the region, ranging from direct inculcation of Western ideas and values in the schools to exposure to a whole panoply of new technologies: steamships and trains, machine-guns and mills, telephone and telegraph, electric lights, radio and the cinema. Southeast Asians responded in many different ways, from complete acceptance to total rejection, with all varieties of adaptation in between. It is possible that the decline in mortality was perceptible enough to contribute, as some say it did in Europe, to the gradual secularization of life, since it became less necessary to invoke supernatural explanations for otherwise unpredictable and inexplicable catastrophes.[70] The apparent success of modern medicine in preventing and curing infectious disease may have helped to foster what David Marr describes as 'the growing conviction that one's life was not preordained' and that society could be changed.[71] The legitimacy of the colonial state might have been enhanced in Southeast Asian eyes by the life-saving actions of imperial medicine, or weakened by the excesses of its 'medical police'. Such propositions may never be verified—we certainly cannot verify them now—but they represent the larger arena of inquiry into which these more specialized studies in the history of death and disease may someday open.

In lifting our eyes to these general questions, however, we must be careful not to lose sight of the particular. One danger in grand generalizations is that they tend to imply that cultural change is a mass phenomenon, with entire societies responding in unison to the same situation. In fact the critical decisions about how to respond to disease and death are made by the individual or the family. Choices involve not only perceptions of the nature of the ailment and prognostications as to the nature and efficacy of the various treatments available, but also such mundane factors as accessibility of care and family finances; the situational tactics adopted in making such choices may or may not imply profound alterations in larger systems of thought.[72]

We must also be careful not to limit ourselves to aggregate categories lest the suffering be concealed in the statistics. We need to see the faces and hear the voices of Thai noblewomen chanting to ward off cholera, Javanese fleeing the plague as their houses are burned behind them, Filipinos trying to survive amid war and epidemic and famine, Vietnamese wondering how to pay the healer and the taxman too. Sometimes we can even put names to the faces: Raden Adjeng Kartini dying in childbirth at the age of twenty-three; Marcelo del Pilar, Manuel Quezon and Carlos Bulosan all coughing their lungs out thousands of miles from their native Philippines. But how can we adequately describe, much less analyse, the sheer carnage of lives lost or wrecked by disease, families shattered, whole villages abandoned? And, everywhere, children dying.

In counting the burials recorded in the parish registers of Oas, a town in southern Luzon, I encountered a sharp rise, from an average of 140 in the surrounding years to 552 in 1790. With 343 of the burials occurring between August and October, it was clearly an epidemic, which other sources reveal to be smallpox. It was only on closer examination of the individual entries that I realized that 303 of those buried were recorded as *angelitos*—'little angels', children under the age of seven[73]—and began to comprehend the human dimensions of this tragedy. As scholars we must try to analyse such events; as human beings we must also be prepared to respond to them with empathy. But can we, with our Westernized, sanitized, twentieth century minds, ever really understand how the people of Oas felt about the death in three months of one-third of all the little children in the parish?

Earlier drafts of this essay were read and commented on by Peter Boomgaard, Lincoln Day, Robert Elson, Lenore Manderson, Davin Marr, Glenn May, Anthony Reid, and F. B. Smith. I would like to acknowledge my gratitude to all of them, while admitting that none would be completely satisfied by my revisions.

1. Of particular inspiration has been the work of the Annales school in France and of the Cambridge group of English historical demographers; see Hubert Charbonneau and André Larose (eds), *The Great Mortalities: Methodological Studies of Demographic Crises in the Past* (Liége, Ordina, 1979); Robert Forster and Orest Ranum (eds), *Biology of Man in History: Selections from the Annales: Économies, Sociétés, Civilisations*, trans. Elborg Forster and Patricia M. Ranum (Baltimore, Johns Hopkins University Press, 1975); E. A. Wrigley (ed.), *An Introduction to English Historical Demography: From the Sixteenth to the Nineteenth Century* (London, Weidenfeld & Nicolson, 1966); Peter Laslett, *The World We Have Lost* (2d ed.; London, Methuen, 1971); E. A. Wrigley and R. S. Schofield, *The Population History of England 1541–1871: A Reconstruction* (London, Edward Arnold, 1981). The rest of the world is not far behind these European pioneers, with scholarship on North America and Japan particularly distinguished. Even in African studies the social history of wealth is coming of age: see *African Historical Demography: Proceedings of a Seminar held in the Centre of African Studies, University of Edinburgh, 29th and 30th April, 1977* (Edinburgh, University of Edinburgh, Centre of African Studies, 1977); Gerard W. Hartwig and K. David Patterson (eds), *Disease in African History: An Introductory Survey and Case Studies* (Durham, N. C., Duke University Press, 1978).

2. For reasons of space and thematic coherence the papers on drug use in Southeast Asia have been omitted from this volume: two have been published in *Journal of Asian Studies* 44, 4 (1985): Anthony Reid, 'From Betel-Chewing to Tobacco-Smoking in Indonesia', and James R. Rush, 'Opium in Java: A Sinister Friend'.

3. See H. J. Jusatz, 'Changes in the State of Infectious Diseases in South and South-east Asia', *Journal of Biosocial Science* 6, 2 (1974), 269–76; N. F. Stanley and R. A. Joske (eds), *Changing Disease Patterns and Human Behaviour* (London, Academic Press, 1980).

4. A Filipino anthropologist points out that the Manobo today define illness as the inability to eat and work normally, thus excluding all *non*-incapacitating diseases, regardless of how visible their symptoms—e.g. children with protruding abdomens—may appear to the 'health worker'; Erlinda Montillo-Burton, 'The Impact of Modern Medical Intervention on the Agusan Manobo Medical System of the Philippines' (Ph.D. dissertation, University of Pittsburgh, 1982), 135–7, 338–9). Another study, dealing with contemporary India, admits a frustration over the fact that 'much of the sickness that does occur is not reported because it is thought to be imbalance, error, or sin'; J. C. Caldwell, P. H. Reddy, and Pat Caldwell, 'The Social Component of Mortality Decline: An Investigation in South India Employing Alternative Methodologies', *Population Studies* 37, 2 (1983), 188.

5. There is also some evidence from the nineteenth century Philippines that boys were slightly more likely than girls to be listed in parish censuses and to have their burials recorded in parish registers, though the differentials appear to be much smaller than those recorded in other Asian societies.

6. See sources cited in Anthony Reid, 'Low Population Growth and Its Causes in Pre-colonial Southeast Asia', below, and in Ramon Pedrosa, 'Abortion and Infanticide in the Philippines during the Spanish Contact', *Philippiniana Sacra* 18, 52 (1983), 7–37.

7. Gerard W. Hartwig, 'Social Consequences of Epidemic Disease: The Nineteenth Century in Eastern Africa', in Hartwig and Patterson, op. cit., 25, 37–41; cf. Anthony Reid (ed.), *Slavery, Bondage and Dependency in Southeast Asia* (St. Lucia, University of Queensland Press, 1983).

8. At the conference the natural sciences were also ably represented by Professors Frank Fenner and Neville Stanley. Rather than turning aside from their own work to attempt original historical research, they contributed to this volume through the expert insights they provided to the rest of us, for which we are most grateful.

9. See in particular John C. Caldwell, P. H. Reddy and Pat Caldwell, 'The Micro Approach in Demographic Investigation: Toward a Methodology', unpublished paper, 1982, which inspired an IUSSP Seminar on 'Micro-Approaches to Demographic Research', Australian National University, 3–7 September 1984.

10. Peter C. Smith and Ng Shui-Meng, 'The Components of Population Growth in Nineteenth-Century South-East Asia: Village Data from the Philippines', *Population Studies* 36, 2 (1982), 237–55; Norman G. Owen, 'Measuring Mortality in the Nineteenth Century Philippines', below.

11. Norman G. Owen, 'Southeast Asia: The Paradox of Nineteenth-Century Population Growth', paper prepared for the Association for Asian Studies meeting, Philadelphia, 22–24 March 1985, provides a more detailed exposition of my views on this topic than the summary included in this introduction.

12. See Reid, 'Low Population Growth'. At 1% growth a year, a given population would have increased over seven-fold in the two hundred years from 1600 to 1800; at 1.5%, nearly twenty-fold. Extrapolating backward from early nineteenth century figures, the Hispanized Philippines would have had a population of 195–235 000 in 1591 at the former rate, just 70–77 000 at the latter—as against the 540 000 actually indicated by the tribute lists of that year. Even more striking discrepancies would be revealed by extrapolating such rates back from nineteenth century Burma and Cambodia to the societies that produced the magnificent monuments of Pagan and Angkor.

13. Recent work in European demographic history suggests the range of possibilities that exist in fact as well as in theory; see Wrigley and Schofield, op. cit., 450–53 and passim.

14. There are some references in the indigenous sources to early enumerations of the population and to other records potentially suitable for demographic analysis, but few such documents have survived the centuries in usable form.

15. Juan de San Antonio, 'The Religious Estate in the Philippines' (translated from chapter 58 of his 1738 *Chrónicas de la Apostólica Provincia de S. Gregorio*), in Emma Helen Blair and James Alexander Robertson (eds), *The Philippine Islands: 1493–1898* (Cleveland, Arthur H. Clark, 1903–9), 28:160; Peter C. Smith, 'The Turn-of-the-Century Birth Rate', in Wilhelm Flieger and Peter C. Smith (eds), *A Demographic Path to Modernity* (Quezon City, University of the Philippines Press, 1975), 87. Cf. Smith and Ng, op. cit., 241, and Norman G. Owen, *Prosperity without Progress* (Berkeley, University of California Press and Quezon City, Ateneo de Manila University Press, 1984), 116, for differing but comparable calculations.

16. Reid, 'Low Population Growth'; M. C. Ricklefs, 'Some Statistical Evidence on Javanese Social, Economic and Demographic History in the Later Seventeenth and Eighteenth Centuries', *Modern Asian Studies*, 20, 1 (1986), 1–32.

17. J. C. Breman, 'Java: bevolkingsgroei en demografische structuur', *Tijdschrift van het Koninklijk Nederlandsch Aardrijkskundig Gennotschap* 80, 3 (1963), 252–303; these figures are roughly in line with those proposed by Peter Boomgaard, 'Bevolkingsgroei en welvaart op Java (1800–1942)', in R. N. J. Kamerling (ed.), *Indonesie toen en nu* (Amsterdam, Intermediair, 1980), 35–52. Calculations of lower rates (1.0% or less) tend to be based on demographic plausibility (e.g. 'the maximum rate of growth of a population living under more or less "natural" conditions in a pre-industrial context') rather than on documentary evidence; Bram Peper, 'Population Growth in Java in the 19th Century', *Population Studies* 24, 1 (1970), 71–84 (quotation from p. 83); Widjojo Nitisastro, *Population Trends in*

Indonesia (Ithaca, N.Y., Cornell University Press, 1970); Peter McDonald, 'An Historical Perspective to Population Growth in Indonesia', in J. J. Fox (ed.), *Indonesia: The Making of a Culture* (Canberra, Australian National University, 1980), 81–94.

18. C. A. Fisher, 'Some Comments on Population Growth in South-East Asia, with Special Reference to the Period Since 1830', in C. D. Cowan (ed.), *The Economic Development of South-East Asia* (London, George Allen & Unwin, 1964), 48–71; Smith and Ng, op. cit., 253; Nicholas N. Dodge, 'Population Estimates for the Malay Peninsula in the Nineteenth Century, with Special Reference to the East Coast States', *Population Studies* 34, 3 (1980), 437–75; Larry Sternstein, 'The Growth of Population of the World's Pre-eminent "Primate City"; Bangkok at its Bicentenary', *Journal of Southeast Asian Studies* 15, 1 (1984), 43–68; cf. Reid, 'Low Population Growth'. (Although Sternstein prefers lower rates, he admits that the trend line which passes through most of the contemporary estimates for the population of Thailand reaches 1.3% by 1860–70 and 3.0% by 1890–1900.) During this period immigration was apparently of little demographic significance, except in Malaya and perhaps Thailand.

19. Surges on the order of 0.8–1.0% have been calculated for England, 1560–1610, for Japan, 1603–1721, and for China, 1700–93; Wrigley and Schofield, op. cit., 182–85; Akira Hayami, 'Population Trends in Pre-industrial Japan', paper presented at 9th Conference of International Association of Historians of Asia, Manila, 21–25 November 1983; Ping-ti Ho, *Studies on the Population of China, 1368–1953* (Cambridge, Harvard University Press, 1959), 277–8.

20. Benjamin White, 'Demand for Labor and Population Growth in Colonial Java', *Human Ecology* 1, 3 (1973), 217–36; Peter Boomgaard, 'Female Labour and Population Growth on Nineteenth Century Java', *Review of Indonesian and Malayan Affairs* 15, 2 (1981), 1–31.

21. See Reid, 'Low Population Growth'.

22. William H. McNeill, 'Migration Patterns and Infection in Traditional Societies', in Stanley and Joske, op. cit., 27–36; Anthony Reid, 'The Structure of Cities in Southeast Asia, Fifteenth to Seventeenth Centuries', *Journal of Southeast Asian Studies* 11, 2 (1980), 235–50; T. G. McGee, *The Southeast Asian City* (New York, Frederick A. Praeger, 1967); Dilip K. Basu (ed.), *The Rise and Growth of the Colonial Port Cities in Asia* (Santa Cruz, University of California, Center for South Pacific Studies, 1979).

23. See, for example, Michael Adas, *The Burma Delta: Economic Development and Social Change on an Asian Rice Frontier, 1852–1941* (Madison, University of Wisconsin Press, 1974); John A. Larkin, 'Philippine History Reconsidered: A Socioeconomic Perspective', *American Historical Review* 87, 3 (1982), 595–628.

24. European historical demographers have been debating for decades the relative significance of these factors; see E. A. Wrigley, 'The Growth of Population in Eighteenth-Century England: A Conundrum Resolved', *Past and Present* 98 (1983), 121–50, for a strong assertion of the importance of fertility change; Thomas McKeown, 'Fertility, Mortality and Causes of Death: An Examination of Issues Related to the Modern Rise of Population', *Population Studies* 32, 3 (1978), 535–42, for a virtual dismissal of it.

25. Peter C. Smith, op. cit., 84, 88; cf. Sternstein, op. cit., 54–55.

26. Smith and Ng, op. cit., 249, calculate a drop of over two years in the singulate mean age at female marriage in Nagcarlan, Laguna, during the second half of the nineteenth century, but the demographic significance of this finding is limited not only by the size of the sample but by the lateness of the shift (at least half a century after the acceleration of population growth) and by the fact that female age at first marriage was apparently already higher in the Philippines than elsewhere in Southeast Asia. Preliminary analysis of marriage records from another Philippine parish (Tigaon, Camarines Sur) indicates that a similar decline

in stated age at female first marriage between 1847–62 and 1863–97 was preceded by a comparable rise from 1820–46 to 1847–62.

27. Paul Alexander, 'Labour Expropriation and Fertility: Population Growth in Nineteenth Century Java', in W. Penn Handwerker (ed.), *Culture and Reproduction* (Boulder, Co., Westview Press, 1986), argues ingeniously for a decline in the duration and intensity in breastfeeding as a result of an increased demand for female labour, but admits that 'the argument is deductive—a polite word for speculative'.

28. Elena Yu and William T. Liu, *Fertility and Kinship in the Philippines* (Notre Dame, Indiana, University of Notre Dame Press, 1980), 137.

29. Another traditional means of population control in Southeast Asia was infanticide; although it actually increases mortality rather than reducing fertility, it might in practice be reflected as a lower apparent birth rate. There is no question of its efficacy, but we have yet to substantiate a decline in its practice comparable to, that suggested for Europe or Japan. See Pedrosa, op. cit., 21–37; cf. Thomas McKeown, *The Modern Rise of Population* (London, Edward Arnold, 1976), 47, 146–7; Thomas C. Smith, with Robert Y. Eng and Robert T. Lundy, *Nakahara: Family Farming and Population in a Japanese Village, 1177–1830* (Stanford, California, Stanford University Press, 1977); Susan B. Hanley, 'The Influence of Economic and Social Variables on Marriage and Fertility in Eighteenth and Nineteenth Century Japanese Villages', in Ronald Demos Lee (ed.), *Population Patterns in the Past* (New York, Academic Press, 1977), 176–83.

30. Peter Boomgaard, 'Morbidity and Mortality in Java, 1820–1880', and Peter Gardiner and Mayling Oey, 'Morbidity and Mortality in Java, 1880–1940', below.

31. Peter C. Smith, 'Turn-of-the-Century Birth Rate', 84–6; parish records, Tigaon, 1881–1905; cf. Peter C. Smith, 'Crisis Mortality in the Nineteenth-Century Philippines: Data from Parish Records', *Journal of Asian Studies* 38, 1 (1978), 51–76; Reynaldo C. Ileto, 'Cholera and Colonialism in Southwestern Luzon, 1902', paper presented at conference on 'Disease, Drugs, and Death: Their History in Modern Southeast Asia', Australian National University, 6–8 May 1983; Glenn A. May, '150,000 Missing Filipinos: A Demographic Crisis in Batangas, 1887–1903', *Annales de Démographie Historique*, forthcoming.

32. In his original conference paper Peter Boomgaard provided numerous examples of epidemics in Java prior to 1820; a similar listing for the Philippines might be culled from the index to Blair and Robertson, op. cit. On the difficulty of assessing the severity of pre-colonial crises in India, see Michelle Burge McAlpin, *Subject to Famine: Food Crises and Economic Change in Western India, 1860–1920* (Princeton, NJ, Princeton University Press, 1983), 194–8.

33. Smith, 'Turn-of-the-Century Birth Rate', 84–6; Wilhelm Flieger, Macrina K. Abenoja, and Alice C. Lim, *On the Road to Longevity: 1970 National, Regional and Provincial Mortality Estimates for the Philippines* (Cebu City, San Carlos Publications, 1981), 19–23. Exact calculations are impossible, not only because of the general unreliability of the 1903 census (see May, op. cit.) but because it was taken before the turn-of-the-century demographic crisis had run its course. In round figures, however, the elimination of epidemics would have reduced the crude death rate from 40 to 30 per thousand, with the birth rate constant near 50. Cf. Michelle B. McAlpin, 'Famines, Epidemics, and Population Growth: The Case of India', *Journal of Interdisciplinary History* 14, 2 (1983), 351–66, who argues that the acceleration of Indian population growth in the three decades after 1921 'is due entirely to the absence . . . of major famines and epidemics'.

34. Cf. Asa Briggs, 'Cholera and Society in the Nineteenth Century', *Past and Present* 19 (1961), 76–96.

35. Census data for Madras presidency indicate annual rates of growth averaging close to 1.7% ('probably too high') for the first half of the nineteenth century and 1.1% for the second half, nearly 1.4% for the entire period; Dharma Kumar, *Land*

and Caste in South India (Cambridge, Cambridge University Press, 1965), 101–24. Thomas W. Merrick and Douglas H. Graham, *Population and Economic Development in Brazil* (Baltimore, Johns Hopkins University Press, 1979), 28–39, calculate that natural increase (excluding immigration and slave imports) averaged closed to 1.25% a year, 1776–1872, rising to around 1.75%, 1871–1900, rates not far below those for Java; cf. Nicolas Sanchez-Albornoz, *The Population of Latin America: A History*, trans. W. A. R. Richardson (Berkeley, University of California Press, 1974).

36. Stanley and Joske, op. cit., 12–23, 154, 234–5, 246–7 and passim.

37. Cf. S. Diaz-Briquets, 'Determinants of Mortality Transition in Developing Countries Before and After the Second World War: Some Evidence from Cuba', *Population Studies* 35, 3 (1981), 399–411.

38. McKeown, *Modern Rise of Population*; F. B. Smith, *The People's Health, 1830–1910* (London, Croom Helm, 1979). Smallpox vaccination (or variolation) is the important exception in Europe, and may have been in colonized Southeast Asia, particularly Java and the Philippines, as well; see Peter Razzell, *The Conquest of Smallpox* (Firle, Sussex, Caliban Books, 1977); Boomgaard, 'Morbidity and Mortality'; Jose P. Bantug, *Bosquejo Histórico de la medicina hispano-filipina* (Madrid, Ediciones Cultura Hispánica, 1952), 144–59.

39. On the basis of labour demand White, op. cit., and Boomgaard, 'Female Labour', argue for an increased value placed on the lives of children in nineteenth century Java, presumably leading to reductions in child mortality (including infanticide), abortion, and contraception, but no one has yet attempted to verify this hypothesis either demographically or culturally. There has been no thorough examination of indigenous texts for indications of changing attitudes toward children comparable to recent studies on the West, e.g., Philippe Ariès, *Centuries of Childhood* (London, Jonathan Cape, 1962); Edward Shorter, *The Making of the Modern Family* (New York, Basic Books, 1975); David E. Stannard, *The Puritan Way of Death* (New York, Oxford University Press, 1977).

40. On Southeast Asian warfare, see Reid, 'Low Population Growth'; cf. William H. McNeill, *Plagues and People* (Garden City, N.Y., Anchor Press, 1976), 205-6, on the broader demographic significance of the rise of 'gunpowder empires'.

41. Alfred W. Crosby, Jr., *The Columbian Exchange: Biological Consequences of 1492* (Westport, Conn., Greenwood, 1972), 165–207; William Langer, 'American Food and Europe's Population Growth, 1750–1850', *Journal of Social History* 8, 2 (1975), 51–66; McKeown, *Rise of Modern Population*, 130–33; Canute Vander-Meer, 'Corn on the Island of Cebu', (Ph.D. dissertation, University of Michigan, 1962); Owen, *Prosperity without Progress*, 137–40; R. E. Elson, *Javanese Peasants and the Colonial Sugar Industry* (Singapore, Oxford University Press for the ASAA, 1984), 246. Some of these 'New World' crops may in fact have been known in pre-Columbian Southeast Asia, though none appears to have been of widespread nutritional significance; see Carroll L. Riley et al. (eds), *Man Across the Sea: Problems of Pre-Columbian Contacts* (Austin, University of Texas Press, 1971), particularly M. D. W. Jeffreys, 'Pre-Columbian Maize in Asia', 376–400.

42. McNeill, *Plagues and People*, 212–15.

43. See Robert I. Rotberg and Theodore K. Rabb (eds), *Climate and History: Studies in Interdisciplinary History* (Princeton, Princeton University Press, 1981); Reid A. Bryson and Thomas J. Murray, *Climates of Hunger: Mankind and the World's Changing Weather* (Madison, University of Wisconsin Press, 1977); Chu Ko-chen [Zhu Kezhen], 'A Preliminary Study on the Climatic Fluctuations During the Last 5,000 Years in China', *Scientia Sinica* 16, 2 (1973), 226–56; Susan L. Swan, 'Mexico in the Little Ice Age', *Journal of Interdisciplinary History* 11, 4 (1981), 633–48. A hypothetical improvement in Southeast Asia's climate could also have contributed to a rise in agricultural productivity and thus to improved nutrition and health.

44. McKeown, *Modern Rise of Population*, 80–90, and 'Fertility', 540–2, rejects the view that reduction in the virulence of micro-organisms was a major factor in mortality decline, in part on the grounds that if such a 'fortuitous' explanation were true, 'we could be anything but confident' about the 'future control' of infectious diseases.

45. See Gardiner and Oey, op. cit.; Lenore Manderson, 'Blame, Responsibility and Remedial Action', below.

46. V. D. Wickizer and M. K. Bennett, *The Rice Economy in Southeast Asia* (Stanford, Food Research Institute, 1941); Ngo Vinh Long, *Before the Revolution: The Vietnamese Peasants Under the French* (Cambridge, Mass., MIT Press, 1973); Ian Brown, 'Rural Distress in South East Asia During the World Depression of the Early 1930s', *Journal of Asian Studies*, forthcoming. On the consequences of malnutrition see N. S. Scrimshaw, Carl E. Taylor, and John E. Gordon, *Interactions of Nutrition and Infection* (Geneva, World Health Organization, 1968); David Morley, *Paediatric Priorities in the Developing World* (London, Butterworths, 1973); Leonardo J. Mata, 'Malnutrition-infection Interactions in the Tropics', *American Journal of Tropical Medicine and Hygiene* 24, 4 (1975), 564–74; McKeown, *Modern Rise of Population*, 128–42; Frederick B. Bang, 'The Role of Disease in the Ecology of Famine', in John R. K. Robson (ed.), *Famine: Its Causes, Effects and Management* (New York, Gordon & Breach, 1981), 61–75.

47. Those Southeast Asians who moved into new middle or upper classes enjoyed health expectations much closer to those promised by Western medicine, though they continued to suffer not only from inadequately funded public hygiene but from exposure to risk from the infected and infectious poorer classes that surrounded them.

48. I. Brown, op. cit.; Christopher Baker, 'Economic Reorganization and the Slump in South and Southeast Asia', *Comparative Studies in Society and History* 23, 3 (1981), 325–49; Norman G. Owen, 'Subsistence in the Slump', paper prepared for conference on 'The Economies of Africa and Asia in the Inter-War Depression', London, 12–14 December 1986. As most of the secondary staples were nutritionally inferior to rice and all were generally regarded as less tasty and prestigious, their displacement of rice in Southeast Asian diets can normally be taken as an index to declining welfare. For parallels in Indian demographic and social history, see McAlpin, *Subject to Famine*, and Paul Greenough, *Prosperity and Misery in Modern Bengal: The Famine of 1943–1944* (New York, Oxford University Press, 1982).

49. Cf. Gavin Jones, 'Population Growth in Java', in R. G. Garnaut and P. McCawley (eds), *Indonesia: Dualism, Growth and Poverty* (Canberra, Australian National University, 1980), 515–37. Official statistics from the Philippines actually indicate increases in morbidity levels for many major diseases, including tuberculosis, influenza, 'infantile beriberi', dysentery, measles and whooping cough, between 1924–28 and 1929–33, though these figures may represent improved reporting rather than declining health; Philippines (Commonwealth), *Annual Report of the Bureau of Health for the Fiscal Year Ending 1938* (Manila, Bureau of Printing, 1929), 64–5.

50. 'Political economy' in the broad sense might also produce significant improvement in health through a reorganization of the medical system to enforce effective preventive measures and to make appropriate treatment available to even the poorest; see Joan K. McMichael (ed.), *Health in the Third World: Studies from Vietnam* (Nottingham, Spokesman Books, 1976).

51. In order to focus the conference (and this volume) on modern Southeast Asian History it was necessary to limit the participation of scholars from other disciplines, some of whom, particularly in prehistory and medical anthropology, might have contributed significantly to our understanding of how indigenous attitudes changed over time.

52. See Susan Abeyasekere, 'Death and Disease in Nineteenth Century Batavia', below; Boomgaard, op. cit.; Barbara Lovric, 'Bali: Myth, Magic and Morbidity', below; B. J. Terwiel, 'Asiatic Cholera in Siam', below; Ileto, op. cit.

53. Ibid.; see also David G. Marr, 'Vietnamese Attitudes Regarding Illness and Healing', below, and Colin Brown, 'The Influenza Pandemic of 1918 in Indonesia', below.

54. George M. Foster and Barbara Gallatin Anderson, *Medical Anthropology* (New York, John Wiley, 1978); Donn V. Hart, 'Disease Etiologies of Samaran Filipino Peasants', in Peter Morley and Roy Wallis (eds), *Culture and Curing* (London, Peter Owen, 1978), 57–98.

55. Peter Morley, 'Culture and the Cognitive World of Traditional Medical Beliefs', in Morley and Wallis, op. cit., 1–18; Montillo-Burton, op. cit., 145 and passim; Richard W. Lieban, *Cebuano Sorcery: Malign Magic in the Philippines* (Berkeley, University of California Press, 1967), 61–4 and passim; Foster and Anderson, op. cit., 67–70; Hart, op. cit., 74–5, 88–9.

56. Marr, op. cit.; Montillo-Burton, op. cit., 330–2.

57. See, for example, Foster and Anderson, op. cit., 70–9, on 'American Folk Medicine'.

58. See Bantug, op. cit.; Abeyasekere, C. Brown, Lovric, Marr, and Terwiel, all op. cit.

59. Charles Leslie (ed.), *Asian Medical Systems: A Comparative Study* (Berkeley, University of California Press, 1976); Donn V. Hart, *Bisayan Filipino and Malayan Humoral Pathologies: Folk Medicine and Ethnohistory in Southeast Asia*, Data Paper no. 76 (Ithaca, N.Y., Cornell University, Department of Asian Studies, Southeast Asia Program, 1969); Lenore Manderson, 'Traditional Food Classifications and Humoral Medical Theory in Peninsular Malaysia', *Ecology of Food and Nutrition* 11, 1 (1981), 81–93; Marr, op. cit.

60. Such physicians, Asian and Western alike, do seem to have had some concept of professionalization (including, in some cases, restriction of the profession to men, whereas other branches of healing had practitioners of both sexes). Prior to the late nineteenth century, however, they enjoyed few substantive privileges as a result of their 'profession'. Cf. F. B. Smith, op. cit., 346–82, on professionalization in nineteenth century British medicine.

61. This is not to deny that some remedies had true therapeutic value, only to observe that all existing medical traditions were essentially powerless before the great lethal diseases of the day; cf. McKeown, *Modern Rise*, 91–109; Foster and Anderson, op. cit., 130–6; Abeyasekere, op. cit.

60. Such physicians, Asian and Western alike, do seem to have had some concept of professionalization (including, in some cases, restriction of the profession to men, whereas other branches of healing had practitioners of both sexes). Prior to the late nineteenth century, however, they enjoyed few substantive privileges as a result of their 'profession'. Cf. F. B. Smith, op. cit., 346–82, on professionalization in nineteenth century British medicine.

61. This is not to deny that some remedies had true therapeutic value, only to observe that all existing medical traditions were essentially powerless before the great lethal diseases of the day; cf. McKeown, *Modern Rise*, 91–109; Foster and Anderson, op. cit., 130–6; Susan Abeyasekere, 'Death and Disease in Nineteenth Century Batavia', below.

62. By this I refer to a tradition of medicine imposed by or borrowed from the West during the late nineteenth and early twentieth century and characterized by an exclusivist ideology and an allopathic 'germ theory' that tended to regard disease as an enemy to be confronted and conquered by 'scientific' means. Foster and Anderson, op. cit., 79, distinguish this tradition from both 'personalistic' and 'naturalistic' systems, limiting the latter to those centring on an 'equilibrium model' of health and disease. Since this tradition has now been globally (though not

universally) adopted, the term 'Western' is no longer adequate to describe it; objections have also been raised to calling it 'modern' or 'scientific' medicine. See Fred L. Dunn, 'Traditional Asian Medicine and Cosmopolitan Medicine as Adaptive Systems', in Leslie, op. cit., 133–58; James Nelson Riley, 'Western Medicine's Attempts to Become More Scientific: Examples from the United States and Thailand', *Social Science & Medicine* 11, 10 (1977), 549–60.

63. Henry Harold Scott, *A History of Tropical Medicine*, 2 vols. (London, Edward Arnold, 1939); Julian Amery, *The Life of Joseph Chamberlain* (London, Macmillan, 1951), 4:222–33; R. N. Chaudhuri, 'Tropical Medicine—Past, Present, and Future', *British Medical Journal*, 21 August 1954, 423–30; Robert V. Kubicek, *The Administration of Imperialism* (Durham, N.C., Duke University Press, 1969), 141–53; Michael Worboys, 'The Emergence of Tropical Medicine', in Gerard Lemaine et al.(eds), *Perspectives on the Emergence of Scientific Disciplines* (The Hague, Mouton, 1976), 75–98; Philip D. Curtin, 'Medical Knowledge and Urban Planning in Tropical Africa', *American Historical Review* 90, 3 (1985), 594–613.

64. See Terence H. Hull, 'Plague in Java', below; C. Brown, op. cit.; Ileto, op. cit.

65. Abeyasekere, op. cit.; Robert R. Reed, *City of Pines: The Origins of Baguio as a Colonial Hill Station and Regional Capital* (Berkeley, University of California, Center for South and Southeast Asian Studies, 1976).

66. Leslie, op. cit., provides a sampling of studies; Foster and Anderson, op. cit., 303–39, provide a good bibliography of work through the 1970s.

67. See Hull, op. cit.; C. Brown, below, op. cit.; Ileto, op. cit.

68. See Lovric, op. cit.; Foster and Anderson, op. cit., 228–9, 245–53; Montillo-Burton, op. cit., 134–51, 175–80. Lieban, op. cit., 97–100, observes that Filipino physicians often lose patients to local shamanistic healers (*mananambal*) when the diagnosed maladies are 'refractory or completely unresponsive to modern medicine', e.g. in cases of cancer. In contemporary Malaysia psychiatric disorders are in general more likely to be referred to traditional healers, somatic disorders to 'Western' medicine; Lenore Manderson, personal communication, 18 June 1984; cf. Montillo-Burton, op. cit., 333.

69. See Marr, op. cit.; Clark E. Cunningham, 'Thai "Injection Doctors": Antibiotic Mediators', *Social Science & Medicine* 4, 1 (1970), 1–24. We may wonder if injections were also somehow symbolically suited to indigenous conceptions of healing and power: cf. Peter Underwood and Zdenka Underwood, 'New Spells for Old: Expectations and Realities of Western Medicine in a Remote Tribal Society in Yemen, Arabia', in Stanley and Joske, op. cit., 280–2.

70. McNeill, *Plagues and People*, 227–8.

71. David G. Marr, *Vietnamese Tradition on Trial: 1920–1945* (Berkeley, University of California Press, 1981), 2, 288–367 and passim. Caldwell, Reddy and Caldwell, 'Social Component', 195–203, associate education with modern medicine and suggest that to Indian villagers today these imply 'a commitment to a different kind of world', more secular and 'modern', for better or worse, than that which surrounds them; this should be set against the view of Harold Gould, 'Modern Medicine and Folk Cognition in Rural India', *Human Organization* 24 (1965), 204, that 'acceptance of scientific medicine . . . resulted in no material changes in basic folk cognitive structure'.

72. Alan R. Beals, 'Strategies of Resort to Curers in South India', in Leslie, op. cit., 184–200, and Caldwell, Reddy, and Caldwell, 'Social Component', indicate some of the complex factors involved in choice of medical systems in South India; cf. Montillo-Burton, op. cit., 152–80, 214–342. The problem for historians is to discover how the kinds of information these scholars obtained by observing and asking questions of living villagers might be derived from the dead documents of the past.

73. The assumption underlying this terminology is that baptized children who died prior to the age of first confession (usually seven) would proceed directly to heaven without spending time in purgatory.

II THE DEMOGRAPHIC EVIDENCE

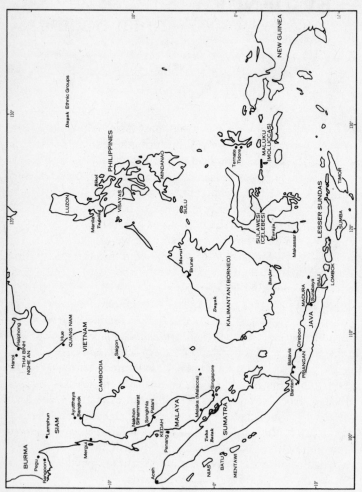

Map 1 Nineteenth Century Southeast Asia

2 Low Population Growth and Its Causes in Pre-Colonial Southeast Asia

ANTHONY REID

ESTIMATING the population of Southeast Asia before the advent of colonial censuses is hazardous, but not inherently more so than for most other parts of the world. Since a rough idea of population size and distribution is essential if we are to understand how Southeast Asia in the seventeenth century fitted into a broader global picture, we cannot afford to give up because the evidence is unsatisfactory. Even though our margins of error may be considerable, we owe the reader the best estimate we can make.

Java, Siam, Burma and Vietnam all had a tradition of counting households within their kingdoms for purposes of taxation and manpower mobilization. 'The Siamese', La Loubère asserted, 'keep an exact account of the Men, Women and Children . . . in this vast extent of Land', recalculating the numbers every year.[1] Unfortunately very few such enumerations have survived, and fewer still have been analysed by modern scholars. People exempt from corvee were moreover not enumerated, such as slaves, religious functionaries, and 'outlaws' outside the areas of permanent settlement. Nevertheless where these estimates have come down to us in indigenous archives or through the enquiries of foreign visitors, they provide a very helpful indication of rises and falls in population. In addition, the Spanish in the Philippines provided periodic estimates of the number of tax-payers (*tributos*) under their sovereignty from 1591 onwards.

If we compare the earliest such estimates available with what appear to be comparably based estimates in the eighteenth or early nineteenth century, just prior to the great modern take-off in population, the following rates of population increase emerge.

TABLE 2.1

POPULATION GROWTH IN SOUTHEAST ASIA, 17th–18th CENTURIES

Country/Region	Population (000)				Growth Rate (% p.a.)
	Year	Estimate	Year	Estimate	
Siam	1687	1 900[a]	1822	2 790[b]	+0.28
Kedah (Malaya)	1614	60[c]	1837	50[d]	–0.08
Banten (West Java)	1696	191[e]	1815	232[f]	+0.16
Mataram (Central & East Java)	1631	3 000[g]	1755	1 035[h]	–0.85
Bali	1597	600[i]	1815	800[j]	+0.13
Luzon & Visayas (Philippines)	1591	668[k]	1735	837[l]	+0.16

(a) La Loubère, *Kingdom of Siam*, 11.

(b) Crawfurd, *Journal of an Embassy*, 452.

(c) A. Beaulieu, 'Mémoires du voyage aux Indes orientales du Général Beaulieu, dressés par luy-mesme', in Melch. Thevenot (ed.), *Relations de divers voyages curieux* (Paris, Cramoisy, 1666), 2:246.

(d) T.J. Newbold, *Political and Statistical Account of the British Settlements in the Straits of Malacca*, (1839; reprint Kuala Lumpur, Oxford University Press, 1971), 2:20.

(e) Th.G. Pigeaud, *Literature of Java* (The Hague, KITLV, 1968), 2:64. The figures for Banten and Mataram are based on multiplying by 6 the number of *cacah*, or taxable households. A Mataram census in 1631 is described as yielding a population of 2.5 million (*Dagh-Register gehouden in 't Casteel Batavia 1631–34*, 37), but I take this to be the same 500 000 *cacah* figure as that of van Goens, multiplied by a factor of 5 rather than 6. Historians of the seventeenth and eighteenth centuries persistently take a minimal reading of the *cacah* estimates, whereas demographers reading back from the high populations of the late-nineteenth century believe them too low. The higher factor of 6, preferred by eighteenth century Dutch observers, has been used here because Javanese households were often large, while some compensation should be made for the non-taxable part of the population.

(f) T.S. Raffles, *The History of Java* (1817; reprint Kuala Lumpur, Oxford University Press, 1978), 1:63.

(g) Van Goens, 114, 225. The manpower figures on p.225 suggest that the conventionalized 500 000 *cacah* were in the heartland of Mataram, excluding coastal *pasisir*.

(h) M.C. Ricklefs, *Jogjakarta under Sultan Mangkubumi, 1749–1792* (London, Oxford University Press, 1974), 71–2, 159.

(i) W. Lodewycksz, 'D'eerste boeck', in G.P. Rouffaer and J.W. Ijzerman (eds), *De eerste schipvaart der Nederlanders naar Oost-Indië onder Cornelis de Houtman, 1595–1597* ('s-Gravenhage, Linschoten Vereeniging, 1915–29), 1:198.

(j) Raffles, op. cit., 2:ccxxxii.

(k) G.P. Dasmarinas, 'Account of the Encomiendas in the Philipinas Islands', in E.H. Blair and J.A. Robertson (eds), *The Philippine Islands: 1493–1803* (Cleveland, Arthur H. Clark, 1903), 8:141.

(l) G.J.H.J.B. Le Gentil de la Galaisière, *A Voyage to the Indian Seas*, trans. W.A.B.M. Fischer (Manila, Filipiniana Book Guild, 1964), 139.

The most spectacular rate of change in these figures is the apparent sharp *reduction* in population in Central and East Java.

This can be partly explained by the lengthy wars of succession prior to the Dutch-guaranteed Gianti Peace of 1755, though some of the lost population may only have migrated to calmer areas in the extreme west or east of Java. All the figures contrast markedly with the rapid growth in all Southeast Asian societies once conditions of internal peace were established, usually by colonial intervention. Continuous rapid growth began first in the Spanish Philippines, with average annual growth rates well over 1% from 1735 onwards. Then came Java, which must also have grown at over 1% per year after the 1755 Peace, to reach about 10 million in 1845 and 20 million in 1880. In most other parts of Southeast Asia, the establishment of colonial rule at some time in the nineteenth or early twentieth century appears to have initiated the extraordinarily rapid growth rates of modern times (between 1% and 3%). The Cakri dynasty in Siam was also able to preserve conditions of relative internal peace from about 1800 onwards, which is probably the reason that Siamese numbers also grew rapidly in the nineteenth century, though not as rapidly as those of the colonially ruled areas.

The low or negative growth rates for the seventeenth and eighteenth centuries illustrated in Table 2.1 suggest that we would not be justified in positing a growth rate higher than 0.2% per annum in extrapolating backwards to estimate populations about 1600 of those areas for which we have no other data. In some countries which had exceptionally high levels of warfare and internal disruption in the seventeenth and eighteenth centuries, such as Cambodia, a lower growth rate of 0.1% or even zero seems more appropriate. Table 2.2 attempts to calculate probable populations for Southeast Asia in 1600 on the basis of first making the best estimate possible for 1800 (on the basis of numerous, though usually unreliable, nineteenth century estimates) and then calculating backwards to a a probable 1600 population in those cases where contemporary sixteenth or seventeenth century estimates (see Table 2.1) do not take precedence. It may encourage the reader to know that the only previous attempt to make such broad and risky calculations, that of the demographers McEvedy and Jones[2], came to surprisingly similar conclusions by different means. Our chief difference is my higher estimates for Vietnam.

Taken as a whole, Southeast Asia was sparsely populated in 1600, especially in comparison with its immediate neighbours. Its

TABLE 2.2

POPULATION ESTIMATES FOR SOUTHEAST ASIA IN 1600

	Estimate for 1800 (000)	*19th Cent. Growth Rate (%p.a.)[a]*	*Estimate for 1600 (000)*	*1600–1800 Growth Rate (% p.a.)*	*1600 Density p/km²*
Burma	4 600[b]	0.83	3 100	0.2	4.6
Siam	3 500[c]	0.78	2 200	0.23	4.3
Cambodia/ Champa/ Mekong Delta	1 500	1.30	1 230	0.1	4.5
Vietnam (North & Centre)	7 000[d]	0.34	4 700	0.2	18.0
Malaya (incl. Patani)	500	1.56	500[e]	0.0	3.4
Sumatra	3 500[f]	0.49	2 400	0.2	5.7
Java	5 000[g]	1.72	4 000	0.11	30.3
Borneo	1 000	0.83	670	0.2	0.9
Sulawesi	1 800	0.45	1 200	0.1[h]	6.3
Bali	700[i]	0.25	600	0.08	79.7
Lesser Sunda Islands	900	0.54	600	0.2	9.1
Maluku	400	0.41	275	0.2	3.7
Luzon & Visayas	1 800	1.30	800[j]	0.4	4.0
Mindanao & Sulu	230	0.98	150	0.2	1.5
Total	32 430		22 425	0.2	5.55

(a) Calculated to the first reliable census, which is not before 1920 in the cases of Borneo, Sulawesi, Maluku and the Lesser Sunda Islands.

(b) H. Burney calculated on the basis of a Burmese enumeration of 1783 that there were then about 4 209 000 people (including 830 000 'wild tribes' and 1 069 600 Shans) in Burma excluding Arakan; see 'On the Population of the Burman Empire', *Journal of the Statistical Society of London* 4, 4 (1842), 335–47. An 1826 enumeration showed a very marginal increase. Details from the same two surveys are set out in F.N. Trager and W.J. Koenig, *Burmese Sit-tàns 1764–1826* (Tucson, University of Arizona Press, 1979), 400–406.

(c) The nineteenth century estimates are conveniently summarized in G.W. Skinner, *Chinese Society in Thailand: An Analytical History* (Ithaca, Cornell University Press, 1957), 68. I have opted for a higher figure than in Table 2.1 to allow for peoples likely to have been outside the purview of the Thai court.

(d) Compare A. Woodside, *Vietnam and the Chinese Model* (Cambridge, Harvard University Press, 1971), 158–9, with Crawfurd, op. cit., 526–8. Even allowing for a million Montagnards outside the tax rolls, other Western estimates appear much too large.

(e) The presumption of a population as high in 1600 as in 1800 is based on high contemporary estimates for the population of Kedah, Johor and Pahang prior to the devastating Acehnese raids of 1618–19 described in A. Reid, 'The Structure of Cities in Southeast Asia, Fifteenth to Seventeenth Centuries', *Journal of Southeast Asian Studies* 11, 2 (1980), 244, and on a large urban population in Patani around 1600.

(f) A relatively low nineteenth century growth rate is explicable in terms of extensive warfare in West Sumatra, Tapanuli and Aceh.

(g) Both Nederburgh's 1795 estimate of 3.5 million and Raffles' 1815 census of 4.6 million are probably underestimates, but not of the magnitude argued by J.D. Durand, 'The Modern Expansion of World Population', *Proceedings of the American Philosophical Society* 3, 3 (1967), 136–60; B. Peper, 'Population Growth in Java in the 19th Century', *Population Studies* 24, 1 (1970), 71–84; and P. MacDonald, 'An Historical Perspective to Population Growth in Indonesia', in J.J. Fox (ed.), *Indonesia:Australian Perspectives: The Making of a Culture* (Canberra, Australian National University, 1980), 81–94—all of whom find the high recorded nineteenth century growth rates unacceptable (see Appendix).

(h) A below average growth is premised on a high outflow of migrants and slaves, in addition to the usual factors.

(i) To accept Raffles' figure (Table 2.1) would give an improbably low growth rate of 0.14% p.a. in the nineteenth century.

(j) Larger than the Church estimates of Table 2.1, to allow for unpacified non-Christians.

overall density of about 5.5 persons per square kilometre contrasts with densities for South Asia of about 32 and for China (excluding Tibet) of about 37.[3] Further away, Europe had about double the Southeast Asian population density. A surprisingly large proportion of this sparse population, moreover, was concentrated in a number of large trading cities and in pockets of intensive wet-rice cultivation—in the Red River delta, parts of Upper Burma and of Central and East Java, in Bali, South Sulawesi and the Central Luzon Plain. Outside these areas Southeast Asia presented the appearance of a vast tropical jungle, upon which the impact of man was largely limited to shifting cultivation in isolated hillside patches, and gathering the varied products of the forest for export. Tigers were a threat even to those who lived on the outskirts of the great cities, such as Melaka, Banten and Dutch Batavia.[4] An envoy to Ayutthaya (Siam) from Golconda in south India is said to have quipped after making the overland journey from Mergui that the Siamese king's dominions might be vast, but they were peopled only by monkeys, not men.[5]

The most extraordinary feature of Southeast Asian population, however, was the very slow rate of growth in the seventeenth and eighteenth centuries, even if compared with China, India and Europe, followed by exceptionally high growth in the nineteenth and twentieth centuries, especially once European colonial rule was established. It does not seem possible to explain this contrast by any improvement in health introduced by Europeans. Southeast Asian health struck European visitors as better than their own in the seventeenth and eighteenth centuries. From the Philippines, Java, Aceh (Sumatra), Siam and southern Vietnam, the impression of foreigners was that 'they reach an advanced age in perfect health'.[6]

Physical stature provides an easily, if inaccurately, observed index of relative nutritional status. Here, too, early European observers found Southeast Asians of 'medium' stature in the seventeenth century, with some exceptions noted as relatively tall—in Siam, Pegu, Makassar and Brunei.[7] Probably this meant only that Southeast Asians averaged about 157 cm (5 ft 2 in) for adult men in the seventeenth century, as they did in the nineteenth and twentieth, but that Europeans were then at least as short and poorly nourished. In the nineteenth century, as Europeans grew rapidly taller, Western observers noted a widening gulf between themselves and Southeast Asians.[8] By the end of the century it is also apparent that Southeast Asians were living shorter and less healthy lives than Europeans. Far from there being a correlation between health and population increase, it appears that Southeast Asian rates of population increase rose to the level of European ones at just that point in the nineteenth century when Southeast Asian health and nutrition was becoming very much inferior to Europe's.

Another factor which must be dismissed is the age of marriage. While European women married exceptionally late in the seventeenth and eighteenth centuries, Southeast Asian women appear typically to have married before they were twenty.[9] If anything, a low age of marriage seems to have an inverse correlation with rapid population growth, since the Philippines had raised its average age of female marriage to twenty in the early nineteenth century when population had already begun to soar.[10] Yet another factor, the attitude of parents to children, can also be discounted. Europeans were frequently struck at the way in which children were indulged and loved for their own sake. John Anderson, reviewing the 'positive checks to population' enumerated by Malthus, insisted that none of them seemed to apply in any way to his healthy Sumatrans, who nevertheless very seldom bore more than six children.[11]

What factors, then, can explain the low population growth rate in Southeast Asia before 1800? Let us begin with some of the more speculative, including the question of royal polygamy.

It appears that the population [of Siam] does not rise . . . and the cause of this is easy to grasp; that comes from slavery and polygamy; a crowd of slaves cannot have wives, and a crowd of wives cannot have children.[12]

The normal domestic pattern of Southeast Asia was certainly monogamous, but the exceptions formed by powerful rulers are so spectacular that they do deserve comment. Throughout Southeast Asia it was common practice for kings to be waited on exclusively by women, and to trust none but women in their domestic quarters. Even if not used as concubines, these royal women were guarded jealously, so that any contact with other men was extremely dangerous. The king of thirteenth century Angkor was said to keep four to five thousand such women in his palace,[13] but was outdone by Sultan Agung of Mataram, who claimed 10 000.[14] Sultan Iskandar Muda of Aceh kept 3 000 women in his palace who were forbidden to talk to any man except the eunuchs of court, though from all of them he was able to produce only one or two male progeny.[15] In the Banten palace, there were said to be 1 200 concubines.[16] The ruler of tiny Tidore had 400 secluded women in his harem, but only twenty-six children. 'Every family is obliged to give the king one or two of its daughters.'[17] Although a few rulers did produce scores of children, the keeping of women on such a scale was 'rather magnificence than debauchery'.[18] Most of them were simply taken out of the reproductive process altogether. What is harder to judge is how far the replication on this regal style by lesser nobles and courtiers was demographically significant. Probably it was at least as much so as were the nunneries of Europe.

Some reports suggest that although Southeast Asian women began childbearing early, they also ended it early. An extreme view was that of Beeckman, who claimed that Banjar women 'are generally past childbearing at 20 or 25; it is rare that a woman holds till 30'.[19] Some authorities, including the Burmese Census Report for 1891, gave as a reason for a relatively early loss of fertility the practice of 'roasting' mothers after childbirth.[20] Though this was believed necessary in many parts of Southeast Asia to restore the 'heat' lost in childbirth, Burmese roasting practice was the most draconian. If there was truth in a relatively early cessation of childbearing in Southeast Asia, however, it is more likely to have resulted from a rigorous life for women, and from deliberate choice to avoid more than a certain number of children.

It has especially been noticed of the animist hill peoples of Southeast Asia, most of them swidden cultivators, that the workload of women is extremely hard. As A. R. Wallace put it:

A [Land] Dayak woman generally spends the whole day in the field, and carries home every night a heavy load of vegetables and firewood, often for several miles, over rough and hilly paths; and not unfrequently has to climb up a rocky mountain by ladders, and over slippery stepping-stones, to an elevation of a thousand feet. Besides this, she has an hour's work every evening to pound the rice with a heavy wooden stamper, which violently strains every part of the body. She begins this kind of labour when nine or ten years old, and it never ceases but with the extreme decrepitude of age. Surely we need not wonder at the limited number of her progeny.[21]

It is certainly the case that married women were more restricted to domestic roles among Muslim and Christian wet-rice farmers and traders. Low gave this as a reason why Dayak women were relatively happy to be taken into slavery (and concubinage or marriage) by Muslims of the coast.[22] Certainly the astonishingly high birth rates of largely Muslim Brunei in the 1950s (between 50 and 60 per thousand)[23] contrast very markedly with those of many upland Borneo peoples. It may therefore be that the moves towards wet-rice cultivation on the valley floors, and towards adherence to one of the world religions, moves frequently stimulated by Western penetration though by no means congruent with it, are further factors involved in a change in fertility patterns.

Twentieth century census figures confirm a picture of remarkably low birth rates and family sizes among a number of animist swidden cultivators. Thus the lowest average family size in the 1903 Philippine census was in the mountain province of Nueva Vizcaya most heavily populated by non-Christians.[24] The 1930 Indonesian Census noted exceptionally low birth rates among animists in the Batu and Mentawei islands off Sumatra, East Sumba (in the Lesser Sundas), West Java (the Baduy), parts of Borneo, and Central Sulawesi (Torajans).[25] Specific surveys of low-fertility areas, cited in that census, gave an average of only 3.9 children ever born and 2.22 surviving for each post-menopausal woman interviewed among animists of Central Sulawesi, while for East Sumba the figures were 3.88 and 2.75. Many substantial samples of Central Sulawesi women interviewed by A. C. Kruyt appreared to have a rate for surviving children well below the basic replacement level.[26] By contrast, recently Christianized peoples, such as the Toba Batak and South Nias in the 1930 Census and the Sa'dan Toraja in the 1971 and 1980 Censuses, show exceptionally high birth rates. Christian Batak and Nias women surveyed in the

1930s averaged 7 or 8 children each and their region had the highest fertility in Indonesia.[27] Christianization, or the changes in physical security, hygiene and agricultural practice frequently associated with it, appears to have vastly increased the fertility of Indonesians in modern times. It seems reasonable to conclude that the much more widespread identification with Islam and Christianity (and Theravada Buddhism?) in the sixteenth to eighteenth centuries may also have brought profound demographic consequences.

Only from the Philippines do we have significant evidence about attitudes to family size in the sixteenth and seventeenth centuries, and this suggests that the Christianization of the Philippines may indeed have caused a major change. The earliest observers of animist Filipinos were impressed at their low birth rate. Around 1580 Loarca reported, 'It is considered a disgrace among them to have many children; for they say that when the property is to be divided among all the children, they will all be poor'.[28] Of Visayans it was said:

Women dislike to give birth many times, specially those who inhabit towns near the sea, saying that in having many children they are like pigs . . . After having one or two, the next time they get pregnant, when they are already three or four months, they kill the creature in the body and abort. There are women for this calling and by massaging the stomach and placing certain herbs . . . the pregnant woman aborts.[29]

In contrast, later Spanish reports insisted that Christianized (and often resettled) Filipinos possessed 'a fertility that causes our wonder'.[30]

Another factor which may have limited the fertility of some peoples little touched by Islam, Christianity or Buddhism was gonorrhea. Studies of the Muruts of Northern Borneo in the 1930s and of Sumba in the 1960s have shown an incidence of gonorrhea in 80 and 90% of those examined, and the resulting infertility in women was as high as 25% in the Sumba survey.[31] Factors which may have spread the infection in such societies were a permissive attitude to sexual relations, especially before marriage, and a belief that the way for a man to free himself of the 'female contamination' represented by venereal disease was to couple with a healthy woman, returning the alien element to her.[32] Although there are numerous references to the prevalence of venereal disease in Southeast Asia from the sixteenth century onward, especially in Java, Bali and Lombok,[33] there is no real way to distinguish gonorrhea from syphilis, or to make any conclusions about fertility, before the twentieth century. It is reasonable to assume, however, that the gradual process of conversion to Islam, Buddhism or Christianity frequently entailed a much stricter attitude to sexual relations outside marriage.

Although some of the above factors may have been a check on rapid rises in population, there seems no doubt that the most important limitation was warfare. Southeast Asian warfare caused relatively few battle casualties. It was the primary objective of war to increase one's manpower, either directly by seizing the enemy's subjects as slaves or captives, or indirectly by so devastating his country that its inhabitants were obliged to move to one's own. Lives were not therefore wasted in fighting. On the other hand, the disruption and uncertainty caused by war cannot be overestimated. The larger states mobilized a substantial proportion of their male population into vast, ill-organized armies, without providing adequate supplies either for the soldiers or for their families left behind. Thousands of captives were marched back home by the victorious armies of Burma and Siam, or shipped home by Aceh and Makassar, with incalculable losses on the voyage. Perhaps even more important a factor demographically was the need to be constantly ready for flight in troubled times. This probably meant avoiding further births at least until older children were able to run by themselves.

Table 2.1 showed a remarkable decline in population in Central and East Java prior to the Gianti Peace of 1755, which put an end to eighty years of almost constant warfare between rival claimants to the throne of Mataram. That warfare was the primary cause of this decline was borne out by numerous contemporary observers. In the interior regions, the Javanese rulers reported to Governor-General Mossel, 'not a quarter of the families which were there before the disturbances are left now';[34] while in the coastal areas 'half the people who were there before the Chinese revolt are no longer there, as the precious, deserted coconut groves along the coast witness'.[35]

In densely settled wet-rice areas much of the loss of population was caused by destruction of food crops—either as a tactic of war or as a result of the passage of thousand of troops. In Sultan Agung's campaigns against the coastal regions of East Java and Madura in 1620–25, 80 000 troops besieged Surabaya and its nearby towns off and on for five years, devastating all the rice crops, and even poisoning and damming up the river water of the city.[36] After these campaigns 'in Surabaya not more than 500 of its 50 to 60 000 people were left, the rest having died or gone away because of misery and famine'.[37] Even on the side of Mataram there must have been enormously heavy losses, not only from the famine and disease that beset the unsuccessful besiegers of Batavia in 1628–29, but also from 'the lack of men, so that they had not been able to bring the water to the rice fields' during the wars against Madura in 1624, with the result that major rice-growing areas of Mataram itself were barren.[38]

The demographic pattern of pre-colonial Southeast Asia, it would appear, was very far removed from the smooth but shallow growth curve resulting from backward projections. When conditions of reasonable stability prevailed, the combination of early marriage, abundant food and relative health probably gave rise to quite rapid population growth, at least among the wet-rice cultivators and urban traders of the lowland and coast. Population must have declined equally sharply when these areas were laid waste by the movement of armies, however. Java probably underwent several such periods of population decline in the three turbulent centuries before 1755, and certainly did so in 1675–1755. Siam must have lost a large portion of its population when it was laid waste by the Burmese in 1549–69 and again in the 1760s, with terrible resultant deaths from famine and disease as well as deportation.[39] Similarly Malaya lost much of its population as a result of the campaigns of Aceh in the period 1618–24.

To conclude, the shift to rapid population growth in the nineteenth century (or earlier in the Philippines and Java) was caused firstly by the *pax imperica*, and secondarily perhaps by changes in values and practices which accompanied the movement of animist swidden cultivators into the orbit of the world religions centred in the cities and lowlands.

1. S. de la Loubère, *A New Historical Relation of the Kingdom of Siam* (1691; reprint Kuala Lumpur, Oxford University Press, 1969), 11.
2. C. McEvedy and R. Jones, *Atlas of World Population History* (Harmondsworth, Penguin, 1978), 190–203.
3. McEvedy and Jones, op. cit.
4. Ma Huan, *Ying-yai Sheng-lan*: '*The Overall Survey of the Ocean's Shores*', trans. J.V.G. Mills (Cambridge, Hakluyt Society, 1970), 113; C. Fryke, 'A relation of a Voyage made to the East Indies by Christopher Fryke', in C.E. Fayle (ed.), *Voyages to the East Indies* (London, Casse, 1929), 76–7; J. Bontius, *An Account of*

the Diseases, Natural History, and Medicine of the East Indies (translated from the Latin of 1629) (London, John Donaldson, 1776), 177–8.

5. Cited in J. Crawfurd, *Journal of an Embassy from the Governor-General of India to the Courts of Siam and Cochin China* (1828; reprint Kuala Lumpur, Oxford University Press, 1967), 453.

6. M. de Loarca, 'Relation of the Filipinas Islands', in E.H. Blair and J.A. Robertson (eds), *The Philippine Islands: 1493–1898* (Cleveland, Arthur H. Clark, 1903–1909) 5:116–17; R. van Goens, *De vijf gezantschapsreizen van Rijklof van Goens naar het hof van Mataram, 1648–1654*, ed. H.J. de Graaf ('s-Gravenhage, Linschoten Vereeniging, 1956), 180; *The Ship of Sulaiman*, trans. J. O'Kane (London, Routledge & Kegan Paul, 1972), 179; *Rhodes of Viet Nam: The Travels and Missions of Father Alexander de Rhodes in China and Other Kingdoms of the Orient*, trans. S. Hertz (Westminster, Md., Newman Press, 1966), 31; C. Borri, *Cochin-China*, trans. R. Ashley (1633; reprint New York, Da Capo Press, 1970), I (alphabetic pagination).

7. *Ralph Fitch: England's Pioneer to India and Burma*, ed. J. Horton Ryley (London, T. Fisher Unwin, 1899), 154; 'The Voyage of Olivier Noort round about the Globe, being the fourth Circum-Navigation of the same, extracted out of the Latin Diarie', in *Hakluytus Posthumus, or Purchas His Pilgrimes* (Glasgow, James Maclehose for Hakluyt Society, 1905), 2:202–3; S. van der Hagen, 'Oost-Indische Reyse', in *Begin ende voortgang van de Vereenigde Neederlandtsche Geoctroyeerde Oost-Indische Compagnie* (Amsterdam, 1646), 3:82.

8. J. Crawfurd, *History of the Indian Archipelago* (Edinburgh, Archibald Constable, 1820), 1:19.

9. A. Lintgens, 'Verhael vant tgheene mij opt Eijllandt van Baelle medevaeren is', in G.P. Rouffaer and J.W. Ijzerman (eds), *De eerste schipvaart der Nederlanders naar Oost-Indië onder Cornelis de Houtman, 1595–1597* ('s-Gravenhage, Linschoten Vereeniging, 1915–29), 3:77; John Barrow, *A Voyage to Cochinchina in the Years 1792 and 1793* (1806; reprint Kuala Lumpur, Oxford University Press, 1975), 226.

10. Ng Shui Meng, 'Demographic Change, Marriage and Family Formation: The Case of Nineteenth Century Nagcarlan, the Philippines' (Ph.D. dissertation, University of Hawaii, 1979), 138.

11. J. Anderson, *Mission to the East Coast of Sumatra* (1826; reprint Kuala Lumpur, Oxford University Press, 1971), 207–8.

12. J. Pallegoix, *Description du royaume Thai ou Siam* (1854; reprint Farnborough, Gregg International, 1969), 1:244.

13. Chou Ta Kuan, *Mémoires sur les coutumes du Cambodge de Tcheou Ta-Kouan*, trans. P. Pelliot (Paris, Librairie d'Amérique et d'Orient, 1951), 15–16.

14. Van Goens, op. cit., 256.

15. Beaulieu, op. cit., 102.

16. Fryke, op. cit., 42.

17. A. Pigafetta, in *Magellan's Voyage Around the World: Three Contemporary Accounts*, ed. C.E. Nowell (Evanston, Northwestern University Press, 1962), 68.

18. La Loubère, op. cit., 101. Cf. Craig Reynolds, 'A Nineteenth Century Thai Buddhist Defence of Polygamy', *Proceedings of the Seventh IAHA Conference* (Bangkok, Chulalongkorn University Press, 1979), 936–9.

19. D. Beeckman, *A Voyage to and from the Island of Borneo in the East Indies* (1718; reprint London, Dawsons, 1973), 42.

20. Sangermano, *A Description of the Burmese Empire*, trans. W. Tandy (1833; reprint London, Susil Gupta, 1966), 164; Shway Yoe [J.G. Scott], *The Burman: His Life and Notions* (London, MacMillan, 1896), 1–3.

21. A.R. Wallace, *The Malay Archipelago* (1869; reprint New York, Dover Publications, 1962), 70; cf. Raffles, op. cit., 1:70.

22. Hugh Low, *Sarawak: Its Inhabitants and Productions* (London, Richard Bentley, 1848), 120.
23. *Brunei Annual Report* (1959).
24. *Census of the Philippine Islands . . . in the Year 1903*, 3:711.
25. *Volkstelling Nederlands-Indië 1930*, 1:17, 4:13, 37, 5:57.
26. Ibid., 5:57.
27. Ibid., 4:48–9; L. Castles, 'Sources for the Population History of Northern Sumatra', *Masyarakat Indonesia* 2, 2 (1975), 189–209.
28. Loarca, op. cit., 5:118-19. The property referred to was probably in slaves or dependants.
29. 'The Manners, Customs and Beliefs of the Philippine Inhabitants of Long Ago' [The 'Boxer Codex'], trans. C. Quirino and M. Garcia, *The Philippine Journal of Science* 87, 4 (1958), 413. There are numerous later testimonies from other regions about similar expertise in producing abortions. See S. St John, *Life in the Forests of the Far East* (1862; reprint Kuala Lumpur, Oxford University Press, 1974), 2:261; C. Snouck Hurgronje, *The Achehnese*, trans. A.W.S. O'Sullivan (Leiden, Brill, 1906), 1:113; G.L. Forth, *Rindi: An Ethnographic Study of a Traditional Domain in Eastern Sumba* (The Hague, KITLV, 1981), 13. Another means of deliberately limiting births was the long period of breast-feeding, from two to four years, which inhibits the recommencement of ovulation.
30. G. de San Agustin, in Blair and Robertson, op. cit., 40:237; cf. F. Ortega, in Blair and Robertson, op. cit, 9:103; D. de Bobadilla, in Blair and Robertson, op. cit., 29:292.
31. K. G. Tregonning, *A History of Modern Sabah (North Borneo 1881–1963)* (Singapore, University of Malaya Press, 1965), 163; D. Mitchell, 'Endemic Gonorrhoea in Sumba', paper presented at conference of Asian Studies Association of Australia, Melbourne, May 1982.
32. Mitchell, op. cit.; M. de la Bissachère, *État actuel du Tonkin, de la Cochinchine, et des royaumes de Cambodge, Laos, et Lac-tho* (Paris, Galignani, 1812), 1:67.
33. Pigafetta, op. cit., 94; 'The Famous Voyage of Sir Francis Drake', in R. Hakluyt (ed.), *The Principal Navigations of the English Nation* (London, Everyman's Library Edition, 1907), 8:73; Crawfurd, *History*, op. cit., 1:33–4; H. Zollinger, 'The Island of Lombok', *Journal of the Indian Archipelago and Eastern Asia*, 5 (1851), 338.
34. Mossel (1757), cited in B.J.O. Schrieke, *Indonesian Sociological Studies* (The Hague, Nijhoff, 1957), 2:152.
35. Hartingh (1759), cited in Schrieke, loc. cit.; see also Ricklefs, op. cit., 159–60, and J.S. Stavorinus, *Voyages to the East Indies* (1798; reprint London, Dawsons, 1966), 3:336–40.
36. H.J. de Graaf, *De regering van Sultan Agung, vorst van Mataram, 1613–1645* ('s-Gravenhage, KITLV, 1958), 77–97.
37. Cited in Schrieke, op. cit., 2:148.
38. Cited in de Graaf, op. cit., 90, 151.
39. W.A.R. Wood, *A History of Siam* (London, Fisher Unwin, 1926), 146; *Turpin's History of Siam*, trans. B.O. Cartwright (Bangkok, Vajiranana National Library, 1908), 156–78; D.K. Wyatt, 'The "Subtle Revolution" of King Rama I of Siam', in D.K. Wyatt and A. Woodside (eds), *Moral Order and the Question of Change: Essays on Southeast Asian Thought* (New Haven, Yale Southeast Asia Studies, 1982), 11.

Appendix
ESTIMATES OF POPULATION
TABLE 2.3
POPULATION ESTIMATES FOR JAVA. 1652–1880

(000)

Year Source	West	Mataram	N. & E. Coast (incl. Madura)	Total	My Estimate Total	% increase p.a.
1652 (Van Goens)[a] (cacah x 6)		3 000			4 000	
1696 (cacah x 6)[b]	191 (Banten)					
c.1720 (Valentijn)[c]	443	2 208	901	3 552		-0.28
1738 (cacah x 6)[d]		1 858				
1755 (Hageman)[e] (cacah x 6)		1 035	474		3 000	1.02
1774 (cacah x 6)[f]	440	1 213				
1795 (Nederburgh)[g]		1 500	1 496	3 500	4 500	1.45
1815 (Raffles)[h]	1 099	1 922	1 593	4 615	6 000	1.70
1845 (Bleeker)[i]	2 411	2 633	4 271	9 551	10 000	2.00
1880 (official)[j]	4 733	6 180	8 879	19 794	20 000	

(a) Van Goens, op. cit., 114.
(b) Pigeaud, op. cit. 2:64.
(c) F. Valentijn, *Oud en Nieuw Oost-Indien* (Doordrecht, 1726). 4:5. 11. 24. 35. 43. 51–2. (NB: The grand total on p. 53 of 31 million must be disregarded as an absurd mistake in totalling.)
(d) Radermacher and Van Hogendorp, as cited in W. Nitisastro. *Population Trends in Indonesia* (Ithaca. Cornell University Press. 1970). 14.
(e) Ricklefs, op. cit., 71–2. 159.
(f) Ibid., 159.
(g) As cited in Nitisastro, op. cit., 14–15.
(h) Raffles, 1:63.
(i) As cited in Nitisastro, op. cit., 32–4.
(j) Ibid., 6.

TABLE 2.4

POPULATION ESTIMATES FOR INDONESIA OUTSIDE JAVA. 1800–1930

Year	Sumatra	Borneo		Sulawesi	Bali	Lesser Sundas	Maluku	Total
		North	South					
1800 (my estimate)	3 500		1 000	1 800	700	900	400	8 300
1815[a]	4 000				800			
1818/23[b]								
1837[c]	4 500							
1845[d]	4 964		1 200	3 175	800	1 949		
1849[e]	3 550					2 005	543	
1849[f]	2 481							
1862[g]		385						
1905 Census	4 067		1 173	835	827		401	
1920 Census	6 298		1 626	3 108	948	1 732	655	14 367
1930 Census	8 255	800[h]	2 168	4 231	1 101	2 358	893	19 006

(a) Raffles, op. cit., 2:ccxxxii.
(b) Based on S. Raffles. *Memoir of the Life and Public Services of Sir Thomas Stamford Raffles* (London. James Duncan. 1835); Anderson. op. cit., 210.
(c) Francis, 'Korte beschrijving van het Nederlandsch grondgebied ter Westkust von Sumatra. 1837'. *Tijdschrift voor Neerlands Indië* 2 (1839). 31, 44. 98.
(d) Temminck in *Moniteur des Indes* 2 (1845), as cited and amplified in S. St. John. 'The Population of the Indian Archipelago'. *Journal of the Indian Archipelago and Eastern Asia* 3 (1849), 379–84.
(e) N.I. official, cited in Nitisastro, op. cit., 60.
(f) J.R. Logan. 'A General Sketch of Sumatra'. *Journal of the Indian Archipelago and Eastern Asia* 3 (1849), 345–65.
(g) St. John. *Life*, 1:378–90; 2:248, 288.
(h) Based on the 1939 Sarawak Census (490 585), and the 1931 North Borneo Census (270 223), with an estimate of 40 000 for Brunci. Official estimates for all three territories suggest very low growth between 1900 and 1940.

3 Morbidity and Mortality in Java, 1820–1880: Changing Patterns of Disease and Death

PETER BOOMGAARD

WHEN a country is characterized during more than half a century by rapid population growth and ever-increasing agricultural exports, it might be expected that its people are at the same time experiencing declining death rates, improving health and a rising standard of living. It is the purpose of this essay to test that expectation against the experience of nineteenth century Java. Ideally, for such an undertaking we should have access to reliable demographic statistics, registration of deaths by cause, accurate information on identifiable diseases and on both public and private health measures, and some clear indicator of changes in the standard of living. Unfortunately, Java in the nineteenth century was still in its proto-statistical phase, and almost all figures are unreliable; moreover, the etiology of most diseases was not discovered before the 1880s, so the medical terminology of the period is frequently ambiguous. Our scanty information consists of dubious statistics on population, births and deaths by residency, miscellaneous reports on epidemics, figures for some years on patients treated by European physicians, numbers of smallpox vaccinations, and statistics on such economic indicators as rice production, imports and exports, land tax, and crop payments.[1] In view of the inadequacies of these data, the task may appear hopeless. Yet we have more information for Java than for any other country in nineteenth century Southeast Asia, and in writing this kind of socio-economic history we must make the best of what we have.

48

Patterns of Mortality

Prior to 1820 we have no systematic information on death and disease in Java, but a few observations may be ventured. With the exception of Batavia, the country had the reputation of being a healthy place, well supplied with food.[2] Certainly Java between 1750 and 1820 did not experience any demographic catastrophe comparable to the Bengal famine of 1770, when one third of the population perished. Yet Java was by no means immune to hardship and disease. Between 1757 and 1760 West Java and the adjacent districts of Central Java were hit by an epidemic that may have taken 100–150 000 lives—2–3% of the population of the island or roughly 10–15% of the population of the affected regions.[3] At least fifteen times between 1750 and 1810 the Governor-General had to forbid rice exports as a result of partial or complete harvest failures.[4] Dutch accounts of the period mention many prevalent diseases, including *Cholera nostras* (probably not the *Cholera asiatica* of the nineteenth century), dysentery, fevers (mostly malaria and typhoid), leprosy, smallpox and yaws. It is impossible, however, to put these diseases into any kind of quantitative perspective or to specify any general demographic trend beyond that of a possible population increase at a rate of around 1% a year throughout this period.[5]

After 1832, however, it is possible to calculate an annual death rate from the available statistics. There are reasons to assume that figures for total deaths are generally worse than those for total population, so the calculated rates would presumably underestimate actual levels of mortality. Both sets of statistics tend to improve during the nineteenth century, but as there is no evidence that data on deaths improved proportionally more or less than those for total population, we may assume a roughly constant differential between the calculated rate and the expected (or actual) one. Between 1832 and 1880 the average calculated rate is 2.3% a year (23 per thousand), to which we might add a constant 1% (10 per thousand) to obtain an estimate of actual mortality.[6] For the 1820s we lack the data to calculate a death rate for all Java, but by extrapolating from figures for twelve residencies and adding in an educated guess as to the number of deaths caused by the Java War (1825–30) we can calculate an approximate average death rate for the decade of 2.8% (28 per thousand) a year. A tabular presentation of these calculated rates by decades shows a clear

TABLE 3.1
CALCULATED DEATH RATE BY DECADE, JAVA, 1820-80

Period	Death Rate
1820–29	2.8%
1830–39	2.2%
1840–49	2.6%
1850–59	2.3%
1860–69	2.1%
1870–80	2.2%
1820–80	2.4%

TABLE 3.2
ESTIMATED EXCESS MORTALITY, JAVA, 1820-80

Year(s)	Number of Deaths	Cause(s)
1821	125 000	Cholera
1825–30	200 000	Java War
1834–35	140 000	Smallpox, cholera, dislocation, migration, and harvest failures caused by the introduction of the Cultivation System
1846–51	600 000	Typhoid fever, harvest failures, famine, cholera, smallpox
1864–65	125 000	Cholera, malaria
1874–75	175 000	Cholera, malaria
1880	100 000	Malaria, harvest failures

decline after 1850, even if we ignore the more speculative calculations for the 1820s (Table 3.1).

A comparison of normal mortality—during years without epidemics, wars of famines—with years of abnormal mortality, crosschecked with evidence from other sources on causes of extraordinary deaths, produces the estimates of 'excess' mortality shown in Table 3.2.

Over the course of sixty years, then, the excess mortality due to epidemics and other disasters amounts to little more than 0.3% (3 per thousand) a year, or just about 10% of total mortality. The other 90% of deaths were presumably due to endemic disease and other 'normal' causes.

In historiographic terms, however, the situation is reversed. The majority of Dutch evidence relates to dramatic epidemic diseases, while endemic diseases tend to be relegated to the background. Apart from epidemics, quantitative information on disease is almost entirely limited to data on patients treated by European physicians, representing less than 0.3% of the population. These data provide provocative, but inconclusive, information on the diseases killing the largest numbers of patients (malaria, diarrhoea and dysentery) as well as some estimates of case fatality (28–35% for dysentery, 14–22% leprosy, 11–16% diarrhoea, 3–5% malaria) within this restricted universe.[7]

They are also a major source of information on the normally non-fatal diseases which afflicted the Javanese, such as scabies, venereal disease and yaws. Scabies provided a high number of patients, because European physicians could actually provide effective treatment for it; against most other ailments they were as powerless as the local *dukun* (healer). Venereal disease (called syphilis, but probably gonorrhoea in most cases) was rampant in the coastal districts of the north, where the larger towns with European residents (civil servants, clerks, soldiers and sailors) were concentrated.[8] Not surprisingly, this evoked much official concern, but there is little evidence that it actually caused many deaths or even that it presented a major health problem in the population at large. Javanese rarely resorted to European physicians for venereal complaints, possibly because they recognized that existing treatments were useless. It is also possible that many Javanese were partially immune to syphilis through having had yaws (Dutch: *framboesia*; Javanese: *patek*), a skin disease caused by a spirochete similar to that which causes syphilis. Yaws, which could be a seriously disabling disease, was widespread, especially in West Java and on the northern coast, but as it was neither lethal (in most cases) nor susceptible to cure, it is all but ignored in the official statistics.

The official statistics on disease, recorded in the Colonial Reports (*Koloniaal Verslag; KV*) after 1855, focus, as indicated above, on epidemic disease. In particular they report on those diseases perceived as the great killers in nineteenth century Java: dysentery, cholera, 'fevers' (malaria and typhoid) and smallpox. The numbers actually reported are undoubtedly seriously underestimated; by comparing these data with the fragmentary figures available from other sources it appears that the epidemic deaths reported in the annual *KV* tables can safely be doubled at least. Nevertheless, they are useful for indicating the order of magnitude of mortality and for showing which of these diseases actually accounted for the majority of epidemic deaths: *Cholera asiatica* and 'fevers'. The other two suspects, dysentery and smallpox, though extensively reported, turn out to be guilty of only relatively limited killing. It is to these major diseases that we must look for understanding the principal developments in nineteenth century mortality in Java.

Gastro-intestinal Diseases (Dysentery and Cholera)

Nowadays we distinguish between bacillary and amoebic dysentery, but in the nineteenth century the two forms were indistinguishable, referred to simply by the Dutch term *rode loop*. Dysentery was never absent from residential reports, but rarely was it considered important. The number of patients treated for diarrhoea was about twice that of dysentery patients, but case mortality was much lower; many cases that were then diagnosed as diarrhoea may in fact have been less virulent attacks of bacillary dysentery. Both are contagious diseases, transmitted through direct contact, or indirect contact by way of infected food, utensils or water. Bacillary dysentery can be precipitated by undernourishment, and both dysentery and diarrhoea are well-known companions of famines.[9] Epidemics of dysentery are hardly mentioned in the sources, and when they are mentioned they are minor. It is possible that in the Semarang famines of 1849/50, however, dysentery was an important cause of death. Only in 1863 did mortality due to dysentery reach the 1 000 mark—yet in the same year over 10 000 victims of epidemic fevers were recorded. Van der Burg's contention that dysentery declined in scope and virulence between the 1860s and 1880s is not supported by detailed analysis of the available evidence.[10]

Cholera is transmitted mainly by water polluted with faeces of people suffering from the disease. Nowadays only *Cholera asiatica* is called 'cholera', but in the nineteenth century there was some confusion as to whether *Cholera asiatica* was a new disease or just another name for *Cholera nostras*, a gastro-enteritic disease endemic in the archipelago before 1820. It was called *bort* by the Dutch, and *cholera* in Latin, French and English. After 1817, when the first pandemic of *Cholera asiatica* visited Asia, the older disease was called *Cholera nostras*, in order to distinguish it from the much more widespread and virulent *asiatica*. Modern textbooks no longer acknowledge *nostras* as a subspecies of cholera; it is now regarded as a kind of summer diarrhoea, which from time to time could attain virulent and epidemic proportions.[11] In 1885 the Dutch physician Semmelink published a collection of reports on cholera-like diseases before 1817, trying to prove that all cholera prior to that date had been either *Cholera nostras* or some other gastro-enteritic disorder, but certainly not *Cholera asiatica*.[12] His conclusions were not universally accepted, yet it should be noted that Semmelink had lived through several cholera pandemics, while modern writers can only have witnessed isolated cases, as epidemic cholera disappeared from Java by 1918.

Cholera started its global career in 1817, when British troops and ships were present during an outbreak of cholera in Bengal, where it probably had been endemic for a long time.[13] In April 1821 it reached Semarang, on Java's north coast, where in eleven days it killed 1 255 people. By 27 April it appeared in Batavia, where mortality was lower: 778 deaths in eleven days. Eventually it was reported in at least fourteen residencies, all but one located on the north coast; within these residencies the epidemic seems to have struck predominantly lowland areas. Three to four months was the modal duration of the epidemic; by December it had almost disappeared from most residencies—for the time being.[14] In 1822 cholera reappeared in at least three residencies, in 1823 only in one, but in 1824 again in three.

This pattern is also typical of the next two outbreaks: a sudden eruption in a large number of residencies, followed by one to three years in which the number of afflicted residencies diminished; then another, far more restricted outburst, after which the epidemic receded. Measured from peak to peak, epidemic cholera hit Java every ten to seventeen years—thirteen on average. Although after the third epidemic it became an endemic disease, it is almost certain that every peak resulted from external reintroduction. Certainly during the first half of the century it could be entirely absent for many years in a row, e.g., 1827–31 and 1835–50. The story of cholera is in fact largely that of a series of global pandemics. The first (1817–24) was restricted to Asia; the other ones were truly global and scourged, for instance, the Netherlands as much as Java. Major pandemics are recorded in 1817–24, 1826–39,

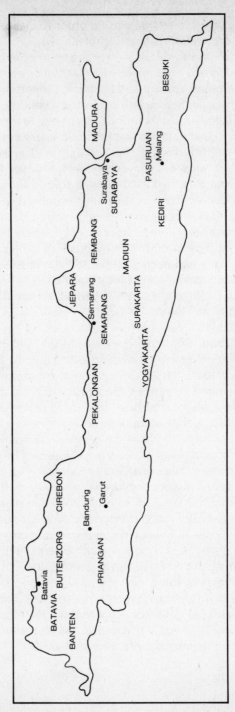

Map 2 Colonial Java

1846–62, and 1863–75; Java was particularly afflicted in 1821, 1834, 1857, 1864, and 1874.[15]

Although all attempts at quantification are necessarily speculative, we might estimate total cholera mortality during peak years 1820–80 at 125 000 in 1921, 25 000 in 1834, 50 000 in 1851, 65 000 in 1864, and 70 000 in 1874. In 1821 cholera hit a virgin population, and a high death rate was to be expected; compared to mortality in other, more populous countries, it was even modest. The slowly increasing peak mortality figures from the other four epidemics might be explained as a balance between increasing population density and better communications on the one hand, and increasing immunity on the other. Estimates for case mortality are only available for the three last epidemics: 40% in 1851, 60% in 1864, and 50% in 1874.

With the exception of Banten, all north coast residencies, including Madura, experienced an above-average incidence of cholera. All inland and south coast residencies, except Bagelen, were characterized by a below-average incidence. The pattern is quite clear: epidemic cholera was always reintroduced from overseas, and the coastal, urban areas were hit first and hardest. Population density played a secondary role: only in sparsely populated Banten and densely populated Bagelen did it overrule that coast–inland dichotomy. Cholera was of course a gruesome experience, well-known for its ability to kill within twenty-four hours. Thus it is not surprising that van der Burg claimed he had never seen a disease that caused so much fear. It was reported that whole villages were deserted when cholera was rumoured to be on its way.[16] There was no cure, although some nineteenth century physicians believed that 'cholera-mixture' was effective. As this 'cholera-mixture' contained opiates, it may have given some relief, but it did little to stop dehydration, cholera's most lethal characteristic.

Fevers (Malaria and Typhoid)

Malaria is caused by the bite of a mosquito, vector of a parasite (*Plasmodium*). There are four species of 'human' malaria parasites, of which three are relevant for Java: *Plasmodium vivax*, *P. malariae* and *P. falciparum*, corresponding to the traditional subdivision of tertiary, quarternary and tropical malaria. The mosquito, *Anopheles*, is also known for its many species, of which four are relevant for Java: *Anopheles maculatus*, *A. sundaicus*, *A. aconitus* and *A. hyrcanus*.[17]

The historiographical problems presented by malaria are huge. The term 'malaria' is rarely used before the second half of the nineteenth century, and as a rule the various manifestations of malaria were collectively called 'fevers' (Dutch: *koortsen*). Malaria is not the only disease to cause fever, and in some cases it can be deduced from the descriptions that other illnesses were responsible for the symptoms. The major disease in the 1846/50 epidemic was apparently typhoid, while in 1873 about half of the fevers reported were probably caused by dengue. Except in these two cases, however, the majority of 'fevers' can be regarded as malarial afflictions.

The official statistics on patients treated by European doctors give us an impression of the influence of malaria. It was the single most important disease treated, rising in proportion between 1853–58 and 1867–80, and despite low case mortality (3–5%) it was the greatest killer. Case mortality was higher in epidemics— normally 5–15%, rising to 25–35% in the 1852–53 Cirebon epidemic.[18]

Before 1850 few malaria epidemics are mentioned, except in the residencies of eastern Java, where the 'usual' (endemic) fevers at the end or beginning of the monsoon were more important than the occasional epidemics. Isolated epidemics occurred from time to time, like those in the town of Cirebon in 1805 and again in 1815–17, and those under Daendels in Banten and on the north coast precipitated by public works.[19] These two typical examples of 'man-made' malaria would unfortunately not be the last, for throughout the nineteenth century large-scale construction projects in the coastal towns of Batavia, Semarang and Surabaya would invariably result in local epidemics.[20] Nevertheless, it was not until the 1850s that epidemic malaria gained more than local importance. The last year of the period under consideration, 1880, was at the same time the absolute peak year for epidemic malaria, when 75 000 of 550 000 sufferers died.

How do we account for this increase during the second half of the nineteenth century? A look at regional variation in the incidence of malaria might help to explain this phenomenon. In the early nineteenth century there were two ecologically distinct types of human settlements where malaria felt at home; the big towns, with their canals and rivers, and coastal swamp areas. During the second half of the century mountainous upland areas were also invaded. It is tempting to suggest that the spread of *sawah* cultivation to the inland districts of Java was responsible for changes in the water economy of these regions, and thus for the creation of an environment agreeable to some mosquito species. Here the disease would strike a virgin population, thereby causing a disproportionate increase in the number of people affected.

To complicate matters, the 1880 epidemic might well be attributed to a different cause. West Java, nuclear area of the epidemic, was suffering from a very severe attack of rinderpest, which caused large-scale mortality among buffaloes. Modern research has discovered that *Anopheles maculatus*, one of the mosquito species responsible for malaria in Java, might actually prefer cattle to man. It is tempting to speculate that a large-scale withdrawal of buffaloes left the *maculatus* no alternative than settling for the less favoured hosts: humans.[21]

There is thus a confusing array of possible causes of increasing incidence and scope of malaria, not surprising in view of the fact that three species of parasites and at least four species of vectors, each with its own specific characteristics and habitat, are responsible for spreading the disease. Java's experience with changing malaria patterns between 1820 and 1880 can be summarized in a schematic recapitulation (Table 3.3):

TABLE 3.3
FACTORS AFFECTING MALARIA IN NINETEENTH CENTURY JAVA

HUMAN FACTORS	Large-scale construction activities in coastal (*A. sundaicus*) or inland areas (*maculatus*)
	Forest clearing by the local population for *sawah* cultivation
	The same, but executed by non-immune migrants (*maculatus*)
	Changing cultivation cycles in *sawah* areas from synchronized rice cultivation (all villagers preparing their *sawah* at the same time, planting at the same time, etc.) to year-round multicropping without synchronization (*aconitus*, *hyrcanus*)
	Increasing seasonal migration due to better communications
NATURAL FACTORS	Climatological
	Rinderpest and increasing number of people without cattle (*maculatus*)
	Introduction of new vectors

Most of these factors point toward an increase in the incidence and scope of malaria, which is what the logic of epidemiology indicates. There were, however, three countercurrents. The first is a more or less natural one: after some time most areas would have reached the stage of holoendemicity—the perennial transmission of the pathogen—which meant that only children (between the disappearance of their congenital immunity and the age of five) would have been at risk, with the adult population remaining symptom-free.[22] Second, the colonial government was aware of some connections between stagnant water and malaria even before *Plasmodia* and *Anopheles* were identified as pathogens and vectors. The *KV*s of the 1870s and 1880s mention attempts to eradicate swampy areas by drainage, though it is not likely that at this stage such rather haphazard efforts had any real effect.

Third was the growing availability of quinine. Quinine had already been used against fevers on Java in the late eighteenth century, but it was expensive and its supply was inelastic. In the 1850s cinchona plantations were introduced on Java, and from about 1870 onward quinine production increased enormously.[23] The administration of quinine must have already had a moderating influence on both duration and virulence of malaria before 1870, but thereafter Java supplied its own quinine in ever increasing quantities. It is, again, not easy to assess the impact of quinine, in part because it is impossible to guess how many people actually took quinine (not necessarily equivalent to the numbers for whom it was available). We know that quinine was distributed in large quantities during epidemics, but due to a lack of medical personnel it was impossible for the Dutch to supervise its distribution within the village (European physicians gave it to village headmen), let alone its regular consumption. In some cases the population actually resisted the European drug. That situation improved in the 1870s when the so-called *dokter-djawa*—Javanese with some 'modern' medical training—were deployed to supervise the distribution of quinine.[24]

Our analysis is also complicated by the fact that quinine was not equally effective against all three species of *Plasmodium*. It is only against *P. falciparum* that quinine is fully effective (if taken regularly during an attack). Against *P. vivax* and *P. malariae* it seems to be effective during the first attack, but as not all parasites are killed during the attack, short and long term relapses cannot be prevented.[25] It is impossible to strike a balance between availability of quinine and its effectiveness against one species on the one hand, and imperfect reception and limited effectiveness against two species on the other. Apparently quinine had some effect, however, as many reports testify that the population was getting used to it, and results were quite good in many districts over a number of years. This would seem to refute Peper's assertion that there was no treatment of any kind for malaria in nineteenth century Java.[26]

The history of typhoid fever (*Typhus abdominalis*) on Java between 1820 and 1880 is a bit of a riddle. In no report between 1820 and 1846 that I have seen is typhoid (or 'putrid fever') even mentioned. Between 1850 and 1880 it receives only occasional mention. It seems to have been so rare that some physicians emphatically denied that typhoid fever even existed on Java.[27] There can be, however, no doubt about the epidemic of 1846: it is called *typhus* (typhoid) in Dutch, and the rather extensive description is that of typhoid fever.[28] We know that in the late eighteenth century typhoid was a regular visitor in Batavia, and probably in most seafaring towns of the north coast.[29] It is likely that most inhabitants of these towns were immune, because of frequent contact with infected surface water. The 1846 epidemic broke out first in mountainous upland regions, previously regarded as very healthy and in all probability inhabited by a 'virgin' population. The epidemic raged on for five years, killing or immunizing everybody. This could explain the virtual absence of typhoid fever after 1850. It is, however, not easy to understand why western and eastern Java were almost entirely spared in 1846, nor why they did not experience typhoid after 1850.[30]

In 1844 harvest failures and rice shortages occurred in at least ten residencies. In 1845 harvest failures and rice shortages were reported in six residencies; during the same year seven more residencies were hit by heavy rainfall and flooding, damaging the crops. During the first four months of 1846 seven residencies were flooded again. The (Short) Monthly Report of February 1846 reports an 'illness' in Kedu, which by June assumed epidemic proportions; by the end of the year the epidemic had spread to three adjacent residencies and to Surakarta. All these residencies had experienced harvest failures or flooding in 1844–45. The link between shortages and the epidemic was established in 1847 by two high-ranking officials of the civil medical service, Bosch and Fromm.[31]

In 1847, eight residencies were affected by the epidemic, and in

1848 it continued to rage in six. Case mortality was highest in 1847 (47%), but also very high in 1846 and 1848 (30% and 41% respectively). In 1848 there was a rather good rice harvest, but that did not stop the epidemic, though it may have helped to abate its spread and virulence in 1849. It is possible, however, that other illnesses joined the epidemic: a description of an epidemic breaking out in Jepara (Pasisir) in 1848 does not look like typhoid fever.[32]

In 1849 the stage was set for the last and perhaps most lethal phase of the disaster. In the eastern districts of Semarang, hit by typhoid in 1846 and 1847 and either by typhoid again or the Jepara-epidemic in 1848, a series of harvest failures ensued. This led to a large-scale famine, resulting in an exodus of starving peasants to adjacent residencies, which in their turn had to face epidemics and food shortages.[33] In 1850 both rice shortages and epidemics continued, but by now this epidemic had run its course. Java, however, was allowed no rest; in April 1851, the third cholera pandemic reached the island.

It is hard to specify the ultimate causes of the series of disasters that hit Java. In 1841, after a decade of uninterrupted growth, the first drop occurred in the value of agricultural exports from Java. The downswing in the value of agricultural exports continued in 1842 and 1843 and, after an improvement in 1844, deepened until it hit bottom in 1848. The same development can be seen in the rice-production statistics. It seems reasonable to conclude that expansion of agriculture, due to the ongoing implementation of the Cultivation System, had gone too far, resulting both in actual famine and in increased susceptibility to such diseases as typhoid fever.[34]

Smallpox

The historiographical problems surrounding smallpox are not of the same order as the ones that make life difficult for the researcher studying cholera and malaria. Smallpox was already well-established in Java at the beginning of the nineteenth century, and there are no apparent terminological problems surrounding the disease. With smallpox, the central question is whether or not Dutch health care measures were effective.

There seems to be a scholarly consensus that in Java vaccination was the 'only public health measure in the nineteenth century', but that it had minimal influence on the death rate because it did not reach enough people, the population was not co-operative, the preservation of vaccine was extremely difficult, and there were never enough vaccinators. It is also argued that as smallpox was only one disease among many, vaccination could not in any event have had a major effect on mortality.[35]

Quantitative proof for these assertions is not provided by the authors, apart from one figure quoted by Widjojo and White, who state that even as late as 1880 only 2.5% of the native population was vaccinated.[36] Here we shall try to find out from the— admittedly rather unreliable—statistical data what the impact of smallpox and vaccination could have been. Statistical information on the epidemic incidence of smallpox is not available before 1850, so we shall have to start with the *KV* statistics for the period 1851–80. It is soon clear that smallpox, except for one or two years, was a relatively unimportant epidemic. In 1869 and 1870 about 6 500 and 5 000 deaths respectively were reported; during two other years the number was more than 500 but less than 1 000. For all other years, the number of deaths due to smallpox epidemics was around or below the 100 mark. Even if these figures are doubled it will be clear that smallpox could not be compared to cholera or malaria, or even dysentery, as a killer. If we take the figures for 1869 and 1870 together and double them, we get an average of 11 500 deaths per year, just 0.07% of the population of Java around that time. Case fatality was about 15%. How does that compare to mortality around and before 1815, when vaccination cannot have played any role at all?

Between 1775 and 1815 smallpox is mentioned in several coastal towns, Buitenzorg, the Priangan, Yogyakarta and Surakarta.[37] W. van Hogendorp, writing around 1780, estimated that case fatality for Buitenzorg and the Priangan was around 20%.[38] A 1798 report from the Resident of Pekalongan states that smallpox hit the area every two or three years.[39] Carey regards smallpox as the most important endemic disease in Yogyakarta and Surakarta before 1820. In stating that smallpox 'never reached epidemic proportions because of the scattered nature of the population', however, he underestimates the potential of smallpox for spreading into even sparsely populated areas.[40] In a most fascinating article John Crawfurd, British Agent at the Court of the Sultan of Yogyakarta under Raffles, gave the results of a detailed investigation which he personally carried out by interviewing 141 aged women, living in or around the city. It appeared that 10% of all children born to these women had died of smallpox, which accounted for 16% of all causes of death before the age of fourteen.[41]

Leaving Java, but not the Archipelago, we find that when a *prahu* sailing from Nias to Padang in 1832 transmitted smallpox to an unsuspecting and as yet unvaccinated population, 17% of these people were killed by the disease. But for the activities of Dr Willem Bosch, who did his utmost to vaccinate as many people as possible, that percentage could have been much higher.[42] Case studies in Africa show that 20% of a population living in dispersed settlements could be affected by smallpox epidemics, of which again 20% might die.[43] On the other hand, mortality resulting from smallpox should not be overestimated either. If, as is likely, smallpox had been present on Java for centuries, a high degree of immunity must have developed, especially in the more densely populated areas. The fact that in the eighteenth century, and probably earlier, smallpox was mostly referred to as 'children's disease' (*kinderziekte*), proves that it had been there for a long time: only 'old' diseases hit children predominantly. So Carey's hypothesis should perhaps be inverted: sparsely populated areas were probably affected most by smallpox mortality. If we assume a figure of 20% of the population affected and a case mortality of 20%, total mortality in one year due to a smallpox epidemic would then amount to about 4%—more than fifty times as high as our rather inflated estimate for 1869–70. A plausible explanation for this enormous decline in mortality is, of course, vaccination.

Vaccination was not the first attempt by the Dutch to control smallpox; around 1780 variolation was introduced in Batavia on a very limited scale.[44] Vaccination—inoculation with infectious matter from cowpox—was introduced on Java in 1804. It probably did not spread much further than the large coastal towns, and only when Raffles took the matter in hand in 1815 did vaccination seriously get under way.[45] Judging from the published vaccination figures, it was not until 1835 that 25% of the total population had been vaccinated.[46] In some residencies vaccination had slowed during the Java War, but there is no evidence for Breman's assertion that vaccination during that period came to a virtual standstill.[47] Although the disastrous years of 1846–51 slowed down the vaccination programme, in 1851 more than 40% of the entire population had been reached.[48] Around 1860 vaccination must have hit the 50% mark. Even if the figures presented were a bit inflated—which may very well have been the case—they were never absurd.[49]

Overall immunity only partly depended upon vaccination; people who survived an attack from smallpox could expect to possess a lifelong immunity. It was therefore good policy that vaccination, after the first years, was concentrated almost entirely upon very young children. Although no doubt an impressive achievement, this programme by itself might not have been effective in the long run, as 'the protection afforded by vaccination is very effective but relatively transitory and . . . we owe its control much more to surveillance and containment . . . than to mass immunization'.[50] Reporting the outbreak of smallpox and isolation of patients was already a feature of the first Dutch vaccination regulations of 1820, and the instructions of 1821 stressed the need to vaccinate everybody in a region where smallpox had appeared.[51] When in the 1850s the necessity of revaccination became apparent, the population did not take kindly to this new requirement; they resented revaccination as much as they had vaccination in the 1820s and 1830s. If, however, smallpox broke out in a region, everybody submitted obediently to both vaccination and revaccination.[52]

In summary, we may conclude that the campaign against smallpox was characterized by permanent surveillance and isolation of outbreaks, a programme of routine vaccination resulting in a temporary protection of at least 50% of the population by around 1860, and the start of a routine revaccination programme around the same date. It should be clear that such a programme still left considerable scope for the natural smallpox to find enough unprotected victims, as the 1869–70 epidemic testifies. Such epidemics were, however, quickly suppressed, and as an additional advantage the 85% or so who survived an attack were immune for life.

Population density seems to be an important variable in explaining the incidence of smallpox; if one counts the number of times an attack of smallpox is mentioned in the sources by residency, an interesting pattern emerges. Generally, smallpox-prone residencies were either densely populated (which would be conducive to easy transmission) or very sparsely populated (which implies poor implementation of the vaccination programme). The pattern is, however, a bit more complicated: several sparsely populated Residencies were characterized by a very *low* incidence of smallpox. These residencies might have possessed the required mix of incomplete vaccination and difficult transmission of the pathogen that optimized reinforced immunity.

A frequency table of references to smallpox between 1820 and 1875, combined with the statistical data from the *KV* after 1850, provides a rather elegant seven-year cycle, sometimes combined with the two- or three-year cycle found in eighteenth century Pekalongan. Peaks are to be found in 1820, 1835, 1842, 1849 (preceded by a lower peak in 1846), 1857 (lower peak in 1854/55), 1862 (lower peak in 1860), and 1869/70. Only during the Java War is information lacking, so the peak that could have been expected in 1827/28 must remain hypothetical, unless one accepts a small-pox epidemic in Bali in 1828 as proof of smallpox in Java during the same year.[53]

Conclusions

Patterns of mortality and morbidity in Java were clearly shifting over the period 1820–80, but no strong trend or single dominant factor is visible. At this stage we can enumerate a host of factors which may have influenced this process, but cannot with any certainty evaluate their effect. Some purely biological factors are apparent, particularly in the appearance of a new disease (*Cholera asiatica*) in 1821, which accounted for much of the high mortality over the next thirty years, and possibly also in new malaria vectors, which may help to account for the upsurge in that disease after 1850. Environmental changes may also have contributed to the spread of disease, particularly improvements in transportation, which allowed pathogens (as well as people, animals, and mer-chandise) to travel new roads; the flare-up of typhoid fever in remote and healthy areas is partly attributable to such ease of transmission. The spread of *sawah* cultivation, which may have much to do with the increase in malaria after 1850, is another example of the environmental factor in the history of disease of Java.

The role of European medical science in nineteenth century Java is an ambiguous one, as it involves questions about both the efficacy of medical technology and its actual accessibility to the Javanese. There is some evidence that the Javanese gradually lost some of their mistrust of European medicine, particularly in those situations where it offered genuine help, such as vaccination, quinine, and scabies treatment. But against the other great killers—dysentery/diarrhoea, cholera and typhoid—medical science could only offer palliatives. Improvements in hygiene, either within hospitals or in terms of public health (swamp drainage, etc.) can only have had marginal effects during this period.[54]

Food consumption is often an indicator of improving or declining health in pre-industrial societies, but there is no direct evidence of its levels in nineteenth century Java. Three indirect indices may be applied: production of rice per capita, the export/ import ratio of rice per capita, and the difference between landrent and crop payments per capita. These three rough measures are broadly consistent with each other; they suggest that food consumption failed to increase and may actually have declined during this period.[55] We have even less evidence on the consumption of various drugs (including alcoholic beverages and tobacco) which may have had a deleterious effect on health, though there is tantalizing correlation between the lower mortality of the 1830s and 1860s and a combination of administrative and economic factors which would have made it more difficult for poor Javanese to buy opium in those decades.[56] Finally, we have at present no index, even indirect, of mental well-being for nineteenth century Java, a factor which might have affected bodily health as well.[57]

The net result of all these positive and negative factors seems to have been a real, but slight, decline in mortality and morbidity between 1820–50 and 1850–80, with improvements in medicine all but counterbalanced by deteriorating environmental conditions and a declining ability to purchase food. If these calculations are correct, it means that the high population growth rate (1.0–1.5% a year) of Java during this period may owe as much or more to increasing fertility as to declining mortality—but that must be the subject of a separate study.[58]

Research in the National Archives in Jakarta was made possible by grants of the Netherlands Foundation for the Advancement of Tropical Research (WOTRO), and the Vrije Universiteit, Amsterdam. I am indebted to D. De Moulin, Anne Heavy, Wouter Hugenholtz, Robert Papstein, Heather Sutherland, Lucia van der Drift, Wouter van der Weyden, Judith van Oosterom, and J. D. Vervoorn for their historical, linguistic, and medical comments and suggestions.

1. Data on population can be found in the annual Residential Reports (1823–1890; Algemeen Verslag: AV), Political Reports (1851–1873; Politiek Verslag: PV),

Cultivation Reports (1836–1851; Cultuurverslagen: CV) and the printed Colonial Reports (1849–1930; *Koloniaal Verslag: KV*). Data on diseases can be found in AV, CV, *KV*, PV, the annual Summary Civil Disease Reports (Summier Civiel Ziekenrapport: SCZ) and the (Short) Monthly Reports (Kort) Maandelijks Verslag: (K)MV). Economic statistics can be found in CV and *KV*, and also in P. Creutzberg (ed.), *Changing Economy in Indonesia: a Selection of Statistical Source Material from the Early 19th Century up to 1940*, Volumes 2 (*Public Finance*) and 4 (*Rice Prices*) (The Hague, Nijhoff, 1976, 1978). (Hereafter cited as *CEI*.) Copies of AV and PV may be found in the Arsip Nasional (ARNAS), Jakarta, Indonesia, in the collection Arsip Daerah (AD). CV and (K)MV are both to be found in the Algemeen Rijks Archief (ARA), The Hague, Netherlands, in the collection Archief Ministerie van Koloniën (AMK). The *KV* was published yearly; the SCZ for several years can be found in the *Geneeskundig Tijdschrift van Nederlandsch-Indië (GTNI)*.

2. T. S. Raffles, *The History of Java* (1817; reprint London, Murray, 1830), 1:74; P. B. R. Carey (ed.), *Babad Dipanagara: An Account of the Outbreak of the Java War (1825–1830)* (Kuala Lumpur, Malaysian Branch of the Royal Asiatic Society, 1981), xxxviii.

3. F. de Haan, *Priangan: de Preanger-regentschappen onder het Nederlandsch bestuur tot 1811* (Batavia, Bataviaasch Genootschap van Kunsten en Wetenschappen, 1910–12), 3:522–7.

4. The edicts (*plakkaten*) forbidding rice exports can be found in J. A. van der Chijs, *Nederlandsch-Indisch Plakaatboek* (Batavia/The Hague, Landsdrukkerij/Nijhoff, 1885–1900), vols. 7–15.

5. P. Boomgaard, 'Bevolkingsgroei en welvaart op Java (1800–1942)', in R. N. J. Kamerling (ed.), *Indonesie toen en nu* (Amsterdam, Intermediair, 1980), 35.

6. Cf. Norman G. Owen, 'Measuring Mortality in the Nineteenth Century Philippines', below, for analogous estimates.

7. *KV* and SCZ. Though case fatality for leprosy was high, it was not an important disease in the population as a whole. An 1853 report on leprosy indicates that there were only 2 239 lepers in all Java in that year; ARNAS, Besluit (Decree) 26.8.1853, 14.

8. C. L. van der Burg, *De geneesheer in Nederlandsch-Indië* (Batavia, Ernst, 1882–87), 2:385.

9. W. Kouwenaar et al. (eds), *Leerboek der tropische geneeskunde* (Amsterdam, Scheltema & Holkema, 1951), 329–35; F. McFarlane Burnett & D. O. White, *Natural History of Infectious Disease* (1940; reprint Cambridge, Cambridge University Press, 1972) 46; A. K. Sen, 'Famine Mortality: A Study of the Bengal Famine of 1943', in E. J. Hobsbawm et al. (eds), *Peasants in History: Essays in Honour of Daniel Thorner* (Calcutta, Oxford University Press, 1980), 204.

10. Van der Burg, op. cit., 2:291.

11. Oral communication from D. De Moulin.

12. J. Semmelink, *Geschiedenis der Cholera in Oost-Indië voor 1817* (The Hague, Nijhoff, 1885).

13. Van der Burg, op. cit., 171; Kouwenaar, op. cit., 446; W. H. McNeil, *Plagues and People* (1976; reprint Oxford, Blackwell, 1979), 262. See also B. J. Terwiel, 'Asiatic Cholera in Siam', below.

14. J. Johnson, *De invloed der keerkrings-luchtstreken op Europesche gestellen . . ., naar het Engels door J. M. Daum* (Amsterdam, Van Kampen, 1824); M. J. E. Muller, 'Kort verslag aangaande de Cholera Morbus op Java', *Verhandelingen van het Bataviasch Genootschap* 13 (1832), 1–11; H. Schillet, 'Eenige waarnemingen omtrent de Cholera Orientalis', *Verhandelingen van het Bataviasch Genootschap* 13 (1832), 115–81; ARA, AMK, Verbaal 18.10.1831, 15: Reports from the Governor-General on the 1821 cholera outbreak.

15. See Peter Gardiner and Mayling Oey, 'Morbidity and Mortality in Java, 1880–1940', below, on cholera in Java after 1880.

16. Van der Burg, op. cit. 2:221–2. Cf. B. J. Terwiel, op. cit., and Barbara Lovric, 'Bali: Myth, Magic and Morbidity', below, on the great fear created by cholera among the Siamese and the Balinese respectively.

17. L. J. Bruce-Chwatt, *Essential Malariology* (London, Heinemann, 1980), 11, 163–64.

18. *KV* and SCZ. The construction of harbours, fortresses and highways (like Daendels' post-road) was normally carried out by *corvée* labourers, who often came from hypo-endemic areas (where the incidence of malaria was very low). As most of these construction activities were undertaken in coastal and therefore holo-endemic areas (incidence of malaria ubiquitous, resulting in immunity for the local population), malaria epidemics among the *corvée* labourers were unavoidable.

19. De Haan, op. cit., 3:528; B. Feist, 'Beschrijving der epidemie in het Cheribonsche, 1852/4', *GTNI* 4 (1855), 666–701; D. Schoute, *De geneeskunde in Nederlandsch-Indië gedurende de negentiende eeuw* (Batavia, Kolff, 1934–35), 45.

20. Van de Burg, op. cit., 2:27.

21. Bruce-Chwatt, op. cit., 163; D. Driessen: 'Bijdrage tot de rinderpest-geographie', *GTNI* 21 (1881), 309–510; *KV*, 1881.

22. Bruce-Chwatt, op. cit., 135–40; E. J. Pampana, *A Textbook of Malaria Eradication* (1963; reprint London, Oxford University Press, 1969), 82–92. The susceptibility of children would increase if they were poorly nourished, which is likely to have been the case in many parts of Java.

23. D. Schoute, *De geneeskunde in den dienst der Oost-Indische Compagnie in Nederlandsch-Indië* (Amsterdam, De Bussy, 1929), 316; K. W. van Gorkom, *Oost-Indische cultures* (1884; reprint Amsterdam, De Bussy, 1917-19), 3:270.

24. *KV*, 1880-81; SCZ, 1857.

25. Bruce-Chwatt, op. cit., 177.

26. B. Peper, 'Population Growth in Java in the 19th century: A New Interpretation', *Population Studies* 24, 1 (1970), 80.

27. E. P. Snijders, *Bijdragen tot de kennis van het typhoied-paratyphoied-vraagstuk in de tropen* (Amsterdam, De Bussy, 1922).

28. SCZ, 1846; F. W. F. Scholl, 'Erinnerungen aus Indien, 1843-'64' (manuscript, 1881; private collection).

29. Schoute, *De geneeskunde. . . .der Oost-Indische Compagnie*, 294; Semmelink, op. cit., 193.

30. SCZ, 1846; van der Burg, op. cit., 2:378–9.

31. AVs and (K)MVs, 1845–47; SCZ, 1846; ARA, AMK, Verbaal 4.6.1849, 14: Correspondence on the epidemic of 1846–50.

32. AV Jepara, 1849.

33. Cf. R. E. Elson, 'The Famine in Demak and Grobogan in 1849-50', *Review of Indonesian and Malaysian Affairs*, 19, 1 (1985), 39–85.

34. *CEI*, 1:34; CVs, 1837-50.

35. Peper, op. cit., 79; J. C. Breman, 'Java: bevolkingsgroei en demografische structuur', *Tijdschrift van het Koninklijk Nederlandsch Aardrijkskundig Genootschap* 80, 3 (1963), 252–303; B. White, 'Demand for Labor and Population Growth in Colonial Java', *Human Ecology* 1, 3 (1973), 217–36; Widjojo Nitisastro, *Population Trends in Indonesia* (Ithaca, Cornell University Press, 1970).

36. It is not clear whether the authors are aware of the fact that, presupposing revaccination, a percentage of 2.5 per year is sufficient to keep everybody protected, given an average growth rate of the population of 1–2% per year.

37. De Haan, op. cit., 3:528–30; Schoute, *De Geneeskunde . . . negentiende eeuw*, 45; see also sources cited in next four notes.

38. But not, as Breman (op. cit., 273) states, 20% of the total population. W. van Hogendorp, 'Redevoering der inenting tot de ingezetenen van Batavia', *Verhandelingen van het Bataviasch Genootschap* 1 (1781), 201–16.

39. ARNAS, AD Pekalongan, 47.

40. Carey, op. cit., xxxviii.

41. J. Crawfurd, 'Notes on the population of Java', *Journal of the Indian Archipelago and Eastern Asia* 3 (1849), 42–9.

42. ARA, AMK, Verbaal 8.3.1845, 1: Reports on vaccination.

43. E. W. Herbert, 'Smallpox inoculation in Africa', *Journal of African History* 16 (1975), 545.

44. Variolation — inoculation with infectious matter from human smallpox pustules — was already practised about 1750 in many parts of the world, where it often appeared to be an indigenous 'invention'. In Java, however, there is no evidence for an indigenous tradition of inoculation, and variolation seems to have been limited to Batavia, where it was far from universally acclaimed. Herbert, loc. cit.; McNeill, op. cit., 249–55; R. W. Nicholas, 'The Goddess Sitala and Epidemic Smallpox in Bengal', *Journal of Asian Studies* 41, 1 (1981), 27; J. van der Steege, 'Berigt nopens den aard kinderziekte te Batavia . . .', *Verhandelingen van het Bataviasch Genootschap* 1 (1779), 49-65; Van Hogendorp, op. cit., 207.

45. Schoute, *De Geneeskunde . . . negentiede eeuw*, 85.

46. ARA, AMK, Verbaal 8.3.1845, 1; ARA, AMK, 3042: Statistiek van Java en Madura, door Van Beusechem, 1836; C. G. C. Reinwardt, *Reis naar het Oostelijk gedeelte van den Indischen Archipel in het jaar 1821* (Amsterdam, Muller, 1858), 280; cf. Susan Abeyasekere, 'Death and Disease in Nineteenth Century Batavia', below. The percentages (of population vaccinated) presented here take into account that a high proportion of vaccinated children would have died from other diseases.

47. Breman, op. cit., 272.

48. ARA, AMK, Exh. 19.9.1845, 5; (K)MV, April 1845; W. Bosch, 'Vaccine verslag 1851', *GTNI* 2 (1853), 55–6.

49. After the revision of the vaccination regulations in 1831 (*Indisch Staatsblad* [*IS*] 1831, 48), vaccinators had to hand in lists of people vaccinated by name!

50. T. McKeown, *The Modern Rise of Population* (London, Edward Arnold, 1976), 12.

51. *IS*, 1820, 17; *IS*, 1821, 23.

52. ARA, AMK, Verbaal, 8.3.1845, 1; *KVs* of several years; J. Idsinga, 'Eenige mededeelingen over de koepok-inenting op Java en Madura', *GTNI* 23 (1884), 121.

53. ARNAS, AD Bali, 73; I thank Barbara Lovric for this reference. Note the parallel six- or seven-year cycles calculated for eighteenth century Bengal and nineteenth century Bali; Nicholas, op. cit., 28, 33–4; W. Weck, *Heilkunde und Volkstum auf Bali* (Stuttgart, Enke, 1937), 166–7.

54. Cf. Abeyasekere, op. cit.

55. *CEI*, Vols. 2 and 4; all CVs and *KVs* for 1849/80. Data on the period before 1835: ARA, Collection Schneither, 84–100: Statistical Reports of Residencies, 1820–22; ARA, Collection Du Bus de Gisignies, 371: Cultivation Report 1829. Note, however, that the possibility of improved food supplies and distribution in nineteenth century Java is taken seriously by Gardiner and Oey, op. cit.

56. J. C. Baud, 'Proeve van eene geschiedenis . . . van Opium . . .', *Bijdragen tot de Taal-, Land- en Volkenkunde* 1 (1853), 79–220; E. de Waal, *Aanteekeningen over koloniale onderwerpen*, Volume 1: *De Opiumpacht op Java* (The Hague, Nijhoff, 1865); J. T. Canter Visscher, 'Memorie omtrent de werking der opiumpacht op Java', *Handelingen en Geschriften van het Indisch Genootschap te 's-*

Gravenhage 5 (1858), 107–74; cf. James R. Rush, 'Opium in Java', *Journal of Asian Studies* 44, 3 (1985), 549–60.

57. See K. R. Pelletier, *Holistic Medicine* (New York, Dell, 1979), 96–126.

58. Boomgaard, op. cit.; idem, 'Female Labour and Population Growth in Nineteenth-Century Java', *Review of Indonesian and Malayan Affairs* 15, 2, (1981), 1–33.

4 Morbidity and Mortality in Java 1880–1940: The Evidence of the Colonial Reports

PETER GARDINER and MAYLING OEY

Overall Mortality

NUMBERS of deaths and death rates by residency, derived from village registers, were regularly published in the Colonial Reports (*Koloniaal Verslag; KV*) between 1874 and 1894, and crude death rates alone were published by province during the period 1915 to 1929. The data for both periods are difficult to analyse, not only because of substantial underreporting of numbers of deaths, but also due to considerable confusion about the accuracy of the population base.[1] For the nineteenth century, however, some informed speculation is possible by disregarding the death rates and looking only at reported numbers of deaths.

Apparently mortality in the latter part of the nineteenth century fluctuated fairly widely, not so much from year to year, but through peaks and troughs which coincided reasonably well with periods of major epidemics (Fig. 4.1).[2] If the numbers can be trusted, they imply that the major epidemics of the early 1880s and 1890s contributed to increases in mortality of as much as 40–50% over levels prevailing during non-epidemic years.

Estimating the overall impact of epidemics during the entire period is more difficult. Taking the sum of 'epidemic deaths' as a percentage of the sum of 'native deaths' over the period 1874 to 1894, one arrives at a figure of about 5%. However, this is hardly tenable—it is certainly a gross understatement of epidemic impact—due to differences in coverage and completeness of the reporting systems. An alternate estimate can be made by assuming an underlying (non-epidemic) level of mortality. We should not take the lowest figure (323 000 deaths in 1887), as one would expect at

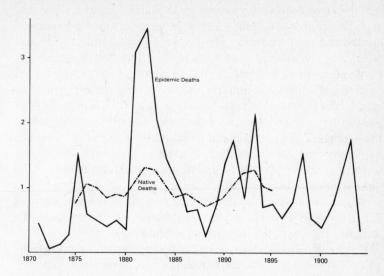

Fig. 4.1. Indices of Reported 'Native Deaths' and Epidemic Deaths, Java and Madura, 1870–1903

Source: KV, 1871–1904
Notes: Index, Native Deaths: 1874–94 average = 1.00
   Index, Epidemic Deaths: 1870–1903 average = 1.00
   Epidemic Deaths include a small proportion of non-Indonesian (European and Chinese) deaths.

least some fluctuations in non-epidemic deaths due to a variety of ecological factors. Somewhat arbitrarily we might take a simple average of the 'native deaths' in the eleven years for which the index value is under 1.0.[3] This gives a figure of 375 000 deaths. If we take this as an estimate of average annual mortality due to non-epidemic disease and compare it with the total number of 'native deaths', it implies that epidemic diseases contributed about 1.25 million *reported* deaths during the period; that is, about 14% of the total.[4]

We can also derive some information on mortality trends. Thus, if we assume that the quality of village registration remained fairly constant and the population grew at an annual rate of approximately 1.5% over the period,[5] the data suggest a secular decline in mortality of around 10% between the late 1870s and the early to mid-1890s.[6] While the assumed growth rate is still open to some question, the assumption regarding the relative quality of registration may be reasonable. It is true that the beginning of the quinquennial census programme in 1880 did lead to a more for-malized reporting system. Concern also began to be expressed around this time for increasing the use of health officials (*inspecteurs*) and government physicians in reporting health conditions, particularly those related to the incidence and prevalence of epidemic disease. It is unlikely, however, that these factors had much effect on the village reporting system. Throughout this period the primary interest of the colonial authorities remained the collection of data on population and their use in programmes of commercial exploitation. The statistics on births and deaths were thus used primarily to update the population figures on an annual basis. Concerns with health centred on epidemics, and were more heavily biased toward ensuring the health and safety of the European population, the indigenous aristocracy and the military, than with the broader population base.[7]

Regional variations are more difficult to explain. Occasionally there was some coincidence between levels of mortality reported through the village registers and areas where epidemics were reported as most severe. Thus, in the 'fever' epidemic of 1880, of the 75 000 deaths reported by the civilian and military medical services for Java, 45 000 occurred in Banten Residency in West Java. The 1880 crude death rate for Banten, based on village registration and the population recorded in the 1880 administrative census, was a staggering 70 per thousand population. How-ever, for other areas and time periods the relationships are not so clear. Residencies with the highest levels of mortality based on village registration in a given year were frequently not those cited in the medical service reports as centres of epidemics. Differences in coverage (annual figures, particularly for the medical service reports on epidemics, seldom included all areas of Java) may explain part of the problem. In any case, extreme caution must be used in interpreting any of these data, except perhaps on a broad regional basis.

The twentieth century material is even more difficult to inter-pret. The data for the early part of the period are dominated by the influenza pandemic which caused an apparent doubling of the death rate in Central and East Java in 1918 (Table 4.1). Beyond this, there is only limited variation in the reported death rates, although the somewhat higher mortality in the period 1919 to 1921 may be related to reported widespread epidemics of malaria and plague. The implied annual growth rate between the last quin-

TABLE 4.1

CRUDE DEATH RATES IN JAVA (VILLAGE REGISTRATION). 1915–29

Year	West Java	Central Java	East Java	Java and Madura
1915	20.5	19.0	19.3	—
1916	17.8	17.1	17.1	—
1917	20.4	20.9	20.2	—
1918	26.9	39.1	42.0	—
1919	20.2	32.5	27.7	27.8
1920	23.7	25.0	23.6	24.1
1921	21.2	26.3	22.0	23.7
1922	20.7	20.7	18.8	20.0
1923	18.8	20.0	16.8	18.2
1924	18.6	20.0	17.0	18.7
1925	20.4	21.7	17.3	19.9
1926	19.6	23.6	19.0	21.0
1927	19.6	19.8	16.8	18.9
1928	20.8	19.9	18.0	19.5
1929	20.6	22.9	17.1	19.8

Source: *KV*, 1916–30.

quennial census in 1905 and the 1920 census was low, on the order of 1.1%, but it rose to about 1.7% between the censuses of 1920 and 1930. The earlier growth rate was certainly affected by the influenza pandemic, but the reported increase would still suggest somewhat lower general mortality in the 1920s. Unfortunately, the relative accuracy of the population counts, particularly that for 1920, remains in doubt.[8] Thus we are forced to use more fragmentary evidence as a basis for speculating on broader trends in mortality during the early twentieth century.

Data on Disease and Cause of Death

Statistical data and written reports on diseases and causes of death, particularly those deriving from epidemics, were more or less regularly provided by medical institutions and by individual health officials and physicians. These reports were far more limited in coverage than those from the village registers, but had the advantage of considerably greater detail. Between the mid-1860s and 1903, summaries published in *Koloniaal Verslag* included both numbers of cases and deaths classified by cause. The summaries were further broken down by region and, for much of the period, by reporting source (European doctors or *dokter-djawa*).[9]

After 1904 detailed published statistics were based on reports from health institutions. The only major exception to this was plague which, after its initial outbreak in 1910, was monitored and reported in considerable detail.[10] Summary statistics on other epidemic diseases also continued, albeit in a less concise and satisfactory statistical format. Throughout the period, the emphasis of the reports was on a select set of diseases classified as 'epidemic' by the colonial authorities. During the latter part of the nineteenth century, cholera, smallpox and 'fever' were reported with great regularity. There were also sporadic reports for a few other diseases: dysentery during the 1860s and 1870s; beri-beri after 1885; and 'syphilis and other venereal diseases', which first appeared as a separate classification in 1899. A further category was provided for 'other epidemic diseases', but few attempts were made in the *Koloniaal Verslag* to quantify or qualify this category in terms of specific causes of death.

'Fever', of course, encompassed a wide variety of illnesses, and attempts were gradually made to refine this category, at least to the extent of separating out malaria from other fevers. Thus in 1888 the broad category for fever (*koorts*) was split into *Febris intermittens* (intermittent fever) and three other types, *Febris biliosa*, *Febris gastrica* and *Febris catarrhalis*. In 1895 four illnesses, *Febris intermittens*, *Febris remittens*, *Febris intermittens perniciosa* and *Cachexia paludosa* became classified as 'malarial diseases' (*malariazieken*). If this represents a true quantification of malaria, which is open to some question, then its overall predominance—90 to 95% of all reported fevers—suggests that malaria would also have dominated the category of 'fever' in earlier years as well.[11]

After 1903, some general information on epidemics, including rough estimates of numbers of cases and deaths, continued to be reported. The diseases to be covered were specified in a series of regulations issued in 1910 and 1911 which also reorganized the civilian and military medical services and reinforced the role of health inspectors in the area of epidemic surveillance and control.[12] The emergence of plague was a major impetus for these actions, but the regulations also included instructions to report on other diseases, including smallpox, cholera, typhoid fever, bacillary dysentery and diphtheria. Subsequently other diseases were added to the list, notably paratyphoid A, epidemic cerebrospinal meningitis and, for a few years, poliomyelitis. Malaria, although not listed in the regulations, continued to appear regularly in the reports. By the 1930s regular reference was also being made to trachoma and tuberculosis. The latter was viewed with some alarm as it not only constituted the largest single cause of death in hospitals, but was also blamed as a major factor in wastage (sick leave, absenteeism, etc.) among indigenous civil servants and students.[13]

Considerable caution must be exercised in interpreting the reports of the colonial medical service on the incidence and fatality of various diseases. While reporting was virtually complete for the European population, and was probably also nearly complete for the group regularly classified as 'other foreigners' (almost entirely ethnic Chinese), it was very poor for the remainder of the population. Among Indonesians, reporting would have been biased toward the élite, both because of the limited supply of medical services and because access to such services would have been prohibitively expensive for the mass of the population.[14] It is also likely that incidence would have been more poorly reported than mortality and that reporting of the latter would have been better during epidemic periods, when there were increased pressures on the medical service to certify causes of death.

In the following sections we look at the impact of a few major epidemic diseases: cholera, smallpox and malaria or 'fever'. A further section deals with other endemic and epidemic diseases, notably typhoid fever, dysentery and tuberculosis, although quantification of their impact on mortality is difficult. Plague and influenza, notable epidemic diseases of the twentieth century, are dealt with elsewhere in this volume.[15]

Cholera

Cholera is perhaps the most striking of epidemic diseases. In non-epidemic periods it tends to exist at relatively low levels, perhaps limited to a few endemic areas. Then incidence suddenly increases, not only in endemic areas, but spreading with remarkable rapidity to surrounding communities and further afield. In populations where control mechanisms are limited and resistance low, it can have a devastating impact. Case fatality rates of 50% or even higher are not uncommon and, although incidence tends to be lower than for other diseases such as malaria or typhoid fever, epidemics can still result in a large number of deaths in a very short period of time. Within a matter of months the epidemic runs its course and a situation of relatively low incidence returns.[16]

In Indonesia the pattern of extreme fluctuation between epidemic and non-epidemic periods is clear (Fig. 4.2). Outbreaks did occur in the intervening periods between major epidemics, but they tended to be locally contained and were, in any case, dramatically overshadowed by the major epidemics that spread over large parts of Java. Fatality was also high. For cases reported by the civilian medical service, 1864–1903, roughly 60% resulted in death, and there is no evidence from the fragmentary data subsequent to this period that this condition in any way improved. Recorded fatality rates from 'fever' and smallpox, the other two epidemic diseases regularly covered over the latter part of the nineteenth century, were closer to 10–15%. Only plague in the twentieth century was a more consistent killer, with reported case fatality of well over 90%. [17]

Major epidemics occurred in 1881–82, 1889, 1892, 1897 and 1901–02, with the first and last of these apparently being the most substantial.[18] Another major epidemic occurred in 1909–10, which led to a reported 60 000 deaths in Java and Madura in 1910. A somewhat smaller epidemic was reported in 1919, but this was overshadowed by the lingering effects of the world-wide influenza pandemic that hit Indonesia in the latter months of 1918. These were the last substantial outbreaks of cholera during the colonial period. Cholera vaccine became available in 1912 and this was accompanied by more concerted efforts at isolation, disinfection and provision of clean drinking water in areas where outbreaks occurred. These efforts even went as far as destruction of housing units where cholera cases were reported, a practice more commonly associated with attempts to control the spread of plague.[19] Although the selective impact of specific measures remains uncertain, the underlying conclusion is clear. By the early 1920s cholera had been effectively eliminated as a significant factor in mortality in Java.[20]

By and large the epidemics were most severe in the densely populated residencies along the north coast and, according to the reports, they frequently started in the major port cities of Batavia, Semarang and Surabaya. This supports contemporary theories that the disease was brought in on ships from other parts of Asia. Quarantine regulations were in effect from early in the nineteenth

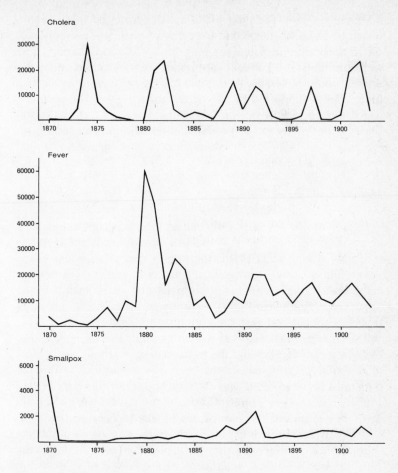

Fig. 4.2. Reported Deaths by selected Epidemic Diseases, Java and Madura, 1870–1903
Source: KV, 1871–1904

century but were generally ineffective, perhaps due to the almost impossible task of monitoring sea traffic within a multi-island nation. However, it may also be a partly spurious correlation, as some epidemics might have arisen locally within the crowded and unsanitary conditions existing in these urban centres.[21]

The inability to control the rapid spread of cholera once it took hold is interestingly documented by reports on the epidemic of 1881–82. This placed the start of the epidemic in Surabaya on

5 September 1881 and linked it to a sailor from the ship *Curacao*
which had recently docked in the port. Cholera was also reported
on 10 September in Semarang and on the 20th in Batavia. These
were probably independent outbreaks, as it is unlikely that the
disease could have spread this far from Surabaya in so short a
time. This is supported by the pattern of spread of the epidemic
which moved rapidly outward from these centres during the following months. By the end of November, within three months of
the first case being reported, cholera had managed to spread
systematically throughout Java.[22]

Malaria

Even with the myriad of difficulties in interpreting the data, it
seems safe to conclude that malaria was a significant factor in
mortality during most of this period. It was a consistent killer,
never falling away to insignificant levels as cholera did periodically. It also surged enormously in particular years, mainly in the
north coast residencies and frequently in areas where combinations of drought and abnormal flooding had occurred.

The causes of malaria were not discovered until the very end of
the nineteenth century and the term *malariazieken* did not appear
in *Koloniaal Verslag* before the early 1890s. Because of this the
data must be interpreted with caution. Up to 1887 the data used in
Fig. 4.2 reflect reports on deaths due to 'fever'. Between 1887 and
1892 they represent the sum of deaths due to *Febris intermittens*
and 'other fevers', with close to 90% of the total generally being
reported in the former category. After 1892 only deaths due to the
four illnesses defined as *malariazieken* are presented.

There was a major upsurge in reported cases and deaths due to
'fever' in 1880.[23] Between the mid-1860s and 1880, reported
deaths averaged only about 3600 annually. From 1880 to 1903 they
averaged over 16 000. Whether this increase was due in part to
improved reporting is unclear; reports on deaths due to smallpox
and cholera show no similar discontinuity, but these diseases were
already perceived by the colonial authorities as clear-cut threats to
the foreign population. The data can thus be taken as broadly
symptomatic, suggesting, but not quantifying, malaria's role in
overall mortality. Within local areas epidemics could be particularly severe. In 1902, for example, 23 149 deaths due to malaria
were reported for Semarang alone. In one sub-district of Cirebon

Regency, malaria was estimated to have wiped out 3.5% of the population in 1903.[24]

Because of the change in reporting procedures, it becomes more difficult to follow trends in malaria after 1904. It seems to have remained a major problem, at least up to the mid-1920s, with occasional outbreaks of epidemic proportions. Thus, Semarang continued to report large numbers of malaria cases and deaths until 1910, as did the belt of north coast residencies extending from Cirebon to Pasuruan. In 1908 a total of around 550 000 cases and 60 000 deaths were reported, with about 60% of these totals being accounted for by only three residencies: Semarang, Pasuruan and Besuki.

After 1911, references to malaria are even more sketchy, although authorities continued to recognize its importance. The *Koloniaal Verslag* for 1917 noted that malaria not only affected mortality directly, but also made survivors weaker and more susceptible to other diseases. This linkage also appeared in descriptions of the 1918 influenza epidemic, which noted its relative severity in areas where malaria was strongly endemic.

By the late 1920s, however, the tone of the reports changed dramatically. Malaria was said to be declining, thanks to drainage of mosquito-breeding areas and improved distribution of quinine. By the early 1930s, it was claimed to be largely under control.[25] This was almost certainly an overstatement, as the ability to enforce mosquito-eradication schemes at the village level would have been difficult in many areas and the quinine distribution programme was far from a complete success.[26] Nevertheless, any substantial reduction in malaria, particularly in areas where it had been highly endemic before, could have had a noticeable impact on overall mortality, certainly greater than that which would have been achieved through control of other epidemic diseases.[27]

In fact, the relation of the incidence of 'fever' with environmental conditions had been recognized from a fairly early date. Even during the 1880s there were frequent references in the *Koloniaal Verslag* to possible linkages between 'fever' epidemics and abnormal floods, and of increases in incidence associated with the opening up of new land in swampy terrain. Swamp drainage (*assainering*) was undertaken to control malaria in the latter years of the nineteenth century, even before the precise etiology of the disease was known, although this was only on a small scale in and around the major cities and towns. Efforts continued in the early twentieth century and were assisted by the knowledge that mosquito breeding places constituted the primary target.[28] However, the programme remained small and was frequently hampered by lack of funding, at least until the late 1920s and 1930s, when public works projects aimed at malaria control began to receive sufficient priority to have a noticeable impact on the incidence of the disease.[29]

Quinine was made available on a widespread basis for the indigenous population in the late 1870s, but it was not until 1906 that it began to be heavily subsidized. It was distributed free after 1909 but it is unclear if even this had much effect, as there were complaints about the difficulty of getting people to take it for any extended period of time.[30] Part of the problem may lie with side effects, which can be frequently uncomfortable.

Smallpox

Smallpox was perhaps the only disease subject to attempts at prophylactic control throughout all of the period under discussion. Smallpox vaccine was discovered in 1798, and by the 1860s was being manufactured on Java for local use. In the 1880s around 600 000 primary vaccinations and a similar number of revaccinations were being carried out annually. Numbers, particularly for revaccinations, increased steadily into the early years of the twentieth century with around 800 000 primary vaccinations and 2 million revaccinations reported annually, 1900–1908. After marked fluctuations during the period 1909 to 1914, these numbers increased slowly into the 1920s when a noticeable upsurge occurred in both categories. By the late 1930s there were around 1.4 million primary vaccinations and 5 million revaccinations a year.

There is no evidence, however, of change in the general level of mortality due to smallpox between 1880 and the 1920s. This was undoubtedly due in part to problems of effectiveness of the vaccination programme: inadequate numbers and quality of personnel, popular ambivalence toward vaccination, and frequent spoilage of the vaccine. In fact, it seems quite likely that the virtual elimination of smallpox in Java in the late 1920s (if the rather incomplete reports can believed) was due as much to improvements in the effectiveness of vaccination as to the upsurge in numbers of vaccinations.[31]

Nevertheless, the data suggest that smallpox played only a marginal role in explaining overall mortality in Java. Deaths reported by the civilian medical service in the latter parts of the nineteenth century were often only a few hundred a year and there were none of the violent upsurges characteristic of cholera and 'fever' (Fig. 4.2). The most significant single smallpox epidemic appears to have occurred in 1912–13, resulting in a reported total of only 8 000 deaths on Java in the latter year. Undoubtedly smallpox mortality was underreported, but this was also true of other epidemic diseases. In this respect, the 'relative' insignificance of smallpox may still be proof that the vaccination programme, despite its shortcomings, was effective prior to the 1920s in preventing more violent outbreaks of the disease than actually occurred.[32]

Other Diseases

Besides plague, which was extensively documented following its emergence in Java in 1910,[33] detailed reports on other diseases are more difficult to find. Reported cases of beri-beri and venereal disease were often fairly high, although mortality was always low. These diseases tended to be endemic among subgroups of the population and in areas which were of particular colonial concern: beri-beri among military personnel, prisoners and estate workers; venereal disease in the larger urban centres, particularly the major ports.[34] Quantification of their impact among the broader rural population is impossible, but it is clear that neither of these diseases was a major factor in mortality in Java.

Other diseases for which some material is available include bacillary dysentery and typhoid fever (*Typhus abdominalis*). The reported numbers of cases and deaths were small, but it is likely, given general levels of sanitation and hygiene, that the true levels of incidence and resultant mortality were considerably higher than is suggested in the reports.[35] A survey of hospital cases and deaths conducted in 1930 ranked dysentery sixth and typhoid seventh among twenty-four listed causes of death, with each contributing about 5% of the deaths observed.[36]

In any case, typhoid and dysentery were apparently widespread, although reports of outbreaks tended to centre on the north coast residencies. Their impact on overall mortality remains indeterminate, although it is interesting to note a report on

Batavia for 1912 which gave a death rate of 3.1 per thousand population due to dysentery (compared with a rate of 4.6 per thousand for malaria), certainly not an insignificant figure.[37]

The same report gave a death rate of 3.5 per thousand population in Batavia from tuberculosis. This disease frequently represented the largest single cause of death among hospital patients, and from about 1910 on it was increasingly recognized as a substantial health problem. It is likely that tuberculosis, as a disease of poverty and crowded and insanitary living conditions, particularly in the cities and towns, may have been as significant a factor in mortality in Java as it was in some other Third World countries at the time.[38]

Some diseases, like measles and diphtheria, were occasionally mentioned, and others, like trachoma, were apparently extremely widespread, although as a group their impact on overall mortality was probably small. Far more important is the group of air-borne respiratory illnesses including pneumonia, bronchitis and influenza, diseases regarded by some experts as critical in explaining pre-transition mortality levels and early stages of mortality decline in less-developed countries.[39] Unfortunately the colonial reports hardly mention the first two at all, and influenza was reported mainly in and after 1918.[40]

Direct Interventions

To try to tie these fragmentary data into a cohesive theory of mortality levels and trends is a difficult proposition. Some diseases, particularly the more striking one such as cholera and plague, were heavily reported, but others that may have had a far more continuing impact on mortality were, like tuberculosis, poorly covered or, like pneumonia and infantile and weanling diarrhoeal diseases, hardly mentioned at all. Even so, a few speculative propositions will be attempted.

With the possible exception of smallpox vaccination, it seems likely that medical interventions had only a limited impact on mortality at any time during this period. For example, even though cholera vaccine was claimed to be a factor in epidemic control in the 1920s and 1930s, it is more likely that the effect was minimal due to problems of introducing vaccination quickly enough once an epidemic had broken out. Other interventions may have been more important: efforts to isolate individuals and seal off infected areas, and vector control through the provision of uncontaminated supplies of drinking water to infected and surrounding areas.

Public health programmes aimed at modification of personal practices related to hygiene and sanitation also probably had only a marginal impact on mortality. Some exception might be postulated for those major cities where improvements in water supply systems did occur late in the period, although the degree to which diseases like dysentery and typhoid fever remained endemic in these areas attest to a less than total success.

This does not mean that some of the basic issues of public health and linkages between living standards, personal hygiene and disease were not recognized. As early as 1880 a manual on popular medicine and public health urged the boiling of drinking water. During the 1930s the Public Health Service was involved in several projects to expand rural medical and public health services.[41] Many of these emphasized the benefits of disease prevention—vaccination, hygiene and sanitation—over epidemic control. In his discussion of the high level of infant mortality in Batavia, de Haas paid special note to what he called the 'complex of social-hygienic factors' contributing to high mortality, and argued that improvements in living standards, education, nutrition, water and sanitation were what was really required to dramatically lower mortality rates.[42] Yet he also noted, perhaps somewhat in desperation, that:

local authorities thus far have not allowed health officials to establish this alliance (of hygiene and pediatrics) on a broader basis. Evidently the authorities are more concerned with the slight financial consequences of such improvements than with the judgment of future historians.[43]

In summary, as far as the period under consideration is concerned, it was a case of too little, too late. Not only were resources (money and personnel) limited, but, as other critics noted, there remained difficulties of motivating changes in long-standing traditions related to personal hygiene and health care.[44]

Nevertheless, control of major epidemics of cholera and malaria, along with virtual eradication of smallpox, was apparently achieved in the 1920s, and this must have had some impact on overall mortality. The higher observed growth rate in the 1920s should therefore be viewed as indicative of at least some improvement in mortality over previous decades. If medical interventions (with the exception of smallpox vaccination) and improvements in standards of personal hygiene are largely discounted, the major explanation is likely to be found in an increasing effectiveness of programmes aimed specifically at vector control.

Swamp drainage was mounted on an increasing scale during the 1920s and 1930s, reflecting an increasing dominance of programmes dealing with malaria (both in the field and in the laboratory) in the work of the Public Health Service. In some local areas the effects of these efforts seem to have been dramatic.[45] Expenditures were also high (some three million guilders were expended on a single project in Batavia in 1931–33), a situation which can be contrasted with the apparent lack of financial concern for programmes aimed more specifically at improving personal hygiene standards among the mass of the population.

On the other hand, there is no evidence that any of these types of interventions (medical, public health, vector control) had any impact before about 1920. The end of the nineteenth and first two decades of the twentieth century were characterized by frequent and often severe epidemics and there is no indication that these declined in either frequency or intensity during this period. It is difficult to link these epidemics to broader underlying patterns of mortality, but the inability to control even the few diseases that were regularly reported suggests general ineffectiveness on the part of the colonial authorities.

Social and Economic Change

If these direct interventions were ineffective prior to the third decade of the twentieth century, what does this imply about previous levels of mortality? The question has historical importance in the light of the continuing debate over the demographic determinants of the remarkably high (for a pre-transitional society) population growth rate observed for Java during the nineteenth century.[46] In this sense we should be asking if it is still possible that general underlying mortality levels in Java underwent some moderate decline before 1920 and, perhaps more significantly, if throughout all of the period under study they may have remained at somewhat lower levels than in most other countries of the region.

Here we are drawn to possible direct and indirect effects of colonial policy, most notably in the economic sphere. This is also an area of intense debate, centred, in recent scholarly writings, around the impact of the Cultivation System (which lasted from 1830 until the late 1860s), and of the plantation system which succeeded it, on the material well-being of the Javanese peasantry. Of particular interest are questions related to levels of nutrition and food supply and their impact on mortality, largely through the mechanism of increasing resistance to disease as a life-threatening event. At the extreme end of the scale is famine, which, for example, was one of the main causes of death in nineteenth century India.[47] More subtle are the lingering effects of malnutrition, which has been increasingly recognized as a major underlying factor in mortality due to a host of other causes.[48] Thus, if basic food supplies increased during or immediately following the Cultivation System, or systems of food distribution from surplus to deficit areas improved, this might have had a salutary effect on mortality levels during the period.

Somewhat contrary to conclusions reached by earlier writers about the 'impoverishment' of the Javanese peasantry under the Cultivation System, statistics (along with contemporary descriptions) utilized by some recent researchers suggest that conditions may have actually improved during at least part of the nineteenth century. Even with the vast amounts of labour expropriated for the production of export crops, the acreage, productivity and per-capita output of rice land under peasant cultivation all rose significantly in the period 1837 to 1851.[49] In the latter year, production was apparently about 3.52 piculs (218 kg.) of *padi* per capita, a figure almost exactly the same as that for Java (excluding the special districts of Jakarta and Yogyakarta) in 1980.[50] The amount of land under peasant rice cultivation in Java continued to increase during the latter part of the nineteenth century. Between 1878 and 1887 harvested rice area increased by about 1.7% per year compared with a recorded population growth rate closer to 1.4%. Average production (excluding Batavia, Madura, Surakarta and Yogyakarta) was 3.74 piculs per capita.[51] However, scarcity of new land suitable for wet-rice cultivation was becoming an increasing problem by the end of the period.

Besides food production there is also the more general question of commercialization and monetization of the economy. For example, increased revenues at the national level would have permitted increased food imports. It is this mechanism which Meegama claims related commercialization of agriculture and increased population growth rates in Sri Lanka around the turn of the century.[52]

Rice imports into Java did not start until after the end of the Cultivation System. Nevertheless, the rapid earlier growth in imports of consumer goods, particularly textiles, may still be indicative of developments in a cash economy.

Elson also notes the influx of cash resulting from payments under the Cultivation System. In many areas, particularly where sugar and coffee were produced, these often substantially exceeded land rent obligations, leaving at least a moderate cash surplus in the hands of the cultivators.[53] For some, at least, this would have meant increased flexibility in marketing food crops and, with expansion of the overall market economy, increased access to consumer goods.

A key factor in all of this was undoubtedly the pace of development of basic economic infrastructure, notably in irrigation and transportation. Irrigation was fundamental to the expansion of sugar-cane production and also for other export crops such as indigo. Roads and, later in the century, railroads were equally important in facilitating movement of goods and people. Admittedly, these improvements were selectively applied to the production of export crops and, in many areas, through expropriation of limited water resources, excessive labour demands, etc., disrupted patterns of domestic cultivation. On the other hand, these facilities almost certainly had a broader impact on the overall expansion of cultivation and on the development of markets for a wide variety of commodities.

There is also the effect of improved transportation on the ability to shift surplus food crop production to areas where shortages had occurred. Davis places great emphasis on improvements in irrigation and transportation in his discussion of the amelioration of widespread famines in India after 1900.[54] In Java there also seems to be ample evidence that improvements in food supply and distribution did occur. Elson and Knight note that for at least some areas where the Cultivation System caused chronic food shortages, the gap could largely be filled by surplus production from adjacent areas.[55] For later periods, the *Koloniaal Verslag* contain frequent references to government sponsored shipments of food to areas hit by crop failures and epidemics, notably to areas of chronic high mortality such as Banten. It must be kept in mind that these are macro-level observations. They obscure what must have been often severe maldistribution of benefits and hence considerable levels of personal suffering due to the vagaries of the colonial economic system.

In any case, the principal conclusion of the paper remains clear: it seems highly unlikely that the limited direct intervention by the colonial authorities had any noticeable impact on overall mortality. If one wants to justify arguments of 'relatively' low or declining mortality in the latter part of the nineteenth and early twentieth centuries in Java, explanations must be sought in the broader, primarily economic sphere rather than in medical or public health innovations designed to reduce mortality or control the impact of specific epidemic diseases.

1. On the controversy surrounding the size and growth of Indonesia's population during the nineteenth century, see Widjojo Nitisastro, *The Population of Indonesia* (Ithaca, Cornell University Press, 1970); B. Peper, 'Population Growth in Java in the 19th Century: A New Interpretation', *Population Studies* 24, 1 (1970), 71–84; and P. Boomgaard, 'Bevolkingsgroei en welvaart op Java (1800–1942)', in R. N. J. Kamerling (ed.), *Indonesie toen en nu* (Amsterdam, Intermediair, 1980).

2. The data in Fig. 4.1 on deaths due to epidemics came from reports of the colonial medical service, which generally covered fewer than 10% of the number of deaths compiled from the village registers. To simplify the comparison, Fig. 4.1 is presented in terms of index number rather than total numbers of deaths.

3. The years are 1874, 1877–79, 1884–89 and 1894 (see Fig. 4.1).

4. Cf. the estimate of Peter Boomgaard, 'Morbidity and Mortality in Java, 1820–1880', above, that epidemic disease accounted for just 10% of all deaths during the period he is analysing. While the calculations seem to imply an *increase* in the significance of epidemic disease in late nineteenth century Java, a situation which would parallel the better-documented pattern in the Philippines—cf. Peter C. Smith, 'Crisis Mortality in the Nineteenth Century Philippines: Data from Parish Records', *Journal of Asian Studies* 38, 1 (1978), 51–76—given the crudeness of both data and methodology, it seems safer to use this result to reaffirm the relatively minor role played by epidemic mortality in nineteenth century Java.

5. Peper, op. cit.

6. This can be easily seen by calculating crude death rates (deaths per thousand population) for each year. As long as the assumptions as to registration quality and the population growth rate hold true, the conclusion is valid irrespective of the actual size of the population.

7. For a more detailed discussion see Peter Gardiner, *Vital Registration in Indonesia: A Study of the Behavioral Determinants of Registration of Births and Deaths*, (Ph.D. dissertation, Canberra, Australian National University, 1981); cf. Susan Abeyasekere, 'Death and Disease in Nineteenth Century Batavia', below, for differential public health care within the colonial capital.

8. Widjojo Nitisastro, op. cit., 68.

9. *Dokter-djawa* were Indonesians holding medical certificates granted by indigenous medical training institutions. The programme was designed to provide persons with a general knowledge to service the needs of the indigenous population. However, the number remained small and never exceeded the number of European-trained physicians in the country.

10. Cf. Terence H. Hull, 'Plague in Java', below.

11. Although there is evidence (see below) that malaria was quantitatively less important in the earlier part of the nineteenth century; cf. Boomgaard, 'Morbidity', and note 23 below.

12. The most important of these was *Bijblad* 7276, 27 January 1911. This ordinance introduced a system of 'weekly death statistics' at the subdistrict level in

Java, Madura, Bali and Lombok. Responsibility for maintaining the system was assigned to the health inspectors (*inspecteurs*) who were located at the regency level.

13. *KV*, 1936.

14. Even by the 1930s, there were fewer than 1000 doctors, or about one per 60 000 population. Most of these medical personnel were located in towns; in Java and Madura almost 40% were in the port cities of Batavia, Semarang and Surabaya. Some private estates in the twentieth century did provide free clinics for workers and their families; prophylactic interventions, notably smallpox vaccination and distribution of quinine, were carried out at low or no cost to acceptors; public health programmes were introduced in the 1930s. Their overall impact, however, would have been small.

15. Cf. Hull, op. cit., and Colin Brown, 'The Influenza Pandemic of 1918 in Indonesia', below.

16. See, for example, A.S. Benenson (ed.), *Control of Communicable Diseases in Man* (Washington D.C., American Public Health Association, 1965), 71; W. H. Mosley, 'Biological Contamination of the Environment by Man', in S. H. Preston (ed.), *Biological and Social Aspects of Mortality and the Length of Life* (Liège, Ordina Publications, 1980).

17. Cf. Hull, op. cit.

18. Cf. Boomgaard, 'Morbidity', on the impact of cholera before 1880.

19. Cf. Hull, op. cit.

20. Minor outbreaks continued to occur, but their impact was limited. For example, when cholera, said to have been imported from Singapore, broke out in Tanjung Priok in early November 1927, an immediate programme of prophylactic vaccination was instituted. Only 12 cases were reported.

21. Note, however, that Boomgaard, 'Morbidity', fully supports the view of foreign intervention, stating that 'epidemic cholera was always reintroduced from overseas'.

22. *KV*, 1882.

23. Boomgaard, 'Morbidity', also notes this upsurge and suggests that, among other factors, it reflected the expansion of *sawah* into previously uncultivated areas.

24. These figures are from the text of the reports and exceed the number of officially certified deaths (reported in the appendix tables of *KV*) which underlie Figure 4.2.

25. Substantial outbreaks were reported in 1931 and 1937 and were linked to flooding attendant on abnormal rains. Due, it was claimed, to improved quinine distribution, total mortality was less than in earlier years.

26. While Boomgaard, 'Morbidity', notes that quinine was distributed in large quantities during epidemics, he also notes that the lack of medical personnel made it impossible to effectively supervise implementation at the individual level. This latter problem would have remained relevant throughout the colonial period.

27. The impact of malaria eradication on mortality has been documented in a few countries where adequate data is available, notably Ceylon; S. A. Meegama, 'Malaria Eradication and Its Effect on Mortality Levels', *Population Studies* 21, 3 (1967), 207–38.

28. For example, there were attempts to get people to periodically drain fish ponds (which were viewed as a particularly inviting source of stagnant water) and to put fish in open wells to eat the mosquito larvae.

29. Eradication programmes would also affect mortality from other diseases, both through the simultaneous elimination of parasites or vectors, and through increased resistance (of a population less weakened through continual bouts of malaria) to mortality from other causes; see S. H. Preston, 'Causes and Consequences of Mortality Decline in Less Developed Countries During the 20th Century',

in R. A. Easterlin (ed.), *Population and Economic Change in Developing Countries* (Chicago, University of Chicago Press, 1980), 289–359.

30. Boomgaard, 'Morbidity', also notes this problem. Overall, however, he takes a more optimistic view, suggesting that quinine did have some effect, particularly in the latter part of the nineteenth century.

31. By the 1930s vaccine was being produced and stored under controlled conditions in an number of centres on Java; methods for transporting and administering vaccine had also improved.

32. Cf. Boomgaard, 'Morbidity', on the efficacy of nineteenth century vaccination in Java.

33. Plague was perhaps the best documented of all epidemic diseases during the colonial period; cf. Hull, op. cit.

34. Cf. Boomgaard, 'Morbidity'.

35. As the Dutch themselves suggested as early as 1910, typhoid might well have been frequently hidden under the general 'fever' classification in the nineteenth century; cf. Boomgaard, 'Morbidity', on the 1846–50 epidemic.

36. *KV*, 1931.

37. *KV*, 1913.

38. In Havana, Cuba, between 1900 and 1931, respiratory tuberculosis was consistently the second largest cause of death (following cardiovascular diseases) and represented 20% of total mortality. F. Diaz-Briquets, 'Determinants of Mortality Transition in Developing Countries Before and After the Second World War: Some Evidence from Cuba', *Population Studies* 35, 3 (1981), 399–411.

39. S. H. Preston, 'Causes and Consequences of Mortality Decline', and S. H. Preston and V.E. Nelson, 'Structure and Change in Cause of Deaths: An International Summary', *Population Studies* 28, 1 (1974), 19–51.

40. Cf. Brown, op. cit.

41. The most famous was probably the Demonstration Health Unit set up in Purwokerto in 1933. It included birth and death registration, immunization programmes, pre- and ante-natal care, and efforts to improve basic hygiene and sanitation. For a discussion of the history of these efforts, see J. H. Hydrick, *Intensive Rural Hygiene Work and Public Health Education of the Public Health Service of Netherlands India* (Batavia, Batavia-Centrum, 1937).

42. J. H. de Haas, 'Infant Mortality in Batavia for the Years 1935 and 1936', *Indian Journal of Pediatrics* 6 (1939), 32.

43. Ibid., 34.

44. This was reflected both by low rates of use of medical facilities and lack of development of improved sanitation at the local level; see W. F. Wertheim, *Indonesian Society in Transition: A Study in Social Change* (The Hague, van Hoeve, 1956), 253–62.

45. Following a programme of drainage and use of insecticides in Cilacap (West Java) in 1920, the recorded death rate fell from 45 per thousand population to 28 in 1925 and continued falling gradually, reaching 23 per thousand in 1930 and 20 in 1934; A. Jonkers, *Welvaartszorg in Indonesia* ('s-Gravenhage, W. van Hoeve, 1948), 20.

46. See references cited under Note 1, above.

47. K. Davis, *The Population of India and Pakistan* (New York, Russell and Russell, 1958).

48. The effect of food supply and nutrition on illness and mortality, particularly that of infants and young children, has been a major focus of recent literature: see W. H. Mosley, 'Will Primary Health Care Reduce Infant and Child Mortality? A Critique of Some Current Strategies with Special Reference to Africa and Asia', paper presented at IUSSP Seminar on 'Social Policy, Health Policy and Mortality Prospects', Paris, Feb.–Mar. 1983.

49. R. E. Elson, 'Peasant Poverty and Prosperity Under the Cultivation System

in Java', paper presented at conference on 'Indonesian Economic History in the Dutch Colonial Period', Australian National University, 16–18 December 1983, 18.

50. Calculated from Biro Pusat Statistik, *Buku Saku Statistik Indonesia 1982* (Jakarta, Biro Pusat Statistik, 1983), Tables II.1.2 and IV.1.4.

51. Calculated from data in *KV*, 1889.

52. S. A. Meegama, 'The Decline of Mortality in Sri Lanka in Historical Perspective', *Solicited Papers*, Vol. 2 (Manila, IUSSP General Conference, 1981), 143–64.

53. Elson, op. cit., 12.

54. Davis, op. cit., 38.

55. Elson, op. cit., 19; G. R. Knight, 'Capitalism and Commodity Production in Java,' in H. Alavi et al. (eds), *Capitalism and Colonial Production* (London, Croom Helm, 1982), 119–59.

5 Measuring Mortality in the Nineteenth Century Philippines

NORMAN G. OWEN

DEATH is ubiquitous in the Southeast Asian past. It is most evident in the great mortality crises described by travellers, assessed by bureaucrats, and remembered in myth and legend by those who suffered, but it can also be seen in the day-to-day struggle for survival throughout the region. No historian can ignore it. Yet if we are to do more than note its inexorable pressure and lament its sudden and cruel manifestations, we must find some means of measuring it, a singularly difficult task. We know that life was short in pre-modern Southeast Asia, but we do not know how short. We know that many people died in epidemics and other crises; sometimes there is even a tally—however derived—of corpses; yet it is all but impossible to get any sense of proportion. Without some estimate of normal mortality we are hard put to judge the relative significance of crises or to discern any changes which may have occurred gradually over time.

Thanks to the Roman Catholic church, the Philippines has by far the most voluminous and detailed evidence for demographic history of any country in Southeast Asia. Wherever parish priests were established—throughout more than half the country by the early seventeenth century—they attempted to count all tribute-payers and 'souls' and to record all baptisms, marriages and burials. Nearly all aggregate population figures are derived directly or indirectly from these parochial accounts. Most of the original records have disappeared over the centuries, and those which have survived are often incomplete and almost always of questionable reliability in one regard or another. Nevertheless, if there is anywhere in the Southeast Asian past a hope for more precise understanding of pre-twentieth century mortality, it is in the Spanish Philippines.[1]

This paper is an attempt to utilize some of these sources to specify the dimensions of a mortality crisis in the Bikol region of southeastern Luzon in the mid-1840s.[2] The Spanish authorities did not perceive this as a single crisis, but as two essentially distinct, though related, events. First there was a severe food shortage caused by two consecutive bad harvests due to untimely typhoons; the government took notice of this only after the second typhoon (3 November 1845) and over the next six months demanded regular reports on food prices and relief efforts.[3] Later came an epidemic of 'cholera', which first struck the region in February 1846 and claimed (according to official reports) nearly a thousand lives over the next two months. The identification of this disease cannot be certain, for at that time the Spanish used the term to refer not only to the virulent and lethal '*cólera asiática*' which we know as 'cholera' today but also to weaker enteric disorders, known as '*cólera común*'.[4] In any event, malnutrition undoubtedly decreased resistance to whatever infectious agent caused the illness, so any distinction between deaths caused by famine and those caused by cholera is to some extent artificial.[5]

The official reports suggest some of the human suffering that occurred in this crisis, as well as some of the ways in which Bikolanos attempted to cope with it. Prices for grain were exorbitant, up to three times usual pre-harvest levels. Those who could not pay were 'faint from weakness', living on roots and forest plants, seeking subsistence in other districts, or dying of 'great mad hunger'. A few months later officials were 'alarmed . . . by the appearance of so terrible a blow' as the cholera which 'attacked the needy and well-to-do classes' alike and killed them 'in the space of a few hours of sickness'.[6] Yet these reports provide very little by which we might actually begin to assess the magnitude of mortality. For this we must turn to demographic sources, beginning with the annual aggregate figures assembled by church and state authorities.

Annual Aggregate Sources

Although from time to time over the previous two hundred years Manila had summed up parish or provincial totals to arrive at nominal enumerations of tribute-payers or 'souls' in the Philippines, from the late eighteenth century onward such aggregations became much more demographically useful. Not only were they compiled more frequently, but most of them included the parish or municipal figures on which national totals were based. Even more significantly, in the early nineteenth century listings of annual baptisms, marriages and burials by parish began to accompany population totals.

For the period from 1818 to 1865 the best known of these compilations, and the most accessible to scholars are those which found their way into the annual *Guías (Guides)* and the published works of such authors as Yldefonso A. de Aragón, Manuel Buzeta and Felipe Bravo, and, for districts administered by Franciscan friars, Félix de Huerta.[7] Occasionally the religious orders or diocesan prelates would publish an *estado* (statement, account) of the population in their jurisdictions, but these *estados*, often issued in broadsheet form, are not easy to locate.[8] Even less accessible are the manuscript *estados* of orders and dioceses, though a considerable number of them have been preserved in the archives of the Philippines and Spain. Finally, there are some annual aggregate figures in the parish records themselves, at least for those few parishes with surviving *padrones* (annual censuses). Each *padron* is normally accompanied by a short *estado* that sums up the parish population by age/status categories of uncertain boundaries and records the number of baptisms, marriages and burials in the preceding year.[10] Since these parish *estados* are presumably the originals from which other aggregations ultimately derive, they are an invaluable demographic source, but they are too rare to serve as the primary basis for evaluating national or even regional mortality.

As we have available to us dozens of listings of population and burials by parish for the period,[11] it would seem simple to calculate both normal and crisis mortality rates. Most of these sources are individually plausible, though in quite a few instances some of the parish death rates appear abnormally low. The real difficulties emerge only when the sources are juxtaposed with each other. Suddenly we discover that data for one year are simply copied from the previous year (so that we have no new information at all), or we find two or more sources for the same year with completely different figures for population or burials, or we observe huge and inexplicable contradictions between population totals for one year and the next. Perhaps the most dramatic example of this last problem is the town of Albay (later Legazpi), which is recorded in four different sources between 1838 and 1848 as having between 12 400 and 14 600 inhabitants and in four other sources for the same period is said to have 23 600 to 25 600![12] Similar, if not as conspicuous, discrepancies are found for many other parishes and years.

At the same time, however, combining several aggregate sources can also provide clues as to how to select and clean the data for analysis. It allows the identification, and thus the elimination, of data which are simply copied from one year to the next. It generally clarifies the parish and year to which figures pertain, information often ambiguous in any single source. Similarly, it reveals the numerous cases in which *tributantes* (individual tribute-payers) have been misidentified as *tributos* (pairs of *tributantes*) and vice versa. In a few instances the combination of sources makes it possible to identify and correct typographical or copying errors as well.[13]

Even after such cleaning, the aggregate data retain many of their contradictions, vitiating the value of any conclusions based on unselective analysis. The available sources for the period 1818–65 show a mean parish crude birth rate (CBR) of 36.0 (Standard Deviation 12.2) and a mean parish crude death rate (CDR) of 22.7 (S.D. 14.2), but as these means include rates based on such vastly differing population totals as those noted for the town of Albay, it is obvious that they are of limited utility. To make the analysis more precise it is necessary to make some qualitative distinctions among the conflicting data.

At first it may appear that given two figures purporting to be exact enumerations (rather than estimates) of population, the higher ought to be more correct. It is easier to imagine priests and officials overlooking large numbers of residents than 'counting' up to 10 000 people who were never there! The breakdown of population figures in some parish *estados*, however, shows how an overcount was in fact possible. The total number of 'souls' was obtained not by direct enumeration but by summing up the categories into which the population was divided: tribute-payers, infants, etc. And in the 1840s and 1850s (perhaps after a new format for parish *estados* was introduced in 1842?) there was clearly great confusion over these categories, particularly one called *adultos de comunión*. This could be interpreted in two different ways: as all residents of an age to take communion (i.e.,

12 or older) or as only those who took communion but were not yet of an age to pay tribute (i.e., from 12 to about 21). What seems to have happened in many cases is that these *adultos* were initially enumerated in the broader sense (all adults in the community) but then added into the total as if they were a separate category from tribute-payers and those exempt from tribute—with the result that they were counted twice, increasing the nominal size of the parish by as much as 50% or even more.

The lower of two conflicting population figures is thus generally to be preferred, a choice that also tends to raise both birth and death rates to slightly more plausible levels and eliminates some of the more exaggerated ratios of 'souls' to *tributos*.[14] In most cases the preferred totals also bring the parish population figures into line with apparent trends before 1840 and after 1860. None of this means that the lower figures are necessarily closer to the 'truth', as there is good reason to suspect consistently high levels of underenumeration, especially of children, in all Philippine demographic data. But they are apparently more representative of the actual enumerations of population, so must be used in any attempt to analyse these refractory data.

In putting this general principle into statistical practice, we must deal not just with cases where there are two or more conflicting figures, but with others where we have just one figure which is manifestly—in terms of vital rates, *tributo* ratios and population trends—too high. Rather than interpolate adjusted figures based on parish trend lines, which would involve further complications in selecting those values to be used in determining the trend, we can simply identify all data resulting in a population/*tributo* ratio of over 5.0 and either eliminate them entirely or impute alternative population figures obtained by multiplying *tributos* by some reasonable constant, such as 4.2.[15] Such adjustments, by removing many of the more obvious cases of mis-enumeration of population, help to improve the general reliability of the data. Over the period from 1818 to 1865, including crisis years, the revised figures give a weighted parish average CBR of 40.0 (S.D. 10.1) and a CDR of 24.5 (S.D. 13.6), implying a natural increase of 1.55% a year, which is consistent with nineteenth century growth rates in the Spanish-ruled Philippines.[16]

Mis-enumeration, however, should be distinguished (at least conceptually) from the more fundamental problem of underregistration. The latter affects not just the reliability—the internal consistency—of the data, but also their validity—how well they measure what they are supposed to measure. By careful comparison of the sources we can identify and correct many of the clerical errors which intervene between the initial recording of events and the data we actually work with: mis-counting, mis-summing, mis-copying and mis-labelling. But we cannot thus identify discrepancies between reality and initial recording: persons not listed in the *padrones*, births and deaths not accompanied by registered baptisms and burials. For this we need to apply tests of demographic plausibility.

By the simplest and most obvious of these tests, a considerable proportion of the aggregate data available for this region are badly flawed. Adapting a rule of thumb from D. C. Eversley, in studying a pre-transitional society we may regard as putatively under-registered all combinations of crude birth and death rates that add up to fewer than 50 events per thousand per year, which would eliminate a fair number of our data.[17] At the same time, when the ratio of burials to baptisms falls below 0.4:1 for significant numbers of parishes or years, it implies either differential under-registration of events or most improbable vital rates.[18] Even with adjusted population figures, some 39% of all cases may be regarded as putatively under-registered by one or both of these criteria.[19]

Where we have more detailed information we find even more demographically implausible data, particularly with regard to age structure. The ratio of children age 7–12 to those age 0–6 is generally far too high for any society with high mortality, averaging around 4:5 (80% survivorship) rather than the 1:2 (50–55%) suggested by standard life tables.[20] Similarly, children under the age of 7 apparently accounted for only 45% of all burials, though by the most apposite life tables the figure should be above 55%.[21]

Faced with such evidence we must resist both total despair and over-reliance on assumptions of demographic plausibility. The former gets us nowhere; the latter, though insidiously attractive, makes it too easy to 'prove', by selection or adjustment of the data, only that which we originally assumed. If, for example, we simply eliminate all combined vital rates below the level of 50 per thousand, we succeed in raising the average to more 'plausible' levels—at the cost of whatever empirical integrity the sources may possess.

Instead we should envisage the crisis we are studying as a peak standing upon terrain of unknown altitude. It may be possible to measure or estimate how high it rises above the surrounding plain without the necessity of determining the height above sea level of either peak or plain. Thus if, for the sake of argument, we can assume relatively consistent levels of registration (or under-registration) for each town,[22] the crisis can be compared with the background 'normality' recorded in the sources, leaving for later any attempted adjustments to demographically plausible levels.

We can begin by calculating for each parish averages for the years surrounding the crisis and comparing them with the rates recorded for 1845–46.[23] By eliminating parishes on the southern coast of Sorsogon, which were apparently unaffected by the crisis, we can compute crisis averages for the rest of the region as a whole. The weighted mean parish death rate was 75% (2.3 S.D.) above normal in 1845 and 172% (5.6 S.D.) in 1846.[24] Birth rates, meanwhile, fell from just 4% (0.2 S.D.) below normal in 1845 to 33% (1.7 S.D.) in 1846, and marriage rates from 41% to 53% below normal over the same two years. The average ratio of deaths to births, normally around 0.6:1, rose almost to unity in 1845 and shot up to 2.75:1 in 1846.[25]

Computation of parish indices also reveals considerable spatial differentiation in crisis intensity. For purposes of analysis the region (without southern Sorsogon) may be divided into nine districts: Camarines Norte, to the far north; Bicol (the Naga plain), Rinconada and Iraya in the central valley; northern Sorsogon to the south; Lagonoy and Tabaco along the Pacific coast of the peninsula; a number of small missions scattered around the hills and isolated coasts; and the offshore island of Catanduanes (see Map 3).[26] The nominal 'background' levels of mortality and fertility, even with adjusted population totals, vary considerably, presumably reflecting different levels of registration. 'Normal' death rates range from 29.3 per thousand in Bicol—old and reasonably populous parishes, most administered by Spanish Fran-ciscan friars, close to each other and to the province capital and diocesan see—to 16.9 in Catanduanes—small parishes, adminis-tered by secular priests (mostly Filipino), remote from higher civil and religious authority. But by comparing each parish with its own 'normality' we can arrive at roughly comparable indices of crisis intensity (see Table 5.1).

The least affected districts were Camarines Norte and northern Sorsogon, with both rates near normal in 1845 and births only

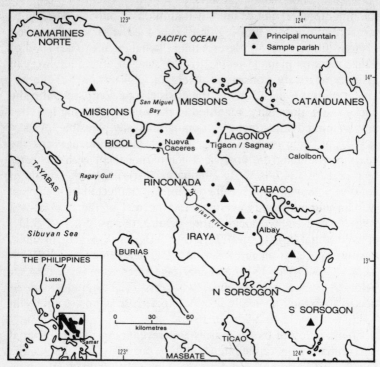

Map 3 Bikol Region

slightly depressed in 1846. A likely inference is that the 1845
typhoon passed between these districts on a westerly course
through the centre of the region.[27] In Bicol, at the northern end of
the central valley, there was also no real demographic crisis in
1845, though official reports describe much hunger and hardship
after the November typhoon. Birth and death rates, though marginally below and above background, respectively, were well
within the range of normal fluctuations. Rinconada was only
slightly more affected. In both these districts, however, the crisis
struck with great force in 1846, and birth rates remained depressed
(24% and 14% below normal, respectively) in 1847, though mortality fell back to normal levels.[28]

Farther up the central valley, mortality reached crisis levels in
populous Iraya in 1845 and worsened in 1846; even in 1847 death
rates remained 28% above normal. Birth rates, on the other hand,

TABLE 5.1

COMPARATIVE CRISIS FERTILITY AND MORTALITY BY DISTRICT. BIKOL REGION. 1845-46

Weighted parish birth and death rates compared with background averages
(Background: mean rates 1818–44, 1847–65)
(Weighting factor: 1845 *tributos*)

District	Pop* (000)	1845 CBR %	S.D.	1845 CDR %	S.D.	1846 CBR %	S.D.	1846 CDR %	S.D.
Camarines N.	19.6	− 2	−0.18	+ 15	+0.52	− 8	−0.43	+ 94	+2.86
Missions	6.4	+ 1	+0.03	+ 80	+1.31	−23	−0.11	+211	+3.74
Bicol	51.3	− 9	−0.42	+ 6	+0.18	−14	−0.74	+160	+5.23
Lagonoy	12.2	−10	−0.64	+ 82	+2.31	N.A.		N.A.	
Catanduanes	13.1	−21	−0.62	+282	+5.54	−55	−2.23	+322	+6.00
Rinconada	26.0	−12	−0.60	+ 20	+0.49	−47	−2.43	+101	+2.54
Tabaco	40.3	− 1	−0.05	+131	+3.80	−33	−1.85	+166	+4.87
Iraya	64.4	+ 5	+0.08	+111	+4.39	−49	−2.57	+231	+9.61
N. Sorsogon	17.4	+ 3	+0.12	− 2	−0.02	−16	−0.67	+ 67	+1.79
TOTAL	250.8	− 4	−0.20	+ 75	+2.28	−33	−1.67	+172	+5.63
S. Sorsogon	15.1	+ 6	+0.28	− 16	−0.38	+20	−0.08	+ 11	+0.30

*1845 population, adjusted.

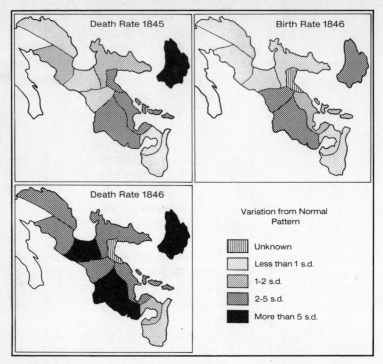

Fig. 5.1. Variation in Vital Rates by District, Bikol Region, 1845–46

were dramatically depressed only in 1846, with 1845 and 1847 near normal. The pattern in Tabaco resembles this (at slightly lower levels of variation) in 1845 and 1846, though in 1847 rates rebounded to normal, with births actually 25% above average. Lacking 1846 data for Lagonoy, we can only surmise that it resembled its near neighbours Tabaco or Rinconada. The data for the missions, though always most questionable, suggest the Iraya–Tabaco pattern, with crisis mortality beginning in 1845.

Official reports in the aftermath of the 1845 typhoon describe the island of Catanduanes as devastated, and the demographic data confirm that it was hit worse than any other district. Both birth and death rates were seriously disturbed in 1845, and though nominal 1846 death rates were marginally lower than those recorded for Bicol (70.8 to 77.0 per thousand) they were substantially higher as a percentage of normal registered levels, while the ratio of deaths to births rose in that year to more than 4:1. It is also the only district for which there is unequivocal evidence of a significant (20%) decline in total population—from 13 100 in 1845 to 10 500 in 1846—though some of this may be accounted for by migration rather than mortality.[29]

Though these comparisons clarify the geographical patterns of the crisis, they do not resolve the question of absolute magnitude. Taken at face value, the adjusted figures show just over a quarter of a million people living in the affected districts in 1845. The death rate rose from background levels of 22 per thousand to 36 in 1845 and 60 in 1846, resulting in some 13 000 'excess' deaths over the two-year period. The birth rate, meanwhile, slipped from a normal 40 to 39 and then to 27, leaving a 'deficit' of around 3 600 births. If we assume a likely infant mortality rate of 25% (250 per thousand) in normal years, this shortfall in births would depress expected mortality by 900 over the two years and thus raise the number of deaths considered 'excess' by the same amount. In sum, the annual aggregate data suggest that this crisis killed nearly 14 000 people (5.6% of the population of the affected districts) *beyond* those who would normally have died in 1845–46, plus at least a few hundred more in 1847.[30]

Here, however, we must re-introduce the problem of plausibility. As noted before, all computed vital rates appear too low for a pre-modern population, and there are other strong indications of incomplete registration. Exactly how these aggregate figures—which clearly have some basis in reality—ought to be converted into more 'valid' totals is more a matter for theory and speculation than for empirical inquiry. In view of the anomalies of age structure it is tempting to suggest that many of the discrepancies are accounted for by substantial under-registration of children and their births and deaths. If we assume, for example, that 20% of all births went unbaptized, that would raise the crude birth rate to 50 per thousand. If the same *number* (not percentage) of child deaths were unrecorded, it would raise the non-crisis death rate to 32 (an increase of 45%)[31] and increase the proportion of all deaths accounted for by children to much more credible levels. Furthermore, if the parish censuses failed to record these children between unregistered births and unregistered deaths, that would help explain why the number of small children listed is almost invariably too low.

All of these assumptions are arbitrary, of course, but as they all point toward more plausible rates and ratios it is likely that they indicate the direction, if not the magnitude, of appropriate adjustments of the aggregate data. Yet even if we accept these conversion factors we could only apply them to the crisis by another quite unprovable assumption, that relative registration rates were unaffected by the crisis. If we posited a constant 45% increase in burials, for example, it would raise death rates to 52 per thousand in 1845 and to 87 in 1846, thus lifting our estimate of 'excess' mortality in the crisis to just over 20 000 deaths (8% of the total population). But with this calculation we have stretched the aggregate annual sources as far as they can reasonably reach—and perhaps beyond.

Parish Registers

We can add another dimension to our understanding of mortality by analysing the monthly totals of burials from surviving parish registers. This technique is well known from its use by historical demographers in other countries, particularly England.[32] The great advantages of this approach, besides those inherent in having monthly rather than annual totals, are the independence and immediacy of the registers (which are prior to all other sources, even parish *estados*) and the putative consistency of coverage over an extended period. The disadvantages include gaps in the area covered (fewer than half the parish registers from the 1840s have survived) and the considerable labour required to count and transcribe events from registers handwritten in Spanish more than a century ago. Moreover, this approach does not resolve two of the fundamental unknowns in Philippine historical demography: the size of the population at risk and the extent of underregistration.

To study the mortality crisis of 1845–46, I utilized burial registers from 15 parishes (out of 66) for the period 1835–56, i.e. ten years before and after the event.[33] The sample of parishes reflects the fortuitous facts of survival and thus is not as representative as we might wish. No pertinent records from Camarines Norte, northern Sorsogon or the missions are available, and only one each from Tabaco and the devastated island of Catanduanes has survived. The remaining registers analysed come from the districts of Bicol (4), Iraya (4), Lagonoy (3) and Rinconada (2). Ten of the 15 are thus from the central valley, and all but one of these 10 is from a parish administered by Spanish friars, whereas most of the coastal parishes were administered by secular priests. While this is

TABLE 5.2

CRISIS MORTALITY BY MONTH, SAMPLE PARISHES, BIKOL REGION, 1845-46

(Mean indices for each parish and month, above/below background average)

Year	Month	%	S.D.	Minimum	Maximum
1845	January	6	0.09	−1.86	1.46
1845	February	12	0.33	−1.14	1.60
1845	March	13	0.13	−1.14	1.36
1845	April	23	0.39	−1.03	1.39
1845	May	−18	−0.24	−1.47	0.86
1845	June	28	0.45	−1.03	2.34
1845	July	42	0.99	−1.01	3.86
1845	August	91	1.62	−0.87	3.71
1845	September	96	1.92	−0.54	7.52
1845	October	177	3.04	−1.18	8.42
1845	November	343	5.94	−0.68	20.72
1845	December	342	5.83	−0.34	27.00
1845	ANNUAL	87	3.06	−0.58	8.90
1846	January	165	3.58	−0.16	14.51
1846	February	193	3.43	−0.33	8.82
1846	March	208	4.77	0.07	15.68
1846	April	121	2.67	−0.61	10.94
1846	May	73	1.67	−1.00	5.01
1846	June	71	2.02	−1.03	12.02
1846	July	133	3.10	−0.29	8.39
1846	August	148	3.57	−0.40	8.34
1846	September	136	2.95	−0.19	7.44
1846	October	134	2.59	−1.45	7.26
1846	November	135	2.61	−0.81	7.68
1846	December	62	1.13	−1.23	4.65
1846	ANNUAL	124	5.35	−0.21	14.37

obviously a very imperfect sample, it should be broad enough to indicate general tendencies in both background and crisis mortality, particularly for the central valley.[34]

If we compare 1845 and 1846 burials for each parish and month with the background averages for the same parish and month,[35] we can derive indices of variation (by percentage and standard deviation) which help to clarify the chronology and geography of the crisis. The mean monthly indices resolve the rather ambiguous testimony of the official reports as to when the crisis actually began (see Table 5.2).

In the first six months of 1845 mortality was well within the range of normality, averaging just 10% above the mean for the surrounding years. Deaths increased sharply from July onward, reaching what might be considered 'crisis' level (more than two S.D. above normal)[36] by October, even before the typhoon that first brought the crisis to the attention of the authorities. Mortality peaked in November and December 1845, declining by January 1846 with the new rice harvest and the arrival of shipments of relief grain; it did not surpass the post-typhoon peak even during the cholera epidemic of February–April 1846. The crisis continued, however, until almost the end of the year, with a secondary peak in August. Thus, although it was at its most severe in late 1845, the dual crisis actually took more lives in 1846, as the average annual indices reveal.

At the same time, the range of readings clearly indicates that the impact of the crisis was very irregular. In each year and in every month but one, at least one parish recorded *fewer* deaths than the background average. Tracing the course of the crisis through individual parish registers reveals not just a wide range of mortality levels but a bewildering variety of local peaks and troughs. The sample parishes may be grouped, however, in such a way as to produce three distinct patterns of mortality corresponding to three geographical zones within the region (see Fig. 5.2).

In the upstream districts of the central valley (Iraya and Rinconada) the pattern resembles that for the sample as a whole: rising mortality from July 1845 onward, with a peak in November–December, then generally high mortality throughout 1846, with secondary peaks in March (cholera) and August.[37] Downstream in Bicol, however, mortality remained moderate throughout 1845, not reaching 'crisis' level even after the November typhoon. Though there was great suffering, as official reports testify, there was apparently no subsistence crisis in the district, traditionally the rice bowl for the rest of the region. Grain prices had in fact fallen from their December peaks by nearly 30% before the mortality crisis began there in February with the coming of cholera. Over the next ten months mortality in this district was sustained at a much higher level than in the other two zones.

The remaining parishes are scattered over three districts in the east of the region: Lagonoy, Tabaco and Catanduanes. This residual 'zone' includes the parish with the highest single monthly index in the sample and two of the three with the lowest indices

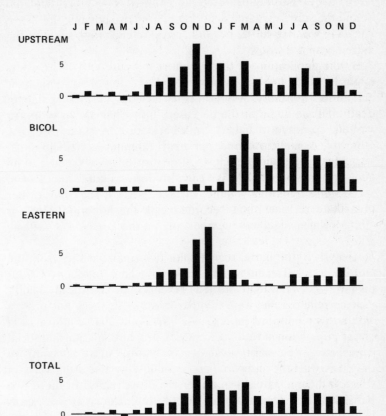

Fig. 5.2. Monthly Variation by Zone, Bikol Region, 1845–46.

over the whole two-year period. Yet collectively these parishes also show a distinctive mortality pattern, with deaths rising rapidly from August to December 1845 (as in the upper valley) but falling even more rapidly in early 1846. By April–June mortality was actually at normal background levels, only to rise again to crisis level over the last six months of the year. Apparently the impact, if any, of cholera on these towns was weak or late. Instead we have what appears to be a classic famine pattern: peak mortality just before harvest, falling almost to normal when food supplies are temporarily restored, then rising again as stocks are depleted before the subsequent harvest, though it is also possible the rise in late 1846 was due to the belated arrival of cholera in some of the more isolated districts.[38]

By the application of further effort the parish burial registers might be made to yield even more information about both crisis and normal mortality. A typical entry includes, besides the date of death and the name of the deceased, his or her age in years (or months, if under a year old),[39] marital status, age/status category, ethnicity, home town and *barangay* (administrative sub-unit), burial fees paid, and the names of nearest relatives (spouse of an adult, parents of a child). We can also derive a crude indicator of social status by noting whether the deceased (or any of his or her immediate relatives) was recorded with the honorific 'Don' or 'Doña' which signified membership in the *principalía* (village élite).[40]

Analysis of the burial registers for two small parishes from the eastern zone—Tigaon/Sagnay (Lagonoy) and Calolbon (Catanduanes)—between 1840 and 1851 reveals some statistically significant correlations, as well as other possible linkages not proven within this number of cases (798).[41] Without reliable information on the population at risk—age and sex structure, marital and social status, etc.—we cannot calculate actual rates, but we can compare the crisis with the surrounding 'normality' to assess the ways in which it diverged from usual patterns of mortality. In these two parishes, where cholera came late, if at all, the crisis was essentially limited to the eight months of famine from July 1845 through February 1846, though we can also examine a second 'crisis' period from March 1846 through February 1847 for comparative purposes.

Perhaps the most important correlation revealed for these two parishes is the exceptional increase in death of male children under seven during the crisis. In normal times this age-group accounted for only 0.86 burials per month, just 34.8% of all male deaths, but in the crisis these figures rose to 6.13 burials per month, 52.7% of all male deaths.[42] Total female mortality rose almost as much as male during the crisis, yet there was no comparable variation from normal age distribution, although there was a slightly higher than average proportion of women dying over the age of sixty, and a statistically significant increase in proportionate mortality among the minority of adult women who were recorded as single.[43] We can easily understand the vulnerability to famine of the very young, the very old, and the socially marginal (although, curiously, there is no crisis correlation at all between legitimacy and child mortality). We are not at all surprised that the *principalía* would survive the subsistence crisis much better than ordinary peasants, accounting for only 7.6% of 'crisis' burials, as against 14.1% in more normal times.[44] But why should the famine strike little boys so much harder than little girls? Four hypotheses come readily to mind: (1) the natural and universal biological superiority of females was simply heightened by the famine; (2) some hitherto unknown local custom favoured girls over boys in the allocation of food in times of scarcity; (3) these two parishes, despite the 'statistical significance' of the findings, were in fact demographically anomalous; (4) girls *died* in as great number as boys but were discriminated against (beyond the customary degree) when it came to *burial*—in spite of the fact that in these parishes 94% of all burial services during the crisis were performed 'gratis'. To raise these possibilities is to suggest some of the strengths and limitations of quantitative analysis: in revealing new linkages it suggests further questions that can be answered, if at all, only by further inquiry.[45]

Conclusions

The measurement of mortality in the nineteenth century Philippines can thus be productive and provocative, in spite of its apparently insoluble central problem: known under-registration, of unknown dimension. Despite computerization, the work is highly labour-intensive, for the collection and cleaning of data cannot at this stage be entrusted to any programme or machine.[46] Once collected and cleaned, however, the data can yield all manner of quantitative comparisons over both space and time.

The most obvious comparisons are international, measuring the severity of this crisis against that of other demographic disasters. Although the cross-cultural data are never precisely equivalent, they are adequate to confirm our suspicions that this was a genuine crisis but not an exceptional one, either in total excess mortality or in percentage of the base population that died (see Table 5.3).[47]

Even within the demographic history of the region it is a comparatively minor event, overshadowed by a number of later epidemics and dwarfed by the terrible years 1900–1905, when to

TABLE 5.3

COMPARATIVE MORTALITY, SELECTED MODERN ASIAN FAMINES[a]

Location	Years	'Excess' Deaths (000)	%of Base Population
Bikol	1845–46	14–20	5.6– 8.0
Java	1846–51	600	6.4
(Demak–Grobogan)	(1849–50)	(80)	(23.8)
North China (five provinces)	1877–78	9 000–13 000?	8.5–12.0?
Bombay Presidency (Gujarat)	1899–1902	585	3.8
	(1899–1901)	(381)	(12.7)
North China (three provinces)	1936	893	4.6
Bengal	1943–46	3 000–3 800	5.0–6.3
Tonkin, Vietnam	1944–45	1 000–2 000?	10.0–20.0?

(a) In each of these crises some deaths were attributed to specific diseases (e.g., typhoid in Java) rather than to famine.

Sources: Bikol: this paper.

Java: Peter Boomgaard, 'Morbidity and Mortality in Java, 1820–1880', above.

Demak-Grobogan: R. E. Elson, 'The Famine in Demak and Grobogan in 1849–50: Its Causes and Circumstances', *Review of Indonesian and Malaysian Affairs* 19, 1 (1985), 39–85.

North China: Ho Ping-ti, *Studies on the Population of China, 1368–1953* (Cambridge, Harvard University Press, 1959), 231–36, 283.

Bombay Presidency and Gujarat: Michelle Burge McAlpin, *Subject to Famine: Food Crises and Economic Change in Western India, 1860–1920* (Princeton, Princeton University Press, 1983), 47–85, 196–97.

Bengal: Paul R. Greenough, *Prosperity and Misery in Modern Bengal: The Famine of 1943–1944* (New York, Oxford University Press, 1982), 299–315.

Tonkin: Vu Ngu Chieu, *The End of an Era: Viet-Nam Under the Japanese Occupation (1940–1945)*, forthcoming; Ngo Vinh Long, *Before the Revolution: The Vietnamese Peasants Under the French* (Cambridge, MIT Press, 1973), 122–35.

the effects of the Philippine–American War were added those of cholera, smallpox, malaria, beri-beri and the collapse of rice production following the death of over half the draft animals by rinderpest.[48] It seems to have been forgotten quickly; I have encountered no mention of it either in archival documents from later in the nineteenth century or in twentieth century local histories. The fact that it was the worst famine recorded in the region over the past two hundred suggests that the Bikolanos (and perhaps most Filipinos?) were normally farther from the subsistence margin than the many Asians who lived under the constant threat of starvation.[49] At the same time, we must not underestimate the scale of human loss caused by even such a minor crisis, one of the routine tragedies that punctuated Southeast Asian life.

The real benefits of quantitative analysis of mortality, however, come not from gross measurement of lives lost but from differentiation: by category of victim (age, sex, marital status, class), by time (year, month or day), by area (parish, district or zone), or even by cause of death, which is recorded in most Philippine burial registers after around 1880. At this stage, most of these benefits are still prospective; they depend on far more extensive internal analysis of the burial records as well as on comparisons with other times and other regions. But eventually they may yield to us much of the secret agenda of death in the Philippines—who was struck down, when, where and by what.

I would like to acknowledge my gratitude to the Roman Catholic Church in the Philippines (particularly Jaime Cardinal Sin, former Archbishop Teopisto V. Alberto of Caceres, former Bishop Teotimo Pacis of Legazpi, Sister Pureza Jimenez, and the parish priests of the Bikol region) for providing access to church records; to the Church of Jesus Christ of the Latter-Day Saints (particularly John Orton, Pearl Evans, John Smith and Joyce Smith) and to the University of Santo Tomas (particularly Juana T. Abello) for providing access to microfilms of these records; to Bruce Cruikshank, Rev. Maximo O. Jacob, Akil A. Pawaki, Rafael G. Roque, Peter C. Smith and James F. Warren for helping in the transcription of data from these and other records; and to Daniel F. Doeppers, Terrence H. Hull, Gavin W. Jones, David G. Marr, Glenn A. May and Anthony Reid for commenting on earlier drafts of this paper.

1. Michael Cullinane and Peter C. Smith, 'The Population of Cebu Province, Philippines, in the Nineteenth Century: A Working Paper in Historical Demography,' paper prepared for Midwest Conference on Asian Affairs, DeKalb, Illinois, 14–15 October 1977; Smith, 'Crisis Mortality in the Nineteenth Century Philippines: Data from Parish Records,' *Journal of Asian Studies* 38, 1 (1978), 51–76; Smith, 'Demographic History: An Approach to the Study of the Filipino Past,' in John A. Larkin (ed.), *Perspectives on Philippine Historiography*, (New Haven, Yale University Southeast Asia Studies, 1979), 27–46; Ng Shui-Meng, 'Demographic Change, Marriage, and Family Formation: The Case of Nineteenth Century Nagcarlan, The Philippines' (Ph.D. dissertation, University of Hawaii, 1979); Smith, Cullinane, and Ng, 'Sources for Family History in the Philippines: Content and Use', paper prepared for World Conference on Records, Salt Lake City, 12–15 August 1980; Smith and Ng, 'The Components of Population Change in Nineteenth-century South-east Asia: Village Data from the Philippines', *Population Studies* 36, 2 (1982), 237–55; Cullinane, 'The Spanish System of Demographic and Spiritual Accounting', unpublished paper.

2. On the history of this region see Norman G. Owen, *Prosperity without Progress: Manila Hemp and Material Life in the Colonial Philippines* (Berkeley, University of California Press, and Quezon City, Ateneo de Manila University Press, 1984.)

3. For details see Norman G. Owen, 'A Subsistence Crisis in the Provincial Philippines: 1845–1846', *Kinaadman (Wisdom): A Journal of the Southern Philippines*, forthcoming.

4. See Fernando Casas, *Memoria sobre el tétano, specialmente interior, y con particularidad de los órganos digestivos, conocido con el nombre de cólera-morbo, y padecido en las Islas Filipinas* (Madrid, Imprenta Real, 1832), 59. Like other

nineteenth century cholera epidemics in the Bikol region—1890–21(?), 1857, 1864–65, 1882–83 and 1889, as recorded in various parish burial registers—this epidemic produced in most affected parishes a rather steep 1–2 month peak in mortality, though the pattern here is complicated (as in the 1880s) by surrounding episodes of high mortality from other causes. The outbreak seems to have raised parochial death tolls to an average of about four times normal for the period of its onslaught, slightly less than in the outbreaks of 1857, 1864–65, and 1882–83, but more than in 1820–21 and 1889. The region does not seem to have had a specific cholera 'season', as apparent peaks occurred in January, March, May, December, September and June in the various epidemics throughout the century. On cholera elsewhere in Southeast Asia, see Peter Boomgaard, 'Morbidity and Mortality in Java, 1820–1880', above; Barbara Lovric, 'Bali: Myth, Magic and Morbidity', below; B. J. Terwiel, 'Asiatic Cholera in Siam', below; and Reynaldo C. Ileto, 'Cholera and Colonialism in Southwestern Luzon, 1902', paper presented at conference on 'Disease, Drugs and Death: Their History in Modern Southeast Asia; Australian National University, 6–8 May 1983.

5. The governor of Camarines Sur, however, pointing out that the epidemic did not strike until after the 'months of greatest scarcity' and was no respecter of classes when it did strike, concluded that its 'cause' was not grain shortages but 'the influence of the atmosphere', which was unusually hot and humid; Francisco de Paula Enriquez to Governor General Narciso Claveria, 26 February, 5 and 12 March 1846, in Philippine National Archives (PNA), Ereccion de Pueblos, Camarines Sur, 1831–83, expediente 28 ('sobre colera morbus').

6. Ibid; PNA, Ereccion de Pueblos, Camarines Sur, 1838–82, exp. 9; PNA, Ereccion de Pueblos, Albay, 1845–64, exp. 3; cf. Owen, 'Subsistence Crisis'.

7. *Calendario manual y guía de forasteros de las Islas Filipinas* (Manila, Imp. en Santo Thomás, 1840); *Guía de forasteros en las Islas Filipinas*, annual (Manila, 1842–65); Aragón, *Estados de la población de Filipinas correspondiente a el año de 1818* (Manila, Imp. de D.M.M. por D. Anastacio Gonzaga, 1820); Buzeta and Bravo, *Diccionario geográfico, estadístico, histórico de las Islas Filipinas*, 2 vols. (Madrid, Imp. de José C. de la Peña, 1850–51); Huerta, *Estado geográfico, topográfico, estadístico, histórico-religioso de la Santa y Apostólica Provincia de San Gregorio Magno . . . desde . . . 1577 hasta . . . 1853* (Manila, Imp. de los Amigos del País, 1855); idem, *Estado geográfico . . . hasta . . . 1865* (Binondo, Imp. de M. Sánchez y Ca., 1865).

8. Titles of these *estados* vary. For the Bikol region the relevant authorities are the Franciscan order (province of Saint Gregory the Great), and the Diocese of Caceres. I used two of the former's published *estados* (1849, 1855) and three of the latter's (1849, 1851, 1864).

9. I used data from *estados* in the Manila Archdiocesan Archives, the Archivo Histórico Nacional and Archivo Franciscano Ibero–Oriental (Madrid), and the Archivo General de Indias (Seville).

10. Unfortunately, it is generally not clear whether these numbers refer to the preceding calendar year, to some other fixed fiscal or canonical year, to the twelve months prior to the date of the *estado*, or simply to the period since the previous *estado* was compiled. The indigenous population was typically divided into six age/status categories (sometimes subdivided by sex): married tribute-payers; unmarried tribute-payers; adults exempt from tribute by office, age, or infirmity; youths who took communion but did not pay tribute; children who confessed but did not take communion; and infants. Spaniards, Christian Chinese, mestizos, and negritos, if any, were recorded separately.

11. The preliminary data for this paper included nearly 3 500 records of individual parish-years, which does not by any means exhaust all possible aggregate sources for the region and period.

12. The lower figures appear in diocesan *estados* for 1838 and 1848, a letter from the Bishop in 1843, and the *Guía* for 1848; the higher in diocesan *estados* for 1845–47 and the *Guía* for 1847.

13. By elimination of duplicated figures and consolidation of jointly administered parishes it was possible to reduce the data actually analysed for this paper to 2 277 records from 66 parishes and parish-pairs. In cleaning the data for analysis I also removed all population figures which were simply derived by multiplying *tributos* by some standard figure, usually 4.5 or 5.0.

14. Normal population/*tributo* ratios tend to fall in the range 4.0–4.5:1, whereas some of these outlyers reach 10:1 or even more. There are several problems inherent in using tribute figures for demographic purposes, including the fact that it was in the interest of most adults to gain exemption from tribute or disappear from the lists entirely. Nevertheless, *tributo* figures do not suffer the particular vagaries displayed by population data in these sources and thus are a useful guide to general trends and orders of magnitude.

15. This is the mean weighted population/*tributo* ratio for data free of other superficial signs of under-registration (i.e., those with combined vital rates over 50 per thousand and burial/baptism ratios of 0.4:1 or higher). The mean ratio for all data, including those suspected of grossly exaggerated population figures, is 4.7:1.

16. If we eliminate, rather than revise, apparently exaggerated population figures, the rates are almost identical: CBR 40.4 (S.D. 9.8), CDR 24.0 (S.D. 12.1); revision has been preferred because it substantially increases the total number of cases for analysis. On the growth of the nineteenth century Philippines, see Smith and Ng, op. cit., 241; for the Bikol region, see Owen, *Prosperity*, 115–17.

17. D. E. C. Eversley, 'Exploitation of Anglican Parish Records by Aggregative Analysis,' in E. A. Wrigley (ed.), *An Introduction to English Historical Demography* (London, Weidenfeld & Nicholson, 1966), 54–5. This level is arbitrary, but clearly on the low side, as it would permit vital rates as low as 30 (CBR) and 20 (CDR), whereas both should probably average at least 5–10 points higher.

18. For example, even if we assume CBRs ranging from 40 to 50 per thousand, this ratio implies CDRs no higher than 16 to 20 per thousand, and thus a highly unlikely 2.4–3.0% rate of natural increase.

19. There is in fact a high correlation (chi-square=55; significance level=0.00000) between low combined rates and low burial/baptism ratios, which suggests that under-registration of deaths was generally greater than that of the births. There is also a positive correlation between birth rates and death rates, somewhat higher (R=0.10, significance=0.00005) than we would anticipate simply from the fact that more births imply higher infant mortality; the obvious inference is that registration of vital events tended to rise and fall simultaneously, if not uniformly.

20. The age brackets are approximate; this is actually the ratio of *mozos de confesión* (children who confess but do not yet take communion) to *parvulos* (children below the age of confession). The sources are scattered parish and diocesan *estados*; standard figures are derived from Ansley J. Coale and Paul Demeny, *Regional Model Life Tables and Stable Populations* (Princeton, Princeton University Press, 1966), especially Model West, levels 5–6, growth rates 1–1.5%. The only parish *padrones* analysed so far for age/sex composition often list *fewer* children age 0–4 than age 5–9; Ng, 199; Smith and Ng, 246; Tigaon parish register for 1820, 1830, 1840 and 1851.

21. Burial registers for Calabanga, Milaor and Libmanan, 1836–65 passim; parish *estados* for Oas, 1837–39; Coale and Demeny, op. cit. Other parish *estados* indicate than an average of 50% of all burials were of children 12 and under, as against the 60% suggested by standard life tables.

22. Small parishes (with fewer than 500 *tributos*) show a statistically significant correlation with indices of under-registration, which is not surprising, as they were

generally more recently converted, more erratically administered, and on terrain which made it more difficult to get to church for baptism or burial.

23. Although in some districts there appear to be after-effects of the crisis in 1847, the average vital rates for that year show it to be normal—less than one standard deviation from the background average—so it has been included in the background series.

24. The principal advantage of measuring variation in standard deviations is that it tends to dampen the effect of less stable series, and thus of erratic registration.

25. On the use of this ratio as a crisis index, see Hubert Charbonneau and André Larose (eds), *The Great Mortalities: Methodological Studies of Demographic Crises in the Past* (Liège, Ordina Editions, 1979), 114, 143; Sherburne F. Cook and Woodrow Borah, 'Mortality in Mexico Prior to 1850', in *Essays in Population History: Mexico and the Caribbean*, 3 vols. (Berkeley, University of California Press, 1972–79), 2:339–40; E. A. Wrigley and R. S. Schofield, *The Population History of England 1541–1871: A Reconstruction* (London, Edward Arnold, 1981), 176–89.

26. These districts differ slightly from the *partidos* described in Owen, *Prosperity*, 14–23, 271–72: Donsol and Quipia here been assigned to Iraya and Pasacao to Bicol.

27. Most typhoons that hit the region in the twentieth century passed through on a west-north-westerly course; Frederick L. Wernstedt and Joseph E. Spencer, *The Philippine Island World* (Berkeley, University of California Press, 1967), 51, 412–13. These districts may also have had access to imported rice from neighbouring provinces and they were relatively distant from the apparent epicentre of the 1846 cholera, reported first in the central valley (Bicol district). The same factors would explain the absence of crisis mortality in southern Sorsogon.

28. In the aftermath such a crisis, of course, even 'normal' CDRs may be regarded as excessive, since many of those most vulnerable (especially the very young and the very old) would already have perished. Continued above-average mortality by age group is thus implied, though we lack the age-specific data to substantiate this assumption.

29. A comparable fall in the number of *tributos* corroborates this decline. Nominal declines for other districts might be accounted for by exaggeration of 1845 population figures or by computational errors. Although there are references in the official reports to people 'scattered' from one town to another in search of food, there is no direct evidence of emigration from the region during the crisis.

30. By combining these aggregate figures with monthly mortality indexes obtained from parish registers (see below), it is possible to conclude that the 'famine' alone took at least 5 500 lives—an approximation of excess deaths between January 1845 and the outbreak of cholera (late February in Bicol, March or later in other districts). This is a minimum estimate not only because it ignores the effects of malnutrition on cholera victims but because it excludes all excess mortality after the initial outbreak, even in those districts which cholera may never have hit. An alternative approach would be to attribute to cholera only two months of four times normal mortality (see note 4, above), which for a population of 250 000 with a normal CDR of 24 would account for some 3 000 excess deaths; this would leave 11 000 deaths primarily due to the famine, a more probable total.

31. Though this estimate of under-registration may appear high, Francis C. Madigan, James Abernathy et al., 'Purposive Concealment of Death in Household Surveys in Misamis Oriental Province'. *Population Studies* 30, 2 (1976), 295–303, calculate that in the present-day province of Misamis Oriental some 75% of urban deaths and 47% of rural deaths are not reported to the municipal authorities. For plausible magnitudes of vital rates, see Peter C. Smith, 'The Turn-of-the-Century Birth Rate: Estimates from Birth Registration and Age Structure', in Wilhelm

Flieger and Peter C. Smith (eds), *A Demographic Path to Modernity: Patterns of Early-Transition in the Philippines* (Quezon City, University of the Philippines Press, for the Population Institute, 1975), 84–7.

32. Eversley, op. cit., suggests some of the possibilities of this approach; Wrigley and Schofield, op. cit., exploit these possibilities to the maximum, using nearly 3.7 million monthly totals compiled from over 400 different registers by their dedicated volunteer assistants.

33. Ending the series in 1856 also prevents distortion of the normal pattern of seasonal mortality by the severe cholera epidemic of April–June 1857.

34. The parishes range in size from under 2 000 to over 12 000 'souls' in 1845. The coverage ranges from the full 22 years (for most registers) to just 12; for two of the parishes we have burial registers for 1845 but not for 1846.

35. Monthly analysis of background mortality shows a curious bipolar modality, with peaks six months apart, in July (the hottest month of the year) and January (the beginning of the harvest season); cf. Ng, op. cit., 102–8, for a different pattern in the southern Tagalog province of Laguna.

36. Wrigley and Schofield, op. cit., 647; cf. Charbonneau and Larose, op. cit., 83–112.

37. This seasonal profile corrects the impression given by the annual aggregate sources that Rinconada, like Bicol, was relatively unaffected by the 1845 famine. Peak mortality in both sample parishes from Rinconada occurred in November 1845, whereas none of the four Bicol sample parishes peaked earlier than March 1846.

38. Cf. note 44, below. One report in the 'colera morbo' expediente (see note 5, above) notes that as of 9 April 1846 at least two towns in Lagonoy—along with one in Iraya, in the central valley—had 'not been invaded by the cholera'.

39. Unfortunately, examination of *padrones* and baptismal registers suggests that age mis-statement was the rule, not the exception.

40. See Norman G. Owen, 'The Principalia in Philippine History: Kabikolan, 1790–1898', *Philippine Studies* 22, 3–4 (1974), 297–324.

41. As these data were transcribed prior to complete analysis of the annual and monthly aggregations, I was unaware that these two parishes were in the same demographic 'zone' or that both showed strong indications of presumptive under-registration. Thus they hardly constitute a representative sample of regional mortality; their analysis is significant more for the questions raised than the answers provided.

42. Cross-tabulation of 'crisis' with four male age-groups (0–6, 7–20, 21–59, and 60+) provides the following statistics: chi-square = 18 (significance=0.00005); contingency coefficient=0.20

43. Chi-square=23 (significance=0.0000); contingency coefficient=0.34. Computations of average age at death (and thus, by implication, of average life expectancy at birth) for the entire period, though not totally trustworthy because of age mis-statement, reflect a similar differential in mortality by sex: male mean 29.8, median 26.9; female mean 35.0, median 32.2.

44. Chi-square=4 (significance=0.04); phi=0.08. Interestingly, in the 'second crisis' in these parishes, this élite actually suffered higher proportionate mortality than usual, which suggests that the major cause of death might have been socially indiscriminate disease (delayed cholera?) rather than famine. The same inference could be drawn from the fact that mortality in the second 'crisis' was disproportionately high in adults age 20–59.

45. The first of these hypotheses might be tested by the study of better-documented famines elsewhere; the second by careful reading of the ethnographic literature; the third by the same kind of quantitative analysis of more parish burial registers; the fourth only by fortuitous discovery of new documentation or extremely detailed

demographic analysis based on nominal linkages (i.e. by family reconstitution). All are beyond the scope of this essay.

46. The establishment of a central computerized data base of aggregate Philippine demographic materials would be a valuable resource for future researchers, but the problems of data cleaning and selection outlined in this paper would presumably remain, as few scholars would choose to utilize figures pre-screened by another.

47. More sophisticated indices of crisis mortality, mostly keyed to European historical examples, are described and discussed in Charbonneau and Larose, op. cit.; cf. Smith, 'Crisis Mortality'; Wrigley and Schofield, op. cit., 645–56. The Bikol crisis can be calculated at 29 (with 20 defining 'crisis' level) on Hollingworths's index, derived from estimates for total population at risk, mortality, and duration, and at level 3 ('crise forte') on Jacques Dupaquier's simpler six-step scale of magnitude, based on standard deviations above normal annual mortality. By comparison, the 1665 plague epidemic in London, which killed over 80 000 (16.6% of the base population) in less than six months, reaches 244 on Hollingworth's index, level 6 ('catastrophe') on Dupaquier's.

48. The demographic consequences of these later Bikol crises have not yet been systematically analysed, but the parish registers examined so far indicate much higher burials rates than were recorded in 1845–46. For mortality elsewhere in the Philippines during the same period, see Smith, 'Crisis Mortality'; Ileto, op. cit.; Glenn A. May, '150,000 Missing Filipinos: A Demographic Crisis in Batangas, 1887–1903'. *Annales de Démographie Historique*, forthcoming.

49. The recurrence of famine in nineteenth century China and India is well known; within Southeast Asia, Vietnam seems to have been peculiarly vulnerable, though this may reflect the superior record-keeping of the Vietnamese court as well as population densities resembling those of south China. The contrast should not be pushed too far, however, as suspiciously high grain prices also accompanied epidemics in the Bikol region in 1857, 1865 and 1900–1903.

III CULTURE AND CURING

6 Bali: Myth, Magic and Morbidity

BARBARA LOVRIC

FEW subjects are more distinguished by their absence from the discourse on Bali than that of morbidity. The myth and magic of Bali, as customarily celebrated in the ethnology of the island, remain strangely separated from the reality of devastating epidemics. Yet the predicament of disease and untimely death appears to have prompted an extensive response which is evident in a vast explanatory mythology that has shaped the themes of literature, the arts and the ritual complex. Textual and cultural evidence suggest that a conspicuous proportion of the most characteristic features of Balinese life, such as temples, offerings, dance and rituals, originate in the experience and conceptions of disease and that these function to a large degree to preserve human well-being in the face of actual or threatened epidemics. Cults of *sakti* (magical power), witchcraft, and demonic deities and magical rites heavily imbued with protective symbolism represent evidence of this response.[1]

In the semi-historical texts which relate the early history of Bali, the *Usana Bali*, a causal relationship is assumed between human welfare on one hand, and the proper enactment of rituals, the care of temples, devotion to the gods, and propitiation of the vast array of demonic beings on the other. It was the duty of the ruling raja to stage large-scale rituals considered crucial to the well-being of subjects and the survival of the kingdom. The religious efforts of the temple priests (*pamangku*) were likewise directed to such pragmatic ends:

> For you *pamangku* should bring offerings to the gods so that there is abundance and Bali is well-populated. The rulers and their ministers are responsible for the enactment of rituals to contain widespread illness and death (*mangda angawe adoh ikang sasab marana*).[2]

The early histories also relate the arrival of religious leaders from Java and their legendary treks across Bali, during which large numbers of their followers perished through disease. The building of temples became one of the earliest means of securing protection against the ravages of epidemic disease.[3] It is related that when a raja named Jayakusunu became ruler of Bali his subjects were few, their numbers having been depleted because of deadly illness. His predecessors had all died prematurely and without heirs. The new ruler sought the protection of Durga, the Goddess of Death, paying homage to her in the graveyard thoughout the night. The Goddess told Jayakusunu that the disease prevailed in the land because temples had been neglected, and rulers had failed to fulfil a particular ritual (*galungan*) prescribed for their ancestors to contain the threat of seasonal illness.[4]

Some understanding of the profound and complex response to disease may be gained through examining how four classical pestilences—leprosy, plague, smallpox and cholera—have been recorded and interpreted in the Balinese tradition. This paper is an attempt to cast light on some of the obscurities surrounding the natural history of disease on Bali, through the use of indigenous magico-medical texts and medical folklore and practices. Such sources are never easy to interpret. The texts conform to a literary convention within which statements and explanations of events are rarely explicit, but contained in cryptic allusions and circumlocutions. Nevertheless, the themes of myth and magic contained in the literate and oral traditions surrounding disease do seem to display what Day has described elsewhere as 'a concrete historical contextuality'.[5]

In Balinese thinking, epidemic disease is something extraneous and identifiable. Each disease entity is given an image, and even a personality. Disease is also seen as a process, the course of which can be modified and the impact of which can be lessened through appropriate magical procedures. It cannot, however, be obliterated. The process whereby each of these diseases has been conceptualized involves complex interrelationships between ecological and geographical determinants, cultural factors and biological and historical variables; hence, the complexity and the varying cultural biographies of the classic pestilences which follow.

Leprosy—The Great Unmentionable

Mayadanawa, a semi-legendary, magically powerful ruler of Bali around the tenth century whose story is related in the *Uṣana Bali*, became so infatuated with the Chinese princess whom he took to wife that he neglected the enactment of prescribed rituals.[6] She is said to have died of 'a disease which could not be treated'. Because the gods refused to cure his wife, Mayadanawa stopped all offerings to them. Bali became desolate and depopulated (*sepi*) as disease raged. After the eventual overpowering of Mayadanawa's *sakti*, the god Indra instructed the village leaders (*punggawa*) and temple priests on the correct observation of rituals and the imperative of preserving ancestral traditions:[7]

> All of you *punggawa* and *pamangku*, I give to you these instructions. Do not transgress the power of the gods. Should you do so, you will be cursed by them. You will be afflicted with *tutumpur agung*. You will not be reincarnated as human beings. Furthermore, should you fail to offer devotion in the temples, each of you and all of your descendants will be afflicted. If you do not make ceremonial offerings, *tutumpur agung* will spread among your kin.

There is no specific Balinese word for leprosy, only terms which refer to the nature of the illness, such as *gering agung* (the great illness), or to signs of the progress of the disease, such as *geseng tumpur* (referring to the burnt or blackish colour of the skin of a leprosy victim), or to the final qualifying symptom of leprosy, the sloughing off of limbs and features, *tutumpur agung*. Leprosy is also referred to metonymically as *Culik Daki*, the name of the spirit who initiates the morbid changes in the tissues leading to the condition. There is no specific term for leprosy because it is, ultimately, an unmentionable. Early or indeterminate forms of the disease are designated by the term *ila* (dangerous). The medical treatises on leprosy, entitled *Usada Ila* and *Usada Gering Agung*, list numerous forms of dermatological afflictions which may be confused with leprosy and warn of the repercussions of failure of the *balian* (healer) to differentiate true leprosy. Once a diagnosis of leprosy is made, radical measures are adopted. The victim may no longer be treated and is banished to the outskirts of the village, to the forest, or to the seaside. The purificatory rites of cremation are denied until a specific lapse of time after death proportionate to the caste status of the victim. Neither the disease itself nor the rules of social ostracism discriminate in terms of caste or social status.

The above references to leprosy in Balinese texts suggest that on Bali, as elsewhere, leprosy is a disease of antiquity which has been endemic for a long time.[8] The facts that leprosy exhibits a wide clinical spectrum and that there is little to distinguish the early cutaneous signs of leprosy from other dermatological afflictions are recognized; hence much cautionary advice to healers. The observation that leprosy is frequently a family infection was perhaps implied in the warnings to village leaders, temple priests and healers that they, their kin and their descendants would be afflicted should they neglect their responsibilities. There is, to my knowledge, no creator-protector demonic deity associated with leprosy and therefore none to whom appeals are made to prevent or contain the incidence of the disease. Leprosy is simply perceived as a curse of the gods; it cannot be cured or alleviated.

Leprosy remains a health problem in Bali today; there are still leper colonies, one just north of a large tourist hotel complex. Known preventive and curative measures are unsatisfactory and the mode of transmission of the disease remains uncertain. The uniqueness of the sympton complex of leprosy—the disfigurement and deformity, the characteristic 'fishy' odour about the afflicted and the high endemicity—doubtless influence the social stigma the disease still evokes. Those afflicted by this ancient scourge must cease to participate in the affairs of the community. They become 'the living dead', a modern term for which an equivalent exists in the *usada*: *urip tan urip*. Death is not the most terrifying aspect of leprosy.

The Calon Arang: An Historical Legend of the Plague?

Reputed to be the most devastating pestilence of all time, the plague or the 'Black Death' of Western history in all probability had its homeland in north and central Asia. The first authenticated record of plague dates from the sixth century. In the eleventh century the plague spread from Asia and climaxed three centuries later, recurring sporadically and less virulently thereafter. Yet the first incidence of bubonic plague in the Netherlands Indies recorded by the Dutch was in 1910;[9] their reports indicate that it was a new disease there. Twentieth century plague epidemics in Indonesia were apparently confined to Java.[10]

As a subject of horror, the plague has been a rich source of literary stimulation. Perceived, at times, as a kind of psychic entity, it is credited with having provided the compost for fear and dread to grow into cults of witchcraft.[11] The *Calon Arang* (Widow-Witch), an Old Javanese semi-historical text, is set on Java during the reign of Erlangga (A.D. 1010–42). The following is a synopsis of the epidemic episode in a version of the *Calong Arang*:[12]

A *rangda* (widow-witch) named Calon Arang, who had acquired great *sakti* through the study of *pangiwa* (magic of the 'left-hand path'), lived on Java during the reign of Erlangga. When the *rangda*'s anger was aroused by the community, together with her pupils in black magic (*leyak*), she went to the graveyard and there offered homage to Durga, the Goddess of Death. She then requested Durga's consent to destroy Erlangga's kingdom by bringing pestilence and decimating the population (*anĕda tumpu-raning wwang sanagara*). Durga agreed to her request but instructed the *rangda* to control her anger and confine the disease to the periphery, not to take it inland to the centre (*aywa pati tĕkeng tĕngah*). Throughout the night the *rangda* and her *leyak* danced in the graveyard and at the crossroads. Shortly afterwards, villagers fell ill. People carried away corpses only themselves to be carried away a short time later. Many people suddenly experienced fever and chills and died (*makweh pĕjah gĕringnya panas-tis*).

Erlangga ordered the *rangda*'s death but all attempts on her life failed. Her *sakti* was such that she could not be killed by ordinary means and consequently an even greater degree of anger was aroused within her. Together with the *leyak* she returned to the graveyard. There they took the corpse of a man who had died on *tumpak kaliwon* (a day of magical portent), tied it to a *kĕpuh* tree (also of magical potency) and, breathing over it, brought the man back to life. They then slit his throat and the *rangda* soaked her hair in the blood which flowed from the body and it became matted with dried blood. The body was then disembowelled and the *rangda* draped the entrails about her neck. The freshly slain corpse was then presented as an offering to Durga and all the *bhuta* (demons) inhabiting the graveyard. Durga agreed to a request from the *rangda* to spread the disease through the whole kingdom including the centre.

Very soon people throughout the kingdom fell ill and died. There were corpses piled up in graveyards, in the fields and on the streets. Others were left in houses to putrify. *Leyak* would enter houses through gaps in the wall when people slept. Some villagers fled their village seeking to escape to villages not affected by the pestilence (*tan kamaranan.*) Observing the people deserting the affected villages, the *bhuta-kala* (demons) called out to them to remain because the pestilence had passed and the village was safe. Many nonetheless chose to flee and they did indeed perish. Those who heeded the warning and remained, escaped death.

The text then relates the overpowering, exorcism and release through death of Calon Arang by Mpu Bharada, a priest of the *Bhairawa* sect of Tantrism.[13] A final episode deals with Erlangga's decision to abdicate and retire to the forest to pursue a life of asceticism.

Is there a possibility that the pestilence described in the *Calon Arang* has some association with the spread of the highly fatal plague bacillus in Asia in the eleventh century? Certain epidemiological and historical facts concerning the plague do seem to fit with the imagery of a horrifying epidemic in the legend, particularly the presentation of the illness (high fever and chills, rapid prostration and almost instantaneous death) and its course (the spread of the disease from the coastal areas to the inland centre of the kingdom). Even the self-contained nature of . plague epidemics—the fact that the plague bacilli die out spontaneously as the population is decimated—seems to be recalled in the pleas to refugees not to leave their villages once the crisis had passed.[14]

In medieval Europe, many interpreted the plague as a manifestation of divine vengeance. This unprecedented scourge aroused two extreme human reactions: complete licentiousness and extravagances of religiosity and superstition. Universally, the plague inspired terror as well as a search for meaning and significance. Paintings and woodcuts of the time reflected a preoccupation with its gruesome and morbid effects, depicting scenes of graveyards, death, dying and putrefaction. The medieval chroniclers evoked images of the rapid course of the disease, almost instantaneous death, streets and fields littered with the dead, terror-stricken people fleeing, decimation of populations, desolation and bizarre behaviour such as mad grotesque dancing in public places, provoked by fear and panic.[15]

Though there are remarkable parallels between the medieval European response to the plague and the imagery of the *Calon Arang*, available sources do not generally allow us to look through the Southeast Asian past with the same degree of clarity. From epigraphic evidence it is known that in 1016 a serious catastrophe (*pralaya*), the nature of which is not specified, led to the destruction of a Javanese kingdom and the death of the king, Dharmavamsa Teguh (Erlangga's father-in-law), and prompted Erlangga to seek refuge in the mountains for four years. The cause of the 'tragic events' remains a matter of conjecture. Coedès feels that the 'most likely' of the 'various conjectures' is a Sumatran revenge expedition against Java. In 1019 Erlangga returned and succeeded his father-in-law as ruler. In 1032 Erlangga is said to have rid the country of a woman 'endowed with formidable power, similar to a *rākshasi* [female demon]'.[16]

Could an epidemiological disaster be one of the historical causes of the collapse of a Javanese kingdom and the retreat of Erlangga? The war–pestilence sequence is frequent in history. It is possible that the events of 1016 and 1032 became merged in the legend, that two separate and unrelated events have been conflated. As subjects were the real political and economic resource in the inland agrarian-based kingdoms of ancient Java and Bali, the role of epidemiological disasters in changes of centres of power and the decline of kingdoms may warrant consideration.

Balinese interest in a great disaster in eleventh century Java is not strange in view of the fact that at the time there were cultural and political ties between the two islands centring on the key figures in the legend. Erlangga was the son of the Javanese queen Gunapriyadharmapatni (Mahendradatta) and her Balinese consort, Dharmodayana (Udayana). The identity of Calon Arang is a more contentious issue. According to contemporary Balinese, she is Mahendradatta, Erlangga's mother, who was banished to the forest under suspicion of killing her husband through black magic. Mahendradatta is believed to be portrayed as Durga in a funerary statue at Kutri in Bali. Given the characteristic fluidity of the mystical mode of thought of the ancient Javanese and Balinese, and the fusion of deities and demons, it was but a short transition for the *rangda* to come to symbolize Durga.

While relatively unimportant in contemporary Java, the *Calon Arang* is of great cultural significance for the Balinese, perhaps seminal in their conceptions of epidemic diseases. Durga, the supreme demonic protective deity, and the cults of *sakti* and witchcraft, prime symbols of disease and the focus of attention in epidemics, appear in context in this semi-historical legend. Sacred masks symbolizing Rangda/Durga are kept in temples throughout Bali and used in ritual dance enactments, exorcistically in times of actual, and prophylactically in times of anticipated, pestilence. There are various versions of the myth in written, oral-dramatic, dance-dramatic, pictorial and *wayang* forms. In all of these the gruesome spectre of a ravaging pestilence and the mystical-magical power, uncontrolled and unleashed, that is believed to have caused it are focal themes.

The *rangda*, in her graveyard garb of blood and entrails, is the characteristic representation occurring in plastic, pictorial and dramatic enactments of the *Calon Arang*. With her panting, flaming, enlarged tongue hanging loose, her protruding, glazed eyes, matted hair and dripping entrails, the *rangda* does seem to suggest an embodiment of Durga, the Haunter of Graveyards and of Kali, the Great Black Goddess, Death Incarnate and smeared with blood.[17] The extent to which the *rangda* recalls and perhaps immortalizes the morbid dimensions of plague may derive from the pathological features sometimes ascribed to plague corpses: the overwhelming haemorrhagic discolouration of the skin; the bulging, blood-shot, wide-open eyes; the protruding tongue and perforated abdomen associated with sudden death. An enactment of the *Calon Arang* dance-drama in temple enclosures on Bali displays features of a grotesque parody of a plague-like epidemic, with an initial scene featuring victims fleeing from villages affected by pestilence. Such enactments are perceived as a magical means of containing the severity of threatening diseases.

There are also larger epidemiological implications. If the plague is the pestilence which prompted the writing of the *Calon Arang*, the date of arrival of the plague on Java must be moved back several centuries. Considering Java's geographical position on the trade-route between India and China and the centuries-old two-way traffic, it seems unlikely that the island could have been by-passed by pandemics of the plague until the twentieth century, as is generally assumed. The case of Bali is more obscure, owing in part to the somewhat marginal role of the island in the history of the archipelago. Lacking good harbours and producing little of interest for merchants, Bali was outside the major circuit of commerce and trade in the archipelago,[18] and thus perhaps removed from the dynamics of plague transmission through the intermediary of infected rats or their fleas from ships. The fact that there appears to be no record of a plague-like epidemic on Bali in indigenous sources, no *usada* on the plague and no Balinese term for the plague could be taken to suggest that this pestilence may never have been part of the disease burden of Bali.

On the other hand, though peripheral to most international commerce, there had always been some traffic between Java and Bali. Moreover, Bali retained some commercial and political ties with Java, even after the Islamization of the latter island and the advent of the Dutch, so plague transmission was by no means impossible. It is conceivable that a first encounter with so horrific a pestilence became a never-to-be-forgotten event, literally unmentionable (like leprosy), unresolvable save by rituals which immortalize its occurrence and function to prevent its recurrence. That there should remain more obscurity than clarity surrounding what is after all a 900-year-old enigma—the pestilence of the *Calon Arang*—is hardly striking.

Smallpox, the Decline of Majapahit and the Rise of Islam

Smallpox, like other diseases, is perceived by the Balinese as a supernatural phenomenon; unlike any other, it is conceived as a divine gift (*paica*) rather than an affliction. The Balinese term for smallpox, *kacacar*, incorporates the perceived cause and the effects of the illness; the verbal prefix *ka-* indicates that the morbid condition, *cacar* (eaten away), is of external or divine origin. In common Balinese language, the word for smallpox is *krawan* (possibly from *ka-rauh-an*, meaning 'possessed by a spirit or deity'), or *kawan* (from *kawuhan* meaning 'what lies to the west'). There is also a legend which describes the disease as part of the 'wares' of Bhatara Kala (The Lord Kala) which were said to have been distributed throughout Bali by a blind man[19]—perhaps an allusion to the fact that, especially in tropical regions, smallpox was known to be a common precipitating cause of blindness. According to medical folklore, Dewa Majapahit, in search of subjects, brought smallpox to Bali. *Dewa* can mean 'god' or allude to a ruler; having the disease was referred to as *madewa* (having the god). Majapahit was the last Javanese Hindu-Buddhist kingdom whose hegemony over the archipelago was broken by the Islamic coastal trading principalities in the fifteenth century. The soul of one dying of smallpox was said to have flown home to the world of Buda.

A Balinese medical treatise on smallpox is entitled *Tutur Wekas ing Majapahit: Usada Kacacar*, meaning 'Secret, Mystical Knowledge Concerning the End of Majapahit: The Treatment of Smallpox'. The term *wekas* also has the meaning of 'legacy' or 'what is left behind'. The section of the text which comprises the *Tutur* (Secret Knowledge) is brief and cryptic:

> Smallpox came to Bali, and the one able to cure it was none other than Siwa-Buda as he was from Majapahit. He knew the way to effect recovery as well as the treatment, and even the advantage (*don*) of the disease, and

the place of the mystical syllables in the body; searching for . . . subjects.[20]

Another section of the same text reads:

> Pondering the fate of man afflicted by smallpox, Sang Hyang Buda decreed that his glow should light up the world. Traditional order (*makrama*) being no longer apparent in the world, the Powerful Demon Trinity brings disease and death.[21]

A more abstruse reference to extraneous events occurs in another smallpox *usada*, in the form of *sarana* (prescribed magical implements) together with a *mantra* (magical formula). After listing the names of some medicinal herbs, the text continues:

> The Dewa of Majapahit becomes the god of smallpox . . . When they came from across the sea they were only nine. They were secretive. A Brahmana arrived from Bali. Man follows a path to safety.[22]

Part of a *Kaputusan Sang Hyang Buda* (The Mystery of Sang Hyang Buda) in an *Usada Kacacar* reads:

> Sang Hyang Buda descends . . . to Bali to gather all the people . . . There is disturbance and fear . . . Sang Hyang Buda desires to counteract the proliferation of malignant forms of smallpox. The people will not submit to these dangerous forms.[23]

A relationship is implied between the arrival of smallpox on Bali, some extraneous influence, a god or deified ruler of Majapahit, Buda, and the breakdown of an old order. Thus, in Balinese conceptualization of smallpox we may see allegorical allusions to matters only briefly commented upon in the Balinese historical tradition, namely the displacement of Hindu-Buddhist traditions, the demise of Majapahit, and the advent of Islam.

In the Javanese *babad* (chronicle) tradition the defeat and violent death of the last ruler of Majapahit is related in terms of his returning to the world of the gods. The kingdom is said to have collapsed while the ruler was in search of 'auxiliaries'. The religion immediately replaced by Islam is referred to as *agami buda* in this tradition.[24]

Historically, the decline of Majapahit is linked with internal dynastic disputes, Chinese interference, the rise of the trading port of Melaka, and the spread of Islam, which began in the western archipelago. Traditional Javanese and Balinese sources stress the role of Islam. A Balinese *babad* states that Majapahit ceased to exist because Java was overcome by the religion of Islam.[25] Another *babad* elaborates, stating that a mission led by a Brahmana was sent from Bali to Java to protest against the subjugation of the Javanese peasantry to the laws of Islam, but seeing Java so 'desolate and chaotic' (*tistis samun panagara aro-ara*), the mission returned immediately to Bali.[26] In the Balinese *Babad Dalem*, the decline of Majapahit is further linked with the emergence of a Demon God, the treachery of officials and their seizure of power, and a populace possessed by a demon and in a state of intoxication. 'Majapahit was ruined', the text states, as if 'sold out' (*tinukwan*).[27] The Majapahit nobility and their followers who refused to embrace Islam fled to Bali, thus strengthening resistance to Islam there. Balinese still consider themselves to be subjects of Dewa Majapahit. Throughout Bali there are shrines to Dewa Majapahit and numerous temples known by the name Majapahit.

Such ideas and associations continue through cryptic allusions in the sections of the smallpox *usada* which deal with diagnosis, prognosis and treatment of the disease. The main types and phases of smallpox (from the fulminating type with 100% mortality to the mild, benign type with initial pyrexia and sparse eruptions) are differentiated in the *Usada Kacacar*. Constitutional symptoms exhibited by smallpox sufferers are given names, usually of animals. The eruptions or pustules themselves are often given names of minerals, metals, precious stones, medicinal and aromatic plants, fragrant woods and spices. Each name is preceded by the word *puuh*, which means 'quail' and, by symbolic extension (the colouring of the quail's plumage perhaps), 'pustule' or 'smallpox'.

The *puuh* are further split into prognostic categories of good (*puuh ayu*), fair (*puuh sedeng ayu*) and grave (*puuh ala*). In the early stages of the illness, effort is directed toward securing survival by ritually manipulating the disease organism to assume a form which is less threatening to the host. Through offerings and *mantra* the dangerous forms are urged to change into more benign varieties designated *ganti* (a herbal spice), *katumbah* (coriander), *nasi-nasi* (a hard wood), *sanggawak* (dried, cooked rice) and *syah/siyah*, an ambiguous term for which the most appropriate translation may be the Islamic title *Shah* (spelt 'Syah' in Malay languages).[28] The other terms refer to items which on one level are similes for the changing appearance of smallpox eruptions, but on another are trade items extracted from islands of the archipelago or exchanged in Islamized Javanese port towns. All these ultimately benign forms are invited to 'come and proliferate' (*teka saak*).[29] Collectively, the signs and symptoms of smallpox are named *candra mahala* (the moon is dangerous)—perhaps an allusion to the crescent moon of Islam? The life-threatening varieties are termed *satus dwalapan* which literally means 'one hundred and eight', but *dwal* also has a meaning of 'the wares', 'selling' or 'decay'.[30]

In order to appreciate fully the significance of these texts, one must understand the role of *mantra* in Balinese thought. There is nothing devotional in a *mantra*; it is not a form of prayer, but a magical formula, part of the power of which lies in the subtle insinuations implied in utterances. As with other forms of magic, *mantra* involve moral ambiguity. Their objective is to confront offending spirits causing disease by addressing them directly, by identifying them and revealing their qualities, their abodes and, most significantly, their origins. The power of *mantra* is believed to lie in the magical effect of the utterance of inherent truths.

In the smallpox *mantra* the challenged spirits bear such titles as *Pangeran*, *Susuhunan* (or *Sunan*) and *Sedah*, apparently Javanese Islamic terms of address. Other spirits are addressed by such titles as: *Ki Pulang Paling*, *Ki Balang Bungalan* and *Ki Kulang-Kaling*, which have a meaning of 'He who Goes To and Fro'; *Mas Kaya* (Wealth and Power); *Pandung Bhuta* (Demon thief); *Giri Prakosa* (Violent Giri/Mountain); and *Giri Suta* (Descendant of Giri), all of which may be symbolically linked to Javanese Islam. The nine *wali*, the proselytizing saints of Islam on Java, were renowned itinerants. Indigenous legends emphasize their commercial interests and trade connections. One, *Sunan Kali Jaga*, was formerly a notorious thief and gambler. *Giri* means 'mountain' but may also refer to the site near Gresik (a major Javanese trading centre and centre to Islam in the fifteenth century)[31] where another *wali*, *Sunan Giri*, established his mosque. *Sunan Giri* is reputed to have been the key vanquisher of the last ruler of Majapahit and to have founded a line of descendants who mounted conversion campaigns on the islands east of Java. It was a descendant of Sunan Giri, named *Pangeran* Prepan, who attempted to propagate Islam on Bali and whose attempts were repulsed by the Balinese.[32]

The immediate origins of the spirits are indicated as *Sabrang* (across the seas), *Kling* (South India, Java, or Majapahit), *Mlayu*

(Malay Peninsula/Sumatra), *Jamur Jipang* (?), *Janur Kuning* (?)[33] and Java. One *mantra* specifically suggests that smallpox reached Bali after having been in these places:

> O Vile Demon, don't make this person suffer. Having been to Jamur-Jipang, Kling, Sabrang and Mlayu, you come to Bali and cause man suffering.[34]

In another *mantra*, the ancient origin of the demon spirit of smallpox is 'exposed' as *Gunung Alah* (Mountain of Allah):

> O you Demons, white, red, yellow, black and five coloured, don't cause man suffering. Your ancient origins are known. You become Ki Ulu Puhun (The One with the Blackened/Burnt Head), *Pangeran* Gunung Alah.[35]

In another *usada* the *mantra* reads:

> . . . *Pangeran* Gunung Alah created you, Pangeran Gunung Alah, the god whose sperm was spilt.[36]

Other smallpox *usada* mention 'Bagenda Ali', perhaps another reference to Islam or its prophet.

Beyond these direct, if cryptic, references to Islamic titles and institutions are other elements of Balinese smallpox lore which may reflect local perceptions of the new ethos associated with Javanese Islam. The *Usada Kacacar*, for example, prohibited the consumption of meat by the smallpox victim for forty-two days, while particularly 'dangerous' kinds of meat, such as pork, were to be presented as offerings. Balinese also would 'secretly' feed a little lizard flesh to children when epidemics first erupted, to prevent them from getting a severe form of the disease. This may be paralleled by Islamic prohibitions of the consumption of certain meats, such as pork and lizard flesh.

In prohibiting smallpox sufferers from consuming the flesh of cocks killed in cockfights and prescribing money won at gambling[37] or exchanged at markets as bedside offerings for smallpox sufferers, the Balinese may also have been mindful of Islamic prohibitions on gambling and some kind of link between trade and Islam. There were also, as noted above, many allusions to trade and trade goods in rituals, and the variety and quantity of offerings at the bedside of a smallpox sufferer were said to have made the atmosphere resemble that of a marketplace; perhaps this too implied an association with Islam, which had raised markets to new heights of activity and prestige in Java. Finally, the effective prohibition on the cremation of corpses of smallpox victims (in accordance with usual Balinese custom) is paralleled by the replacement of cremation by burial in Islamic Java.[38] In all these areas it is apparently implied that resistance to smallpox was facilitated by adoption of certain Islamic practices and proscriptions.

Though they refused to embrace Islam, it is probable that the Balinese were conversant with some of the concepts and practices of their Javanese neighbours who had submitted to the laws of Islam. Also, some Muslims had settled along the west coast of Bali. Certainly, Balinese awareness of Islam and its new kind of magical power is apparent in the magico-medical texts. Does, then, some of the medical folklore surrounding smallpox reflect in part early Balinese encounters with Islam and their antipathy to, or perhaps their awe of, Islamic magic, customs and prohibitions?[39]

Juxtaposed motifs of propagation of Islam, the procurement of modified variants of it, deadly epidemics and peripatetic preachers with healing powers occur in the Balinese, Javanese and Sasak (Lombok) post-Islamic historical traditions. The following is a synopsis of such an episode in the Balinese text, *Dwijendra Tatwa*:[40]

Dwijendra, a Brahmana priest, crossed from Java to Bali at a time of change and disaster (*sanghara kalpa*) which had caused the subjects of Majapahit to flee eastward to Bali. Their fear had been aroused by Islam which had taken hold of Java. On Bali, where a deadly epidemic raged, Dwijendra instructed the people on the use of holy water and the placing of offerings of prepared betel-nut in the four directions as an antidote against further epidemics.

Dwijendra also encountered some Sasak people from Lombok adrift in a boat, half-conscious, afraid and bewildered. Having revived them, Dwijendra returned with them to Lombok and taught them a modified form of Islam named '*gama Salem Wetu Telu*' (Three-Times-a-Day Islam).

In the Sasak version, Dwijendra visits Lombok to find the island in the grip of 'plagues', which had arisen, it was revealed to him, in the embracing of Islam by the populace. Dwijendra then preached the modified version of Islam through which the epidemics are said to have abated.[41]

The cultural response of the Balinese to smallpox is somewhat paradoxical. The lethal forms were recognized and the devastating effects of smallpox epidemics were experienced; epidemics recorded in the nineteenth century virtually paralysed social, politi cal and religious life in some regions.[42] Nevertheless, the disease was not perceived as a scourge. Though its method and effectiveness were understood, there was some cultural resistance to smallpox vaccination.[43] There was also an awareness of the fact that a single attack of smallpox gave life-long immunity which vaccination did not give. Smallpox was viewed as a supernatural problem rather than a medical one. Vaccination was considered an interference with the will of Dewa Majapahit.[44]

On Bali, according to Boon, it was believed that smallpox 'manifested posthumously the religious purity of the deceased', so ritual elevation by cremation was not required. Sometimes the disease was also used by royal lines in claims to legitimacy.[45] Since numerous Majapahit nobles and priests were driven to Bali by Islamic expansion in Java, is it possible they were believed to have brought the disease with them? Elsewhere in the world smallpox, no respecter of class, was often introduced by the nobility, the most mobile element of the population.[46] As the process of conversion to Islam, according to Javanese legend, also began with the ruling élite and worked down,[47] a further parallel might also be seen; the high status ascribed to smallpox may be partially explicable through this curious conceptual equation.

Indigenous attitudes to Islam and proselytism may provide one of the keys to meaning behind the smallpox–gift–wares–Islam symbolism perceptible in Balinese conceptualization of smallpox. The Balinese appear to have had some idea of inoculation (the principle of a modified, less virulent organism with which the host can adapt) as an effective means of producing immunity and ensuring survival. Since it was a gift of the God Buda and of the Dewa Majapahit who was in search of subjects, as well as the wares of a Demon God associated with the destruction of the kingdom of Majapahit, was smallpox also tacitly assumed by the Balinese to be a kind of 'trade-off'—smallpox instead of Islam? Smallpox does seem to represent an apt, albeit inglorious, metaphor for the Islamization of Java, the attempted Islamization of Bali and the legendary tales of attempts to procure modified variants of the powerful new religion on Lombok.[48] Smallpox was a specifically human disease. It could not be cured, but it could be modified. The metaphor may perhaps work inversely. The Balinese, like the Javanese, are known masters of the art of associative thinking and of the juxtaposition of symbols.

Links between smallpox, Majapahit, Siwa–Buddhism, Islam

and trade in Balinese smallpox-related medical texts and folklore, though undeniably tenuous, are too prominent and consistent to be dismissed as meaningless coincidence. In the *usada*, by explicit (if ambiguous) reference, the disease is cast as a legacy of the Javanese Siwa–Buddhist kingdom of Majapahit, decreed by the God Buda to whose abode the soul of the smallpox victim returns. Through connotations in the names (in the form of references to Javanese and Malay Islamic titles) and origins (in the form of references to regions in the archipelago converted to Islam) attributed to the 'spirits' of smallpox in *mantra*, the disease is connected with Islam, which in turn is connected with the decline of Majapahit. In the ritual prescriptions and proscriptions, there are possible allusions to Muslim influences on Javanese customs. Through the naming of the signs and the symptomology of smallpox in the *usada*, there are associations with trade, which in turn is associated with the spread of Islam. The Balinese response to smallpox, not unlike the attitude to Islam in some respects, is paradoxical. Though known to be deadly, smallpox was perceived as a gift from which some benefit and immunity could be secured if contracted in a modified form—analogous with Balinese interpretation and toleration of a modified version of Islam on nearby Lombok.

These linkages do indeed reflect fifteenth century historical events and cultural crises—the expansion of trade and Islam, increased mobility, the spread of smallpox, the displacement of Majapahit as the centre of political and economic power and the threatened annihilation of Hindu–Buddhist traditions—from which the Balinese emerged as the sole retainers of an intact Siwa–Buddhist cultural heritage and political culture. These events were perhaps accompanied by fortuitous smallpox epidemics. Unless these mythic connections and specifically smallpox-related symbols are intended as an elaborate deception (and there remain any number of contradictions and riddles yet to be unravelled), the Balinese appear to have written religious, economic and political change, as well as the biological uniqueness of the virus itself, into their biography of smallpox.

Cholera: The Biography of Ratu Gede Macaling, 'The Great Fanged Lord'

In present day Bali, a demonic, protective deity known as Ratu Gege Macaling or Bhatara (Lord) Dalem Ped is venerated in rituals specifically associated with cholera. Those dying of cholera are sometimes said to have been *kambil Macaling* (taken by Macaling). Legends surrounding the god of cholera suggest that he is of less ancient origin than other cult figures associated with epidemic diseases. His abode is outside Bali, in the temple Dalem Ped on the arid island of Nusa Penida, which lies south-east of central Bali. Curiously, there are no cult images of Macaling, as there are of other demonic, protective deities. Balinese are loathe to utter the name Macaling, and few dare to discuss his origin. Much of the legend around Macaling derives from the oral tradition. To my knowledge there are no *usada* on cholera, only *lontar* (palm-leaf manuscripts) which contain the name Macaling in their titles and consist of *mantra* revealing his origin and the parameters of his power and presence. When drawn into a discussion, Balinese refer to his deeds in vague terms and name him through the honorary Indonesian term of reference *beliau*, always in hushed tones. His awesome presence is perhaps too imminent. Cholera epidemics still occur on Bali.

Within the explanatory mythology which seeks to connect him with the high gods of the Hindu–Buddhist pantheon, Macaling is Bhatara Kala, Bhatara Tengah ing Segara (The Demon God of the Depths of the Sea). His task is to protect the people of Bali, provided they do not neglect prescribed devotional rituals; otherwise he allows cholera to rage and decimate the population. In an *Usana Nusa Pulo* text,[49] Macaling is one of a number of descendants of a magically powerful *Dukuh* (Hermit-Priest), all of whom are accredited with great *sakti* and who occupy magically powerful (*tenget*) sites on Nusa Penida. A long *mantra* lists the lineage of the *Dukuh* and their respective manifestations in temples, together with their weapons, namely kris, whip, machete, sword and *lontar*.[50] In the *babad*[51] tradition there appears an I Macaling, a pupil in black magic of a *balian* named Ki Balian Batur. Together they created a diarrhoeal illness in central and south Bali. Ki Balian Batur eventually 'submitted joyfully to execution by rifle', the only *pusaka* (magically powerful heirloom) potent enough to secure 'his exorcism and release through death'. I Macaling continued using his *sakti* to cause *ngutah bayar*, a cholera-like illness, among merchants who stayed overnight in his village. Finally a ruse was devised whereby I Macaling was tricked into leaving Bali for Nusa Penida, following which trade is said to have increased and Bali to have become well populated.

Julius Jacobs observed that the Balinese were not pleased with the arrival of his vessel, an old Dutch warship. In fact, a cholera epidemic followed his arrival in 1881. Jacobs cited two other cases of cholera outbreaks following the arrival of foreign warships, one in 1868 with a Dutch military expedition against Buleleng, and the other after the arrival of the *Arjoena* in 1871.[52] In the 1930s Weck observed that in the minds of the people in north Bali there was a strong association between war and cholera.[53] They were of the opinion that cholera epidemics always followed the arrival of foreign ships. The people of central and east Bali also perceive an association between cholera and a kind of military invasion. In this case, the invading army takes the form of *bhuta-bregala* (demons), the warring armies of Macaling from across the sea. This army is said to move across Bali like a wave, wielding ropes, machetes, hewing knives, shields, sickles, torches and *lontar*. They enter villages and seek their victim, hack at the belly and seal up the anus so that the abdomen swells up and there is excruciating pain. After a short time, they simultaneously pull out the cork from the anus and the life from the body.[54]

The fear and dread aroused by cholera has apparently led to proliferation of tales involving tall figures wielding sharp weapons with which they attack unwary villagers, who thereupon experience sharp, stabbing pains. Two such cholera stories involve, in one case 'a very tall human', and in another, 'a refined human wearing a hat', Each carries a basket and a long thin knife with which they intend to cut out the insides of the villagers upon whom they chance.[55]

Traditionally, Balinese dance is not performance but enactment, often used to exorcise disease. Part of the response to disease is to externalize it, and one of the functions of dance is to act out the fear which disease provokes and simultaneously to exorcise the offending spirit. A particular Balinese dance form called *baris*, of which there are some thirty types, is enacted by 'armies' of male dancers. *Baris* are often named according to the weapons or implements held by the dancer, or the costumes worn. Weapons include such things as lances, sickles, shields, machetes, ropes, clubs and rifles. When enacting the *Baris Cina* or *Baris Tuan* (both terms signifying 'foreign'), dancers wear shabby, Western-type garments, hats and shoes, and carry ropes and spears.

It is possible that the Balinese conceptualization of cholera is reflected in some forms of *baris*. There are striking similarities

among the weapons used in some *baris*, those carried by the
bhuta-bregala of cholera folklore, and those of Macaling's kinsmen
from Nusa Penida. Certain *baris* costumes such as loincloths, and
black-and-white checked or striped sashes also are worn by the
bhuta-bregala. The characteristic fearful expressions, tense poses
and rigidly outstretched limbs of the *baris* dancer, and the strange
hoarse, high-pitched cries which accompany a change of dance
position all seem to recall the painful muscular limb and abdomi-
nal cramps and voice changes so characteristic of cholera as well as
the cholera imagery in folklore of abdomens being struck with
sharp weapons and the stabbing pain.[56]

Motifs in the cholera myths may indicate the circumstances and
possible era of the arrival of epidemic cholera on Bali.[57] For
example, the practitioner of magic responsible for the cholera-
like disease could only be destroyed by weaponry of foreign origin,
a rifle, which had been added to the sacred regalia of the royal
lineage of Klungkung. In the rifle motif there is not only an
allusion to the association of cholera with war but also perhaps the
idea that cholera is a modern disease which can be more effectively
treated by the use of modern medicines. In contemporary Bali,
balian are generally not inclined to treat cholera. They send cases
to Western-type doctors whose medicine, they say in the case of
cholera, 'is much quicker'. Western-type preventative health
measures are also in evidence in present-day Bali. The magical
rites peculiar to cholera, however, have not been rendered
redundant.

On Bali the wet season is cholera season, referred to as *masan
grubug* (cholera epidemic time). As cholera time approaches,
Balinese make special offerings (*aci-aci*) at local temples; some
wear talismans and construct shrines in front of houseyards. Such
magical measures are intended to dissuade Macaling from claiming
too many victims. In the seaside village of Sanur, the wet season
begins with a three-day ceremony called *Karya Ngusaba Desa:
Panangluk Marana* (A Ceremony to Safeguard the Village: The
Containment of Death). It appears that such a ceremony has been
held in Sanur at the beginning of the wet season for as long as
people can remember. 'Long ago', I was told, 'a cholera epidemic
began in Sanur whence it spread over the whole of Bali. It was as
though a tumultuous war was raging.' The movements of Macaling
during the wet season are documented in a *lontar* [58] which may be
summarized as follows:

On the first night of the *Panangluk Marana*, held on the last day of the fifth Balinese month (November/December, the beginning of the wet season), Macaling and his army arrive on the beach at Sanur from Nusa Penida and sleep on the beaches. During the second night, they sleep in Sanur and check to see that all necessary offerings have been made. Should they have been neglected, Macaling may ask for twenty-five victims. They continue to Denpasar where they may request eighty victims. From there, they move across to Java and then to Sulawesi. On the night of the new moon between the sixth and seventh months of the Balinese year, they arrive back on Bali and another *Panangluk Marana* is held on the beach at Lebih, Gianyar. A similar ceremony is held in nearby Kramas. The end of the wet season is marked by a four-day ritual held throughout Bali, called *Tawur Kasanga*. *Tawur Kasanga*, on the night of the new moon between the ninth and the tenth Balinese months (the end of the wet season), culminates in elaborate offerings at graveyards, crossroads, beaches and village boundaries with noisy purification rites which mark the return of Macaling and his army of *bhuta-bregala* to Nusa Penida

A *Panangluk Marana* is not then, as supposed in some ethnography, simply a ritual to promote good harvests or to ward off plagues of rats.[59] It is another of the many Balinese rituals intended to ward off the devastating epidemic illness. In south Bali at least, *Tawur Kasanga* is not just a random extermination of miscellaneous demons. It has become a ritual send-off for a recent demonic protective deity, the god of cholera, Ratu Gede Macaling. Both these rituals belong to the category of offerings known as *Bhuta Yadnya* (Offerings for Demonic Powers). They mark what is in fact the seasonal pattern of cholera epidemics in Bali and have become associated with the appeasement of Ratu Gede Macaling.

Cholera is certainly the dread epidemic disease of contemporary Bali. The spectacular clinical symptoms of the disease are such that it could not fail to arouse fear and capture the imagination of the closely knit community. Cholera epidemics are, not surprisingly, memorable events for the survivors. The ritual response they have evoked on Bali is equal to the spectacle of the disease itself and the biography of its 'creator' is almost as sensational as the spectacle.

Concluding Remarks

One of the objectives in this paper has been to bring together some of the factual and conceptual aspects of patterns of morbidity on Bali. The nature of the invading disease organism and historical circumstances at the time it was first experienced seem to have contributed to the cultural constructions of four major pestilences. The varying conceptualizations of diseases seem to imply some explanation and perhaps even judgement of past experiences of morbidity. Myths and magical rites which have evolved from the realities of morbidity appear to have historical and biological, as well as metaphysical, levels of meaning.

The reason why the Balinese classify leprosy as a curse of the gods upon ancestors, plague as the gruesome creation of a powerful witch reified in the *rangda* cult figure, smallpox as a gift of a god-ruler, and cholera as part of the weaponry of a warring practitioner of powerful magic, may relate more to facts of history and the natural history of disease than one is prone to assume. In the ethno-medical accounts of each pestilence there is an interesting and at times intriguing interplay between cultural factors and biological and historical variables.

This paper is an attempt not just to illuminate the cultural and medical history of Bali, but to demonstrate the use of indigenous sources in historical epidemiology. Such sources may not display a Western historical attitude and approach to documentation, but they are, nevertheless, more than a phantasmagoria of legend and magic. Conceptions, even mystical-magical ones, are not formed in a vacuum. In short, these sources provide an insight into indigenous perspectives on disease, perceptions which have shaped attitudes and practices in the field of health in the past and will continue to do so in the conceivable future.

I wish to acknowledge with gratitude the assistance of Anthony Day, Tony Milner, Craig Reynolds, Raechelle Rubinstein, Peter Worsley and especially Norman Owen, who offered helpful comments on earlier drafts of this paper.

1. The two genres of traditional literature consulted for this paper are classified as 'historical literature', which includes *Usana Bali* (Ancient History of Bali) texts, *Babad* (Genealogical Histories), the *Calon Arang* and *Tatwa Dwijendra*, and 'magico-medical literature', of which a number include the word 'Usada' (Medical Treatise) in their titles. The manuscripts cited are from the Hooykaas Ketut Sangka (HKS) and Gedong Kirtya (K) collections, Leiden, available at the University of Sydney. Some of the ethnological data concerning smallpox and cholera derive from the writings of two medical officers, Julius Jacobs and Wolfgang Weck, who worked in Bali in the late nineteenth and early twentieth centuries. The paper is also based on participant observation in healing rituals and discussions with traditional healers and village priests as well as with Westernized doctors during field research in Bali in 1981–82 and again, briefly, in 1983.

2. *Gaglaran Pamangku Sane Sampun Mapodgala*, HKS 1959: 2.

3. For example, the story of Rsi Markandheya related in *Bhuwana Tatwa Maha Rsi Markandheya*, compiled by Ketut Ginarsa (Singaraja, Balai Penelitian Bahasa, 1979).

4. An account of Jayakusunu (twelfth century) is found in varying detail in all the versions of *Usana Bali* texts consulted, e.g. HKS 2069, 2987.

5. J. A. Day, 'Meanings of Change in the Poetry of Nineteenth Century Java', (Ph.D. dissertation, Cornell University, 1981), 303.

6. One of the more complete versions of the story of Mayadanawa occurs in *Usana Bali Mayadanawa*, HKS 2020. On the basis of textual and ethnographic evidence it seems possible that huge male and female masked cult figures, *Barong Landung* (tall *Barong*) trace their origin to this Mayadanawa and his Chinese wife, though this does not imply that they are associated specifically with leprosy. For the assumption of R. Goris and P. Dronkers, *Bali: Atlas Kebudayaan* (Jakarta, n.d.), 187, that the ritual parading of these cult figures functions to secure agricultural abundance and animal fecundity, there appears to be no evidence in the Balinese ritual complex. The expressed concern with human survival is a more probable motivation.

7. Another consistantly occurring motif in *Usana Bali* texts, e.g., HKS 2165:31b, 2069:40a, 2020:31b, 2243:19b.

8. Goitre, another endemic disease of probable ancient origin, also prompts relatively little therapeutic ritual. It is also the specific subject of an *usada*.

9. J. J. Van Loghem, 'The Plague Problem in the Netherlands Indies', *Bulletin of the Colonial Institute of Amsterdam* 11, 2 (1939), 131. See also Terrence H. Hull, 'Plague in Java', below.

10. Extract from the Yearly Report of 1919 of the Civil Medical Service in the Dutch East Indies, *Mededeelingen van der Burgerlijken Geneeskundigen Dienst Nederlandsche-Indië* 11 (1922), 94; Hull, op. cit.

11. Allan Schwartz, 'The End of an Era', *Ciba Journal* 43 (1967), 30-8; see also W. L. Langer, 'The Black Death', *Scientific American* 210, 2 (1964), 117.

12. R. Ng. Poerbatjaraka, 'De Calon Arang', *Bijdragen tot de Taal-, Land- en Volkenkunde* 82 (1926), 118-22 (hereafter cited as *BKI*). The only date connected to the text is a date of copying, 1540.

13. The symbolism in the legend is best understood within terms of Tantric mystical techniques of utilizing the ambivalent powers of graveyards and corpses.

14. It would be overly rash to propose some peculiar analogy between the image of *leyak* entering houses through holes in walls and the actual transmission of plague bacillus on Java through rats nesting in walls (see Hull, op. cit.). At most, one could posit some unconscious awareness of the significance of the circumstances of pestilence, expressed metaphorically. *Leyak* are in fact believed to assume animal form when executing their foul deeds. Curious reflections of bio-medical reality have been found elsewhere; see, for example, F. G. Garrison, *History of Medicine* (London, W. B. Saunders, 1929), 71, on a ninth century Indian text which contains a warning to people to desert their houses when rats jump about and die, 'presumably from the plague'. G. Marks, *The Medieval Plague* (New York, Doubleday and Co., 1971), 11, also reports the suggestion of a relationship between the plague and the activity of rats observed by an eleventh-century Arabic physician.

15. Langer, op. cit., 115-21; W. H. McNeill, *Plagues and Peoples* (New York, Penguin, 1979), 170.

16. G. Coedès, *The Indianized States of South-east Asia* (Honolulu, East-West Center Press, 1968), 130, 144-5.

17. Scholars have generally attempted to explicate the *rangda* cult figure in terms of psycho-analytical theories—as an evil, taunting mother-figure or as an image of female senility and male sexuality (finding phallic symbolism in the protruding tongue of the *rangda*) — and the associated rituals in terms of sociological theories—as a means of acting-out suppressed anger or reinforcing social solidarity. See G. Bateson and M. Mead, *Balinese Character: A Photographic*

Analysis (New York, New York Academy of Science, 1942); J. Belo, *Bali: Rangda and Barong*, Monograph of the American Ethnological Society (New York, J.J. Augustin, 1949); M. Le Cron Foster, 'Synthesis and Antithesis in Balinese Ritual', in A.L. Becker and A. Yengoyan (eds), *The Imagination of Reality* (Norwood, Ablex, 1979), 175-96. Such theories seem anachronistic and inappropriate within the context of the culture, the myth and the morbid reality. Obviously, there are many layers of meaning. Above all, the grotesque figure appears to embody the morbid and psychic dimensions of disease, the spirit of pestilence (plague?).

18. As H. Schulte Nordholt, 'The Mads Lange Connection', *Indonesia*, no. 32 (1981), 19-23, has argued, Balinese desire to preserve its Hindu–Buddhist traditions, perceived to be threatened by the presence of Islam and later the Dutch, involved deliberate political isolation from the outside world. Trade contact with Java in the seventeenth and eighteenth centuries consisted mainly of the export of Balinese slaves.

19. Wolfgang Weck, *Heilkunde und Volkstum auf Bali* (Stuttgart, Ferdinand Enke, 1937), 168.

20. HKS 3452:2b:26. The terminology in the text implies a smallpox pandemic: *sasab* (widespread illness) *anda* (world). It is also noted that the times were 'afflicted by deadly disease' (*agering kamaranan*). The religion of fifteenth century Majapahit is generally known as *Siwa–Buda* (Siva–Buddha). Rulers bore the titles of deities, were endowed with divine attributes and were deified in death.

21. HKS 3452:2b. 'Sang Hyang' is a title of a god.

22. *Wisada Cacar*, HKS 3138:15b. The 'nine' could be an allusion to the *wali sanga*, 'nine holy men' of Javanese Islam, and 'secretive' to the *walis*' subversive activities. See G. W. Drewes 'The Struggle Between Javanism and Islam as Illustrated by the *Sĕrat Dĕrmagandul*', *BKI* 122, 3 (1966), 309-65.

23. The complete *Kaputusan* and translation appears in C. Hooykaas, *Agama Tirtha: Five Studies in Hindu-Balinese Religion* (Amsterdam, N. V. Noord-Hollandsche UM, 1963), 80-1. My reading differs from that of Hooykaas in some details.

24. G. W. Drewes, op. cit., 316, 321. On Java it was feared that the spirit of a smallpox victim would be stolen by the dreaded Ratu Lara Kidul (Goddess of the South Seas) whose subjects they became; F. van Ossenbruggen, *Het Primitieve Denken in Pokkengerbruiken* ('s Gravenhage, Martinus Nijhoff, 1916), 28. In texts on Javanese Muslim mysticism, the Goddess was believed to be a daughter of the former ruler of Majapahit, Brawijaya.

25. *Babad Brahmana Kemenuh*, HKS 3233:2a.

26. *Babad Arya Tabanan*, K 1792/13:13b; cf. HKS 3138.

27. HKS 1358:21b.

28. Reigning sultans of the early Islamic coastal principalities of Java, Sumatra and the Malay Peninsula bore the titles *Syah* or *Pangeran* as honorific appositions to their personal names.

29. HKS 3138: 17b.

30. A 'commercial' element, notions of 'buying the pox' and the pricking of smallpox scabs are almost universal in smallpox-related folk medicine. See F. Henschen, *The History of Diseases* (London, Longman Green, 1962), 54. McNeill, op. cit., 225–6, suggests 'the entire ritual looked like an adaptation of commercial customs'. In the *usada*, it was recommended that the scabs be pricked with pandanus grasses purchased from Java (HKS 3138: 29b).

31. See M. C. Ricklefs, *A History of Modern Indonesia* (London, Macmillan Press, 1981), 8–12.

32. The names of other spirits confronted in *mantra* include: *Abu-Abu Saking Jawa, Mega Putih, Celeng Putih, Nadah-Nadah, Ngasu Abang, Sang Hyang Wenang Susuhunan Kidul, Dharma Jati, Amangku Jagat, Tunjung Putih, Janur*

Kuning, Bija Kuning.

33. There was an Islamic kingdom on the north coast of East Java called Jipang. *Kuning* was sometimes included in Javanese Islamic titles; Th. Pigeaud, *Islamic States in Java 1500–1700* (The Hague, Martinus Nijhoff, 1976), 26, 163.

34. HKS 3452: 28a.

35. HKS 3452: 7b.

36. *Usada Kacacar*, HKS. There is no HKS record number for this *usada*; its location is bundle 7, no. 11.

37. One returning from a cockfight was not supposed to gaze upon a smallpox sufferer.

38. The placement of the corpse, under *mabasah* ('allowing to decompose') rituals, in an open grave may even be connected with the Islamic prohibition against allowing earth to fall directly upon the corpse. Cf. B. J. Terwiel, 'Asiatic Cholera in Siam', below, who cites La Loubère as attributing Siamese prohibition against cremation of recent smallpox victims to fear of renewed contagion.

39. Intriguing associations between Islam and smallpox continued into the twentieth century. A practice of hanging white or red flags outside house yards and at the boundaries of villages during smallpox epidemics as a magical means of defence was observed on Java and Bali. On Java the flags were sometimes inscribed with the letters 'SI' (Sarekat Islam), meaning 'Islamic League'. They were sometimes placed on graves as well; Van Ossenbruggen, op. cit., 195.

40. HKS 2632: 22b–25a. Dwijendra lived on Bali during the reign of Dalem Batur Enggong, 1460–1550. His daughter is the goddess of traders.

41. F. D. K. Bosch, *Selected Studies in Indonesian Archaeology* (The Hague, van Hoeve, 1961), 156. See also *Babad Tanah Djawi*, Meinsma edition ('s Gravenhage, Martinus Nijhoff, 1941), 20–1, in which an epidemic is associated with conversion to Islam.

42. Schulte Nordholt, op. cit., 46, quoting from the correspondence of Mads Lange. An 1828 epidemic so decimated the population of Badung that there were not sufficient healthy people available to plant the rice crop; Du Bois Letters, No. 73, 28 August 1828, Arsip Nasional, Jakarta. Julius Jacobs, *Eenigen tijd onder de Baliers* (Batavia, G. Kolff and Co., 1883), 199, estimated that three-quarters of the population of Bali was pock-marked.

43. Jacobs, op. cit. Jacobs visited Bali to observe the progress of the smallpox vaccination programme.

44. Weck, op. cit., 167.

45. J. Boon, 'Dynastic Dynamics, Caste and Kingship in Bali Now' (Ph.D. dissertation, University of Chicago, 1973), 37.

46. G. W. Dixon, *Smallpox* (London, J. & A. Churchill, 1962), 191.

47. Ricklefs, op. cit., 8.

48. The proselytizing saints of Javanese Islam have not been immune to ignoble allegorical judgements in the indigenous literary tradition, as Drewes' work on the Javanese *Sěrat Děrmagandul* illustrates. Drewes shows how the text makes critical allusions to Javanese Muslim customs and through cryptic historiography denounces the *wali* for their self-enriching trade endeavours and for conspiring against the last ruler of Majapahit (Dewa Majapahit?).

49. *Usana Pulo Nusa Ki Dukuh Jumpungan*, HKS 1928. *Pulo* and *Nusa* mean 'island' and refer to Nusa Penida.

50. *Lontar*, as repositories of powerful knowledge, are often conceived of as weapons in Balinese mythology.

51. *Babad Mengwi*, *Babad Dalam Sukawati*, *Babad Timbul Sukawati* (Indonesian translations).

52. Jacobs, op. cit., 4.

53. Weck, op. cit., 153, quoting van Eck (1878).

54. Ibid., 155–6.

55. I Gusti Made Sarpa, *Tektekan di Krambitan* (Denpasar, Proyek, Sasana Budaya Bali, 1976), 12.

56. Epidemics are said to have inspired the development of a form of *gamelan* (*bungbung gebyag*) in which only bamboo instruments are used. *Nektek*, a music and dance form in which the sound 'tektek' is made by hitting together bamboo cylinders, is thought to represent a specific ritual response to cholera epidemics; Sarpa, op. cit., 11–13. Given the exorcistic function of dance, the martial imagery of some forms of *baris* may reflect Balinese conceptualization of the cause and mechanism of cholera transmission, and the symptomology of the illness.

57. *Cholera morbus asiatica* aparently reached Southeast Asia around 1820; cf. Terwiel, op. cit.; Peter Boomgaard, 'Morbidity and Mortality in Java, 1820–1880', above.

58. The contents of the *lontar* (now lost) had been copied into an exercise book and were related to me by a village official.

59. W. F. van der Kaaden, 'Nangloek Merana in Gianjar', *Djawa* 7 (1937), 123–8; C. Hooykaas, *Religion of Bali* (Leiden, E. J. Brill, 1973), 6–7.

7 Asiatic Cholera in Siam: Its First Occurrence and the 1820 Epidemic

B. J. TERWIEL

ASIATIC cholera, *Cholera morbus*, or spasmodic cholera, as it was called at the beginning of the nineteenth century, is of particular interest to the historian. Of all pestilences, cholera has been described as being perhaps the most awe-inspiring. 'It may run so rapid a course that a man in good health at daybreak may be dead and buried ere nightfall.'[1] The incubation period is relatively short and the death-rate, at least in the days when the nature of the disease was not yet clearly understood, was high.

During the nineteenth century various cholera epidemics raged across large parts of the world. What is usually taken as the world's first general cholera pandemic began in 1817 in Bengal. By 1818 it had spread over most of India and by 1819 to Ceylon, from whence it was carried along the trade-routes, both westwards to Mauritius and East Africa, and eastwards to Southeast Asia and China.[2] It is now widely accepted that the bacterium *vibrio cholerae*[3] first developed on the Indian subcontinent. The first recorded epidemic of Asiatic cholera in India may have been that of Pondichery in the years 1769–71, which cost 16 000 lives. In 1783 another such outbreak in the upper reaches of the Ganges River claimed 20 000 victims within a period of eight days.[4] There are many accounts of earlier cases of cholera in India, but upon closer scrutiny they do not usually provide details which would warrant attaching the label cholera, the description often reminding the reader more of dysentery.[5]

If Asiatic cholera had already been in existence for many centuries, the possibility of general cholera pandemics before that of 1817 may not be ruled out. Indeed, there are rumors of cholera in Java during the early seventeenth century, and the possibility of a late seventeenth century cholera epidemic which spread via Melaka to China may not be dismissed out of hand.[6] To this it may be

142

added that specialists in early Siamese history usually take for granted that cholera epidemics occasionally raged in Siam, going back to the fourteenth or even the first half of the eleventh century. If the Siamese accounts of early cholera can be verified they ought to be incorporated into the general history of the disease. It is not within the author's competence to determine whether the alleged outbreaks of cholera in the Dutch Indies, in Melaka or in China are based on conclusive evidence; in this paper it is attempted to bring together and evaluate only the evidence pertaining to Siam. In the first part of this essay all relevant Siamese data are scrutinized; then follows an account of the epidemic which reached Siam in 1820.

When Did Asiatic Cholera First Reach Siam?

In the standard history books which cover events prior to 1820, there are four distinct stories which refer to cholera. The earliest of these can be found in a recent book, in which it is mentioned that some time during the first half of the eleventh century the city of Haripunjaya (Lamphun) was temporarily evacuated because of a cholera epidemic.[7] The author bases this remark upon 'chronicles'. A search in the available sources relating to the history of Lamphun has revealed three reports of this epidemic. In the *Phongsāwadān Yōnok* it is described as an outbreak of *khwāmkhai*, 'a fever', while in the *Tamnān Mū'ang Nū'a* the same event is described as an outbreak of *rōk rabāt*, 'a contagious disease'.[8] The identification of the disease seems to have come from the *Çhāmathewīwong*, where it is called an *ahiwāt* sickness.[9] There can be no doubt that *ahiwāt* disease means 'cholera' in modern Thai dictionaries, and that this has been the case ever since the 1820 epidemic. Unfortunately, we may not assume that mention of *ahiwāt* in older sources refers to a cholera epidemic. The word is derived from a Pali name for a contagious disease, the *ahivātakaroga*, literally 'the snake-wind disease'[10] which has hitherto defied identification. In the most authoritative Pali dictionary the compilers have come no closer than describing it as 'a certain contagious disease (plague? cholera?)'.[11] In fact, when the details of the Lamphun epidemic, as described in the *Çhāmathewīwong*, are examined, it becomes abundantly clear that the chroniclers did not mean cholera when they wrote about *ahiwāt* sickness. The epidemic apparently spread gradually (*dōilamdap*). In each house people would die slowly, one after the other until none were left alive, and if someone entered an infected house and touched only an object or utensil, he would carry the disease to his own home where he and his family would all die.[12] Such a description cannot refer to cholera and fits better some virulent form of plague.

The second mention of cholera prior to 1820 goes back to the very founding of the city of Ayutthaya in 1351. It is mentioned that the ruler of Uthong was forced to leave that town because Uthong's river had silted up and an epidemic, 'believed to be cholera', had decimated the people.[13] Various versions of this story of cholera and the founding of Ayutthaya have found their way into standard Thai textbooks. They are all apparently based on Prince Damrong's reconstruction of a certain legend, which he first proposed in 1903, and which involved not cholera, but an unspecified pestilential disease.[14] Later scholars embroidered upon the theme, giving the pestilence a particular label. In recent years, Prince Damrong's hypothesis has been challenged by Thai historians and archaeologists who have established that the town of Uthong was abandoned in the eleventh or twelfth century and that its abandonment was probably unrelated to Ayutthaya's founding.[15]

As far as could be ascertained, there are only two references pertaining to disease in the primary source material related to Ayutthaya's foundation, both in the seventeenth century Dutch compilation of Siamese historical legends. Apparently 'King Uthong' was told that Ayutthaya's site was uninhabitable because of a swamp in which lived a voracious dragon, who on being disturbed forcefully blew saliva from his mouth. This was so poisonous that all people in the neighbourhood died. 'King Uthong' reputedly had to fulfil three tasks before the local dragon could be killed and the marsh be drained. After performing the tasks, Uthong was told by a resident wizard that he and his followers would suffer little from smallpox. 'King Uthong' filled the marsh and freed the country from the scourge of the dragon.[16] Neither the reference to a sickness coming from a swamp nor that to smallpox can be taken as evidence for cholera.

The third (alleged) mention of cholera in early Siamese history is the report in general histories that cholera was first mentioned in the year 1357.[17] This information is derived from the so-called Royal Autograph Chronicle, edited by Prince Damrong, in which it is stated that in Sakarāt 719, the Year of the Cock, Buddhist era

1900, which corresponds to 1357/58 A.D., a prince died of *ahiwāt* disease.[18] This information was evidently based upon the Phan Cḥanthanumāt version of the royal chronicles, which was compiled in 1795/96, during the First Reign of the Chakri dynasty.[19] We have already established that references to *ahiwāt* sickness in pre-1820 sources do not necessarily refer to cholera. Since the sources do not provide any description of the symptoms, this fourteenth century reference is useless as possible evidence for the early presence of cholera.

The fourth and final mention of cholera prior to 1820 occurs in a work by H. G. Q. Wales, who writes about the 'cholera epidemics of 1811 and 1820' as if these were well-known and accepted facts of Siamese history.[20] While there is ample evidence of cholera in 1820, part of what is often called the 'first pandemic', a search in the contemporary literature yields no reference to a contagious disease for the year 1811. Wales seems to have based his remark upon two well-known Siamese works, Damrong's commentary on the Dynastic Chronicles of the Second Reign and Çhulālongkǫn's *Phrarātchaphithī Sipsǫng Dū'an*. In both these works there is a reference which may have led Wales to assume that an epidemic had occurred in 1811. Damrong and Çhulālongkǫn mention that in the Year of the Goat, third of the cycle, which corresponds to the twelve months between March 1811 and March 1812, a royal ceremony to ward off evil had been held.[21] Both authors imply that the ceremony of 1811/12 was comparable to that which had taken place in 1820. However, neither work states that the rituals were in both cases occasioned by cholera, or indeed any other pestilential disease. Wales apparently has misread his sources. This conclusion is strengthened by references to that particular Year of the Goat in two versions of the Records of the Court Astrologers (*Çhotmāihēthōn*), which provide clues as to why King Rama II decided to order the ceremony to be held. The final entry for the relevant year in the *Pramūnthanarak* version reads: 'Dāohāng mi çhan yamrung', or 'a comet with the brilliance of dawn'; while the version in the *Prachumphongsāwadān* (Collection of Annals) gives further details of the comet, such as that it rose in the northwest, moved towards the northeast, and was seen on Sunday, the seventh day of the waning half of the second month, which corresponds to 5 January 1812.[22] This evidence suggests that it was this unusually bright comet, rather than disease, which prompted the royal ceremony to be held in 1811/12.

The four references to cholera prior to 1820, namely those

pertaining to the early eleventh century, to 1351, 1357/58 and 1811, do not stand up to close scrutiny, and historians should not use them as proof of an early local or international cholera epidemic. In addition to checking these four particular instances where cholera has been mentioned by name, it was decided to scan quickly the standard literature dealing with the period up to 1820 for any other mention of contagious disease, in the hope that a description would be found which would enable us to identify cholera.

The chronicles of cities on the Malay Peninsula were consulted first, for the southernmost Thai peoples would have been more likely than others to have been exposed to an international scourge. The chronicles of the city of Nakhon Sithammarat mention epidemics on six occasions, all of them undated and referring to a legendary period of history. The names given to these epidemics fall under two rubrics. The first type is called *khai yamapana, khai ñamapana* and, in another version *khai yupala*, a term which has been tentatively translated as *khai yamapāla*, or 'the disease of the punisher of creatures in hell'.[23] In one instance, the disease is described as '*khruvana yak* devouring people', which Wyatt surmises as meaning 'thick-forest (P. *Garu + vana*) giants'.[24] A neater translation results from taking the word as *khruwanā*, 'parable' or 'simile', giving 'a disease which appeared like *yaksas* [ogres] devouring people'. Whatever translation is preferred, the references, while indicating sudden and possibly violent death, give insufficient information for hazarding a guess as to what type of epidemic repeatedly raged in the legendary period of Nakhon Sithammarat. The second type of contagious disease in Nakhon Sithammarat is *khai hā*, translated by Wyatt as 'plague'.[25] The term *khai hā* actually means 'a pestilential disease, caused by the *hā* spirits'. It is a general term meaning any epidemic which results in a high mortality, including such diseases as plague and cholera. The six references to epidemics in the Nakhon Sithammarat chronicles therefore give no evidence as to whether or not cholera was involved. A perusal of other southern chronicles, such as those of Songkhla and Patani, yielded no further references to epidemics.[26]

In the chronicles of the far north of the region, apart from the plague (?) in Lamphun, mentioned above, only a single reference to an epidemic was encountered, namely that in 877 Çhulasakarāt (1515/16 A.D.) a large number of people died of *thoraphit*.[27] The word *thoraphit* is of Sanskritic origin, meaning 'virulent, noxious', and in Siamese, when referring to a disease (often with the prefix *khai* 'fever'), it is the most formal word for 'smallpox'.[28]

The information on smallpox and *ahiwāt* in the mid-fourteenth century has already been mentioned above. Another reference to disease in the fifteenth century is found in the Luang Prasoet Chronicle. The entry for Çhulasakarāt 816, the Year of the Dog, identified in the *Prachumphongsāwadān* as B. E. 1997, or 1454/55 A.D. is: 'At that time there was an outbreak of *thoraphit*; a great number of people died.'[29] In one of the versions of the *Çhotmāihēthōn* it is said that in the year Çhulasararāt 925 (1563/64 A.D.) *thoraphit* broke out and many people died, again a likely reference to smallpox.[30] For the years 1621–22 and 1622–23 A.D. it is twice mentioned that there was an outbreak of pustules (*ǫk fī*) and that many died.[31] While in these entries the colloquial Thai word for smallpox (*fī dāt*) is not used, the reference to pustules would again seem to indicate a smallpox epidemic. A massive outbreak of smallpox also occurred later in the seventeenth century. The Director of the Dutch East India Company in Ayutthaya estimated in 1659 that at least one third of the population had, during a period of six months, been killed by smallpox.[32] For the year 1749–50, it is reported that *ǫk hat thoraphit* occurred and that many died — yet another reference to smallpox, which is confirmed in the *Pramūnthanarak* version of the *Çhotmāihēthōn*.[33]

The only other reference to a particular virulent disease was found in Pallegoix's *Description*. He writes that during the year 1769 there was famine, followed by a disease which 'from the beginning took away both the faculty of speech and that of reason. The sick person seemed struck with stupidity; occasionally coming out of his lethargy and recovering his freedom of judgement. Every morning the river was covered with corpses'.[34] This description of a contagious disease, occurring soon after a disastrous war with Burma, fits a typhoid epidemic. Hitherto no indigenous accounts giving further details have been found.[35]

Therefore it can be said that Siamese historical sources do not provide information that would support the notion of 'severe epidemics of cholera' before 1820. This lack of information naturally may not be taken as proof of the absence of cholera; it simply indicates that a cursory reading of the chief sources shows no specific mention of cholera. The only disease which is repeatedly mentioned by name from the fourteenth century onward is smallpox. This is reinforced in the late seventeenth century by La Loubère: 'In a word, there are some contagious diseases, but the real Plague of this Country is the Small Pox: it oftentimes makes dreadful ravage, and then they inter the bodies without burning them.'[36] That the Siamese had long experience with this pestilential disease is borne out by the same author when he adds with obvious surprise that they dare not dig up the interred bodies for cremation 'till three years after, or longer, by reason, as they say, that they have experimented, that this Contagion breaks out afresh, if they dig them up sooner'.[37]

The question of whether or not cholera occurred in Siam before 1820 apparently cannot be satisfactorily resolved by examining historical records. There are, however, other approaches which may assist us in forming an opinion. The most obvious one is an examination of the course of the 1820 epidemic.

The 1820 Epidemic in Siam

The epidemic apparently entered Siam at its southern border. It reputedly passed from Penang to Saiburi [Kedah] and then crossed the Malay Peninsula. In one of the versions of the Annals of Songkhla it is said that a sickness arrived during the fifth month of Çhulasakarāt 1182, which corresponds with the lunar month beginning on 15 March 1820.[38] In another version of these Annals it is further revealed that the disease was *ahiwāt* sickness (a term which at the time of compilation of these Annals was understood to mean cholera), that many died, and that the disease lasted right up to the Year of the Snake (which began in April 1821), after which it subsided.[39]

It is possible to determine with some accuracy when this epidemic reached Bangkok. In one of the versions of the *Çhotmāihēthōn*, among the entries for the year Çhulasakarāt 1182 (March 1820–April 1821) is the following: 'During the period from the eleventh to the fifteenth day of the waxing half of the seventh month and during the first and second day of the waning half, there was a pestilential disease. A large number of people died both on the water and on the land.'[40] These dates, transcribed in terms of the international calendar, correspond to the period from Tuesday 23 May to Monday 29 May 1820. The other version of the Records states that a ceremony involving firing off guns and chanting warding-off sutras was held on Monday 22 May, and that

Buddhist monks scattered sand on Wednesday the 25th. It is added that many people died in an epidemic.[41] It therefore took between one and two months for the sickness to travel from southern Siam to the capital.

A more detailed account of the epidemic occurs in the Dynastic Chronicles of the Second Reign, written by Chaophrayā Thiphākǫrawong (Kham Bunnāk) in the late 1860s, almost fifty years after the epidemic had taken place. Indeed, in May 1820 he was only six years old, so he must have relied upon older informants' recollections. Nevertheless, Thiphākǫrawong's *oeuvre* has generally proven trustworthy, and since the Dynastic Chronicles of the Second Reign have not hitherto been translated, the relevant entries are here rendered into English in their entirety:

An outbreak of cholera
Then, during the waxing half of the seventh moon, in the night-time bright lights were seen in the northwestern sky which were called 'spark-cloud', and at that time there was an outbreak of *puang* disease which came from the sea. That sickness came first from Penang and then crossed over to the western provinces proceeding until it reached the mouth of the River Chaophraya. Citizens of the town of Samut Prakan died in large numbers, and as a result several groups migrated to Bangkok and others went in various other directions. It reached Bangkok on the sixth day of the waxing moon of the seventh month, and until the day of the full moon men and women died. In the cemetery grounds and in the pavilions of Wat Saket, Wat Bānglamphū, Wat Bophitphimuk, Wat Prathumkhongkhā and other monasteries the corpses were heaped up on top of each other like bales of cloth. Large numbers were cremated, but there were also corpses floating in the river and in canals everywhere. The clergy fled from the monasteries and householders abandoned their houses. On the roads and in the alleys there was no more traffic, and the markets did not open for trade. People ate only dried fish, pepper and a bit of salt. The water from the river could no longer be used as a source of drinking water, being contaminated by corpses.[42]

It is unlikely that the cause of the 'spark-cloud' will be ascertained. If Thiphākǫrawong's informants' information was accurate, a puzzling phenomenon occurred some time in mid-May 1820. The Thai words appear to fit a shower of meteorites. In Thiphākǫrawong's account the epidemic raged from Thursday 18 May until 27 May 1820, a difference of just a few days from the time given in the *Çhotmāihēthōn* account. Given the difficulty of judging exactly when an epidemic has started and when it may be regarded as having abated, the two accounts may be regarded as reinforcing each other in the matter of dates. Prince Damrong in his Commentary upon the Dynastic Chronicles of the Second Reign accepts Thiphākǫrawong's dates.[43]

From Thiphākǫrawong's account a clear impression is gained of the route followed by the scourge and the panicky flight from infested areas, a circumstance which must have accelerated the spread of the disease.

Later in the Dynastic Chronicles of the Second Reign there is a second, lengthier entry directly related to the 1820 epidemic:

The holding of a disease-breaking ceremony
His Majesty the King communicated that the disease which unfortunately had erupted among monks, nuns, Brahmans and the populace in general was not confined to Bangkok, but was also found abroad, in Penang, as well as in Saiburi. Apparently the sickness would not respond to careful treatment or to the best medicine. Therefore the king ordered that the chanting of *ātānātiya* sutras be held on Monday the tenth day of the waxing moon in the seventh month. Great cannons would be fired the whole night until dawn. The Emerald Buddha and precious relics would be taken in procession on land and by boat by monks of *rātchakhana* rank scattering sand and sprinkling lustral water. The king exhorted royalty, both with *krom* rank and without, as well as officials both high and low of the Front Palace and the Inner Palace, to suspend all duties and to stop all government work; [so that] all mental work and physical work was suspended. He let them direct their attention to meritorious things, chanting Buddhist stanzas and gift-giving. He ordered all commoners who had duties in the Inner Palace, as well as those working outside, to be released to go to their homes.

The king in his goodness said that in general all creatures value their lives in times of great danger. Parents, spouses, children, relatives and siblings love each other and should be able to nurse each other. If there were devout people who were unable to go and look after the Buddhist monks [without subvention], the royal bounty would pay for it. Also the purchase of fish, quadrupeds and fowls from those who usually kill and trade in them would be arranged. These [animals] would be bought [by the authorities] in the market-places of the province of Bangkok and all be released, the royal treasury being great. All convicts serving sentences were released, with the exception of the Burmese prisoners.

The whole populace was forbidden to travel and to kill animals, regardless of whether they were aquatic or terrestrial beasts. All people had to stay at home unless there was a compelling reason for them to go out; in the latter event they could do so.

The king, with great virtue and full of compassion for all inhabitants of the realm, ordered all people to follow his decree until Saturday the seventh day of the waning half of the seventh month in order to cause the epidemic to abate rapidly.

With respect to all male and female corpses without relatives to bury or cremate them, the royal bounty provided money for the costs, and also some land, and it was ordered that the Burmese prisoners had to burn them all.

Apart from the two senior princesses who died, members of the royal family and executive civil servants in the Front Palace and the Inner Palace were generally in good health. The epidemic killed twice as many women as men. It was reported that the disease was moving up northwards.

While the epidemic was raging, the king allowed the Annamite ambassador to return hurriedly to his own country with gifts and with a letter from the Foreign Minister stating that the ambassador had to return to pay respects to the deceased king and to greet a newly enthroned one, and that he could stay away until the epidemic had ceased.[44]

The first sentence in the king's decree, in which it is pointed out that the epidemic came from abroad, moving from Penang to the southern Siamese town of Saiburi before reaching Bangkok, is probably intended to reassure the people that the suffering was not confined to Bangkok. As Thiphākǫrawong reveals somewhat later in the Chronicles,[45] there was a rumour that the epidemic was caused by angry sea-spirits avenging the removal of large amounts of massive rocks which were being used to build the king's new pleasure-garden. Such a rumour was damaging to the king's judgement and reputation and efforts had to be made to combat it.

In this account of Rama II's decree we find a confirmation of the exact period when the epidemic occurred. The chanting of *ātānātiya* sutras reportedly took place on 22 May 1820, so it may be inferred that at that time the disease must have already reached epidemic proportions. The measures decided upon by Rama II appear to be manifold. In the first place, a traditional state ceremony for warding off evil forces was ordered. The *ātānātiya* sutras are particularly appropriate for such an occasion,[46] and the firing of cannon all around the capital city served the same purpose. The procession with the nation's most revered relics appears to have had the function of not only reinforcing the warding-off ceremonies, but also of 'drawing a protective circle' around Bangkok. While firing of cannon and chanting of warding-off sutras may be regarded as standard procedures when a major threat such as a pestilential disease hung over the city, it is quite possible that the use of Buddhist monks in procession with relics constituted a small innovation. Such processions appear more commonly on happier occasions.

Much of the king's decree consists of a series of measures

directly related to Buddhist ethics. Precepts of virtuous behaviour have always formed an integral part of the Buddhist religion, and in Siam it may be regarded as axiomatic that proper moral action would inevitably lead to happiness, well-being and good health. Examples of moral action are the release of an animal held in captivity, or the donation of a gift. Immoral action, as defined by Buddhist ethics, such as killing, stealing and lying, would invariably bring bad luck and misfortune. This is why the king decided to buy and free captive animals, to release convicts from gaol, and to encourage donations to Buddhist monks. He prescribed a massive 'merit-making', involving the whole population of Bangkok, in order to hasten the moment when the bad times would depart and more fortunate events prevail.

To those unfamiliar with Siamese history it may come as a surprise to read that the Burmese prisoners were not to be released, the only exception to the amnesty granted by the king. This is because the Burmese prisoners had only recently caused an uproar by revolting, killing one of their warders and taking to the streets, where they were overpowered.[47] This event had taken place in March or April 1819 and was therefore still fresh in people's memory. This is probably also the reason why the Burmese prisoners were singled out for the unpleasant task of disposing of many of the corpses.

The king's wish that all government work be halted, that people should remain at home, off the roads and away from marketplaces, seems to be primarily motivated by the wish to free the capital's inhabitants to take part in the proposed massive 'merit-making'. The fact that this measure is in accordance with present-day medical ideas of combatting epidemics by diminishing the chances of further contamination is possibly fortuitous. There is some evidence to show that Siamese medical knowledge in 1820 was quite unable to handle a disaster such as this cholera epidemic. The following paragraph in the Dynastic Chronicles represents the views of the author at the time of writing, after much further information had been obtained and some time after Bangkok had had suffered yet another outbreak of cholera:

At that time people were still very ignorant and stupid, and they whispered among each other that the taking of large rocks from the sea in order to build a hill in the king's garden was the cause of it. Angry powers and angry spirits had caused the disease to occur. This [accusation] was without precedent, unheard of, and totally baseless. I think that this sickness was already in the world during the time of the Buddha when there was an outbreak in the town of Vesali. From the time that this particular epidemic broke out in Hindustan it had travelled from country to country. It was impossible for a country to avoid catching it. In the Year of the Tiger, tenth of the cycle [April 1818-March 1819] it broke out in Burma. As for European countries, some had only a little, but some suffered badly. China was geographically isolated. Wise men speculate that there is no reason to assign a specific cause other than that it seems that the disease thrives where there is filth and dirt. That is where a lot of people will die. Among clean people whose residences are not sullied and filthy there are few who die. This is why Europeans believe so strongly in hygiene.[48]

Thiphākǫrawong had spent some time reflecting on epidemics and in another place he stated that it was exposure to 'bad air' which brought on such sicknesses.[49] In 1820, however, the epidemic was of a severity such as no person could recollect,[50] and local medical practitioners were at a loss as to what to prescribe. Siamese intellectuals were just becoming aware of the fact that some European doctors were experimenting, occasionally with a measure of success, with the use of various potent drugs in the treatment of cholera. It was not until 1822 that Prince Çhetsādabodin, Rama II's trusted son, who represented the king on many occasions and who was already one of Siam's most powerful men, questioned Dr George Finlayson on Western methods of treating cholera. For a period of almost three hours the irate Finlayson was detained while Çhetsādabodin persuaded him to hand over various drugs, together with detailed instructions on their use, which were written down by an attendant.[51]

This appears to be the beginning of an active interest in Western medicine which continued when Çhetsādabodin succeeded his father. Under Rama III a resident American missionary-doctor was paid by the crown to inoculate some ten thousand Siamese, 'principally in the palace and in the families of the nobles', against smallpox.[52] Such innovative action may not, however, be seen as a sign that Western medicine was beginning to replace traditional Siamese practices; the latest Western techniques were simply added to the well-established customs without challenging the validity of the latter.

Estimates of the numbers of victims of the 1820 epidemic vary enormously. Crawfurd, who visited Bangkok only two years after the epidemic, reports: 'The intensity of its ravages continued here for about fifteen days only, during which short time, according to the phrakhlang's statement, it carried off two persons in ten, or a fifth of the whole population.'[53] If, which seems unlikely, the whole population of Siam were meant, this would mean, using Crawfurd's own rough calculations, a death-toll of a million people, or, using more conservative figures, at least some 320 000 deaths.[54] Thompson, probably taking the Phrakhlang's statement to be applicable to Bangkok only, and surmising the city to have had half a million inhabitants (a gross overestimation), puts the number of victims at roughly one hundred thousand.[55] Damrong, specifically referring to Bangkok and its surroundings, but omitting to mention his sources, numbers about 30 000 dead,[56] a figure which corresponds to the number of victims in Saigon, at least according to the Siamese Chronicles.[57] Taking into account that at the time of the epidemic the population of Bangkok and environs may well have been around 150 000, the Prakhlang's estimate turns out to be compatible with that of Damrong. A figure of 30 000 victims may be taken as our most realistic estimate. This, together with Thiphākǫrawong's description, still indicates a much larger toll than has been recorded for subsequent cholera epidemics in Bangkok. In 1873, some 6 660 people died of cholera, and in 1919 some 13 000 deaths were noted.[58] The relatively larger toll for 1820 is in keeping with the notion that this may have been the first time that the bacterium infested the region.

The Dynastic Chronicles of the Second Reign have yet a further entry related to cholera, namely an account of the ritual preventative measure taken upon hearing of the devastating epidemic in Vietnam. The events described below apparently occurred during the months before the New Year ritual during the first months of 1821.

The great chanting session

Reflecting on the outbreak of the pestilential disease in Annam [Vietnam], which closely resembled that of the city [Bangkok], the king's compassion, sorrow and sympathy were aroused. He therefore decided to ask Phraçhaonongyathoe Sasithon,[59] together with Çhaochommāndā Maew,[60] to train the Palace Ladies in dancing and chanting sutras, because they had already practised chanting during the First Reign. He ordered the Palace Sages to come and drill in the Palace Entrance Hall and the Palace Ladies to practise chanting high in the Southern Building, whilst remaining out of sight. He ordered them to train until they knew the sounds of the words and the letter-contractions, the accentuated and the short syllables, so that they could enunciate them clearly and more proficiently than did the Buddhist monks. He chose people with good voices to chant according to the ancient texts. All the sutras to be learnt ranged from the *Phānyak* and *Phānwān* to the *Mahāchaimahāsān*. He let each individual sequence be practised until each sutra could be chanted in a loud voice and until thirty persons could perform the *Phānyak*. When they could chant well together the king ordered them to perform in shifts. During the daytime they chanted in the Palace Hall and at night he went to listen to them in the Theatre. On some nights they chanted the whole sequence twice. After each sequence each person received a quarter of a baht from the royal purse. If the chanting had been done well and neatly without mistakes, the royal remuneration sometimes constituted an increased sum of money or sometimes a gift of goods. The king went every day and every night to listen to the performance. Gradually there were diversions and the chants declined in number, until the time of the fourth month arrived and the royal ceremony of firing the cannon had to be held, during which chanting had to be done in the Theatre.[61]

This account demonstrates a most elaborate set of preventative measures, based upon the traditional notion that epidemics were caused by evil spirits. The sutras mentioned in the text have no other function than to drive away such bad forces. They are very difficult to learn and indeed sound most impressive. The *phānyak*, for example, has only relatively few words, but some of the syllables are held on for long spells by all the chanters, each of them setting up a most forceful ululation. The chanting of *phānyak* and related sutras was performed in Bangkok as recently as 1968 by four venerable Buddhist monks. It was broadcast on the radio and many Thais for the first time in their lives had the opportunity of appreciating the peculiar, eerie and spine-chilling sounds which characterize long sections of this chanting. The effect of a group of well-trained women chanting it must have been even more dramatic.

From the indigenous accounts it is thus possible to reconstruct some features of the 1820 epidemic. It has been possible to give fairly accurate dates for the occurrence and duration of the scourge. The directions in which the disease moved can be mapped out, while the observation that people fled after cholera had reached the town of Samut Songkhram may provide us with at least one of the reasons for the rapid spread of this disease. The Siamese measures to combat the epidemic appear to have been quite effective. To many inhabitants of Bangkok this effectiveness may have been felt to have been the result of the quick enactment of the strongest protective state rituals. To observers in the twentieth century it would seem that there were other factors involved. Apparently people quickly became aware of the fact that the river and canal water was not fit for consumption. Probably the most effective measures were the decisions to close all market-places, to declare a general ban on work and to advise people to remain at home, forcing them to live off their stores of food.

Another feature concerns the number of separate accounts of this event. Of the Siamese sources quoted above, five are independent reports, that of Thiphākǫrawong providing an unprecedentedly detailed account. No epidemic in pre-twentieth century Siam has attracted so much attention. This fact by itself may be a reflection of the shock and horror caused by this highly contagious disease which struck so rapidly and caused so large a loss of life. The accounts fit in with the idea that the 1820 epidemic was essentially a new and alarming phenomenon, and would suggest that no other such pestilence had yet struck within living memory.

The geographical spread of the sources also warrants attention. The disease is identified in Saiburi, but not reported in its local annals. Of all the peninsular cities, only Songkhla mentions the epidemic. We know that cholera reached Bangkok via the coastal town of Samut Prakan, and that it moved further northwards. There are many provincial accounts of events around the year 1820. In Nakhon Sithammarat, these describe a threat from Burma, local alliances and uprisings; and chronicles of the north and north-east also abound in stories of attacks and alliances without a single reference to disease. While this omission may reflect the general bias of Siamese chroniclers towards court intrigues, politics and warfare, it would seem that the epidemic, if it did indeed spread all over the nation, did not strike with uniform severity. The cholera bacillus, which had found such a favourable environment in coastal places such as Songkhla, Samut Prakan and Bangkok, would not have been able to thrive in the less populated, well-drained or relatively dry regions inland.

Finally, it ought to be noted that there are various names given to the disease. Thiphākǫrawong mentions two distinct terms when writing about cholera: *ahiwāt* disease and *puang* sickness.[62] Damrong adds the comment that in 1820 the populace referred to cholera not by the term *ahiwāt*, but as *khai puang yai*, literally 'the major *puang* disease'.[63] In one of the versions of the Records of the Court Astrologers, however, cholera is called *rōk long rāk*, or 'the disease of diarrhoea and vomit'.[64]

In the Siamese language of the Ayutthaya period and after, it is common to have two types of words to describe specific contagious diseases: words obviously derived from Sanskrit or Pali, and words which belong to the indigenous Thai vocabulary. Words of the first type are often polysyllabic and elegant, while the latter are usually monosyllabic words which often describe more directly a major characteristic of the disease. Thus the elegant word for smallpox is *thoraphit*, probably derived from the Sanskrit *dhāravisha*, or 'having a poisoned edge', while the common Thai word for the same disease is *ǭk fi dāt*, or literally 'breaking out abundantly in pustules'. For typhoid and typhus the common words are *khai rāksāt nǭi* and *khai rāksāt yai* respectively, which may be translated as the 'lesser splashing-vomit disease' and the 'major splashing-vomit disease', no elegant form being in use.

Each of the three terms for cholera warrants a few comments. *Ahiwāt* disease was apparently not the word used by ordinary people in 1820. It had up till then been encountered in the Buddhist scriptures as describing some unspecified contagious disease, and it had also been used once in the Chronicles to refer to the death of a prince in the fourteenth century. It is not known exactly when *ahiwāt* came to be used to describe cholera. If cholera had not been in Siam prior to 1820, it seems likely that the formal, elegant term was used not long after the disease had struck. It is quite possible, reading between the lines of Thiphākǭrawong's account, to imagine that the court deliberately chose an old term, one which went back to the time of the Buddha, so as to instruct the populace that the disease had to be seen as a 'natural' and inevitable event; a choice which would assist in countering the rumours of the king's provocation of the gods being the cause of disaster.

The word *puang* appears to have referred to a general class of disorders of the alimentary tract, usually accompanied by diarrhoea and vomiting. Thus there was *puang ling*, 'monkey *puang*', which began with heavy vomiting and which caused the hair of the scalp to stand up in tufts like that on a monkey's head. *Puang lom*, 'wind *puang*', also caused much vomiting, due to an excess of the vital element 'wind'.[65] A description of cholera as the 'major *puang*' seems therefore quite apt. Yet, the term *khai puang yai* seems to have disappeared altogether from the Siamese language, even though the term *puang* survived and continues to indicate certain diseases of the alimentary tract. Not even the 1873 dictionary

ary of the Thai language, compiled by a qualified medical practitioner and therefore particularly strong on medical terms, mentions *khai puang yai*, a term commonly used in 1820 for a disease which continued to plague the country thereafter. *Rōk long rāk*, on the other hand, continued to be used as common name for cholera.

It seems puzzling that one of the popular names for a major disease would disappear so soon without trace at a time when cholera was a well-known and feared illness. The sudden disappearance of the expression *khai puang yai* appears to fit in more with a situation in which cholera, when it reached Bangkok in 1820, was a new and as yet formally unlabelled disease. Since it immediately became a chief concern, various names seem to have arisen, among them a fairly popular classification of it as a major *puang* affliction. The term *rōk long rāk* competed with *khai puang yai* for a position in the language, the former winning and the latter soon being forgotten.

All available accounts of the 1820 epidemic thus strengthen the notion that up till then cholera was unknown in Siam. The king's measures to combat the disease were not specifically intended to fight cholera; basically the same steps would have been appropriate to protect the country from, say, a series of heavy earthquakes. The fact that people were allowed to flee from Samut Songkhram to Bangkok suggests that the nature of the disease was not known, as does the lengthy questioning of a Western physician in order to make him divulge his knowledge of the disease and its possible treatment. To this may be added hints of a death-toll vastly exceeding the figures for later cholera epidemics, as well as the sudden disappearance of one of the common words given to the sickness.

It is a difficult, perhaps impossible, task to prove that cholera did not exist in Siam before 1820. All that we can do here, besides studying the first well-documented epidemic, is to demonstrate that assertions that it *did* exist earlier are based, directly or indirectly, upon a misunderstanding of what the primary sources actually say, often due to inadequate attention to linguistic change across time. Such a demonstration may serve as a cautionary tale for future students of Siamese history, some of whom may, in their own time, write the still unwritten history of disease in Siam.

1. H. H. Scott, *A History of Tropical Medicine* (London, Edward Arnold, 1939), 2:649.

2. R. Pollitzer, *Cholera* (Geneva, World Health Organization, 1959), 19–20; cf. Peter Boomgaard, 'Morbidity and Mortality in Java, 1820–1880', above.

3. It was not until 1884 that the existence of the bacterium was established beyond doubt, when Robert Koch made the result of his researches known at a conference in Berlin. See R. Koch, 'The Etiology of Cholera' in W. W. Cheyne (ed.), *Recent Essays by Various Authors on Bacteria in Relation to Disease* (London, New. Sydenham Society, 1886), 327–84.

4. Information drawn from the entry 'cholera' in A. Winkler Prins (ed.), *Geillustreerde Encyclopaedie* (Amsterdam, Brinkman, 1873), 5:414–19.

5. Thus the intriguing statement in Scott, op. cit., 651: 'The earliest description of the disease in epidemic form was probably the outbreak which devastated Ahmed Shad's military forces in A. D. 1438.' After much searching it became clear that Ahmed Shad was a misprint for Ahmed Shah, or Alau'd-din Ahmad II, one of the Bahmani rulers, and the military setback must have been that of 1446/47. The 'cholera epidemic' in question turned out to be nothing more than the military commander suffering from 'ishalehuni', or blood diarrhoea, a description which does not indicate an epidemic, nor the presence of cholera. I thank Dr S. A. A. Rizvi of the Australian National University for kindly checking and translating the original Persian sources.

6. Pollitzer, op. cit., 12–16.

7. D. K. Wyatt, *Thailand: A Short History* (New Haven, Yale University Press, 1984), 33.

8. *Phongsāwadān Yōnok, chabap Hǫsamuthaengchāt* (Bangkok, Kromsinlapakǫn, B. E. 2504 [1961]), 222; Sanguan Chōtsukharat, *Tamnān Mū' ang Nū'a* (Bangkok, Odian, B. E. 2508 [1965]), 82.

9. *Khamplae Chāmathewīwong Phongsāwadān Mū'ang Haripunchai* (Bangkok, Bannakit, B. E. 2516 [1973]), 192.

10. T. W. Rhys Davids and H. Oldenberg (trans), *Vinaya Texts*, Part I, Sacred Books of the East Series (Delhi, Motilal Banarsidass, 1968), 13:204n.

11. D. Anderson, H. Smith and H. Hendriksen (eds), *A Critical Pāli Dictionary* (Copenhagen, Royal Danish Academy of Sciences and Letters, 1924–1948), 1:536.

12. *Khamplae Chāmathewiwong*, 192–3.

13. E.g., Rong Syamananda, *A History of Thailand* (Bangkok, Thai Watana Panich, 1977), 32.

14. For a summary of his reconstruction, see Damrong Ratchanuphap, 'The Foundation of Ayuthia', *Selected Articles from the Siam Society Journal*, Vol. 3, *Early History and Ayudhya Period* (Bangkok, Siam Society, 1959), 199–202.

15. Charnvit Kasetsiri, *The Rise of Ayudhya: A History of Siam in the Fourteenth and Fifteenth Centuries* (Kuala Lumpur, Oxford University Press, 1976). 55–72.

16. J. van Vliet, *The Short History of the Kings of Siam*, trans. L. Andaya (Bangkok, Siam Society, 1975), 17–18, 57–8. A similar legend may be found in the Jengtung State Chronicle; see Sao Saimong Mangrai, *The Padaeng Chronicle and the Jengtung State Chronicle Translated* (Ann Arbor, University of Michigan, Center for South and Southeast Asian Studies, 1981), 215–16.

17. E. g., V. Thompson, *Thailand: the New Siam* (New York, Macmillan, 1941), 705.

18. *Phrarātchaphongsāwadān chabap Phrarātchahatlēkhā* (Bangkok, Khlang Witthayā, B. E. 2516 [1973]), 1:106.

19. *Phrarātchaphongsāwadān Krungsi'ayuthayā chabap Phan Çhanthanumāt (Çhoem) kap Phra Chakraphatdiphong (Çhāt)* (Bangkok, Khlang Witthayā, B. E. 2507 [1964]), 3, 503.

20. H. G. Q. Wales, *Supplementary Notes on Siamese State Ceremonies* (London, Quaritch, 1971), 33.

21. Damrong Ratchanuphap, *Phrarātchaphongsāwadān Krungratanakosin*

Ratchakān thī 2 (Bangkok, Khurusaphā, B. E. 2505 [1962]), 2:75; Phrabātsomdetphra Çhunlaçhomklāo Chaoyūhua, *Phrarātchaphithī Sipsǭng Dū'an* (B. E. 2454; reprint Bangkok, Khlang Witthayā, B. E. 2514 [1971]), 168.

22. *Çhotmāihēthōn chabap Phrayā Pramūnthanarak* (Bangkok, Cremation volume for Nāng Choi Chuto, B. E. 2464 [1921]), 30; *Çhotmāihēthōn, Prachumphongsāwadān* [Collection of Annals] Part 8 (Bangkok, Khurusaphā, B. E. 2507 [1964]), 8:126–7.

23. D. K. Wyatt (trans. and ed.), *The Crystal Sands: the Chronicles of Nagara Sri Dharrmaraja,* Southeast Asia Program Data Paper no. 98 (Ithaca, N.Y., Cornell University, 1975), 72n.

24. Ibid., 73n.

25. Ibid., 85n.

26. *Prachumphongsāwadān,* Part 3, 3:1–80, and *Prachumphongsāwadān,* Part 54, 30:183–315.

27. Phongsāwadān Yōnok, 393.

28. R. Frankfurter, 'Events in Ayuddhya from Chulasakaraj 686–966', *The Siam Society Fiftieth Anniversary Commemorative Publication* (Bangkok, Siam Society, 1954), 1:49, prefers to translate *thoraphit* by 'pernicious fever', but in my view the term warrants a more specific translation.

29. *Prachumphongsāwadān,* 1:135. The Thai text reads: 'Khrang nan khon thang puang koet thoraphit tāi māk nak'.

30. *Çhotmāihēthōn,* 111.

31. Ibid., 112.

32. G. V. Smith, *The Dutch in Seventeenth-Century Thailand,* Center for Southeast Asian Studies Special Report no. 16 (DeKalb, Ill., Northern Illinois University, 1977), 171, n23.

33. *Çhotmāihēthōn,* 114; *Çhotmāihēthōn chabap Phrayā Pramūnthanarak,* 4.

34. A. Pallegoix, *Description du royaume thai ou Siam* (1854) reprint Farnborough, Gregg International, 1969), 2:259–60 (my translation). This is apparently based on a letter, dated 1 November 1769, by J. Corre; see *Nouvelles Lettres Édifiantes,* 1820, 5:479–80.

35. F. H. Turpin, *Histoire civile et naturelle du royaume de Siam* (Paris, Costard, 1771), 338–9, mentions the famine of 1769, but not the epidemic.

36. S. de la Loubère, *The Kingdom of Siam* (1691; reprint Kuala Lumpur, Oxford University Press, 1969), 39.

37. Ibid. Cf. Barbara Lovric, 'Bali: Myth, Magic and Morbidity', above, on the Balinese prohibition of cremation of smallpox victims, which is tentatively linked to association with Islam.

38. Çhaophrayā Wichiankhirī Bunsang (ed.), 'Phongsāwadān Mū'ang Songkhlā', Part 1, in *Prachumphongsāwadān,* Part 53, 30:212.

39. *Prachumphongsāwadān,* Part 3, 3:61. This seems rather a long time for the disease to continue raging. It may be related to the fact that Songkhla is situated in a marshy region and that the town lacked proper drainage. I thank A. Diller of the Australian National University for pointing out this circumstance.

40. *Çhotmāihēthōn chabap Phrayā Pramūnthanarak,* 37.

41. *Çhotmāihēthōn,* 131.

42. Çhaophrayā Thiphākǫrawong, *Phrarātchaphongsāwadān Krungratanakosin Ratchakān thī 2* (Bangkok, Khurusaphā, B. E. 2504 [1961]), 115–16.

43. Damrong, op. cit., 2:74.

44. Thiphākǫrawong, op. cit., 117–19.

45. Ibid.; the translation follows below.

46. On the *ātānātiya* sutra see K. E. Wells, *Thai Buddhism: Its Rites and Activities* (Bangkok, Suriyabun, 1975), 235–42.

47. *Çhotmāihēthōn chabap Phrayā Pramūnthanarak,* 36.

48. Thiphākǫrawong, op. cit., 119–20. This reflects the general ideas about cholera at that time. Cf. Mrs Beeton: 'To oppose cholera, there seems no surer or better means than cleanliness, sobriety, and judicious ventilation.' J. Beeton, *The Book of Household Management* (London, S. O. Beeton, 1861), 1073.

49. H. Alabaster, *The Wheel of the Law: Buddhism Illustrated from Siamese Sources* (1871; reprint Farnborough, Gregg International, 1971), 8–9.

50. Damrong, op. cit., 2:74.

51. G. Finlayson, *The Mission to Siam and Hue the Capital of Cochin China in the years 1821–2* (London, John Murray, 1826), 198–9.

52. *Chinese Repository*, November 1839, 8:384.

53. J. Crawfurd, *Journal of an Embassy to the Courts of Siam and Cochin China* (1828; reprint Kuala Lumpur, Oxford University Press, 1967), 155; and *Crawfurd Papers* (Bangkok, National Library, 1915), 141–2.

54. *Crawfurd Papers*, 102; the estimate of five million may well be excessive. Roberts places a figure of 3 600 000 upon the total population, of which he considers only 1 600 000 to be Siamese, 1 200 000 Lao and no less than 500 000 Chinese. See E. Roberts, *Embassy to the Eastern Courts of Cochin-China, Siam, and Muscat* (New York, Harper & Brothers, 1837), 308.

55. Thompson, op. cit., 705.

56. Damrong, op. cit., 2:76.

57. Thiphākǫrawong, op. cit., 128. Historians interested in the cholera epidemic in Vietnam may like to know that in the Dynastic Chronicles of the Second Reign there is an account giving a rough breakdown of the victims in various Vietnamese towns and cities.

58. *Siam: General and Medical Features* (Bangkok, Far Eastern Association of Tropical Medicine, 1930), 220, and Thompson, op. cit., 705.

59. A daughter of Rama I, born in 1794/95, Rama II's half-sister. See *Rātchasakunwong* (Bangkok, Cremation Volume for Nāi Sanan Bunsiriphan, B. E. 2512 [1969]), 15.

60. Sasithon's mother. See ibid.

61. Thiphākǫrawong, op. cit., 128–9.

62. Ibid., 115.

63. Damrong, op. cit., 2:73.

64. *Prachumphongsāwadān*, 8:131.

65. D. B. Bradley, *Dictionary of the Siamese Language* (1873; reprint Bangkok, Khurusaphā, B. E. 2514 [1971]), 797.

8 Vietnamese Attitudes Regarding Illness and Healing

DAVID G. MARR

Once upon a time the wealthy head of Hoằng Nông village (Diên Hà district, Thái Bình province), already having reached the age of forty, finally saw his prayers answered by the birth of a son and heir. Even before reaching his first birthday the child was toddling around, treasured beyond measure by both his mother and father, and cared for by a wet nurse.

One day the child suddenly was not able to eat, cried as if hurting in the throat, and began to swell up around the face. The father and mother naturally became very frightened and called in all the well-known local healers to examine the boy. However, as none could figure out the nature of the illness, they pleaded helplessness. The village head then rushed to Hanoi to invite Dr Leroy des Barres to come to Thái Bình. After arriving and examining the boy, Dr des Barres concluded, 'Only in Hanoi are there adequate resources to treat him, and even then there is no certainty he'll recover quickly'.

As the village head thought frantically, wavering back and forth, a friend came in and said, 'This is an illness for which the healer Mr Thạch Cầu ought to be sought. With luck he can cure it'. The village head urged his friend to go to Bắc Ninh to invite Thạch Cầu to come. Arriving the following day Thạch Cầu examined the boy, noting the facial colour and smell of the mouth in particular. He realized the boy had swallowed a snail shell.

After inviting Thạch Cầu to sit down to drink some tea, the village head asked, 'Sir, why is my child sick, and do you think you can cure him?' Thạch Cầu responded, 'I can cure him, but you'll have to give me a lot of money for my troubles'. To this the village head replied, 'Please devote yourself completely to healing our child. We will pay whatever it costs without regret'. Thạch Cầu smiled and said, 'Put together three thousand piastres as a pledge. If you are one piastre short I won't treat him'.

The village head shuddered, since three thousand piastres was a lot of money in those days. Nevertheless, deeply anxious to see their boy recover, both mother and father rushed out to borrow three thousand,

162

carrying the money back and placing it in front of Thạch Cầu. He counted it carefully, then instructed the parents to put it in a safe place pending recovery of the patient.

After that, Thạch Cầu told the parents to purchase ten ducks, tie their wings, and hang each upside down from poles, with the heads dangling about one handspan from the ground. This done, a vessel was placed under each duck to catch saliva. After one hour the ten vessels together contained about one-half a bowl of duck saliva. Thạch Cầu then went out with a house servant to locate a handful of worm turnings. This was mixed thoroughly with the duck saliva and a bit of flour, and the combination packed carefully around the small boy's throat. Finally, Thạch Cầu took a bit of sweet-smelling powder, mixed it with warm water, and instructed the servant to drip it slowly in the boy's mouth.

Thạch Cầu then went out to wait. In less than half an hour there was the sound of a child choking once, then crying loudly. Thạch Cầu rushed in and pulled from the child's mouth a blood clot the size of the head of one's thumb. Placing it on a plate for all to see, he pronounced, 'Inside that blood clot is a snail. Your child's illness is over'. No one believed him, but slicing the clot open did indeed reveal a snail.

Thạch Cầu instructed the family to cook some rice gruel for the child to sip. The next morning the boy was completely recovered and eating normally. Thạch Cầu explained the cause of the trouble for all to hear: 'A servant took the child out to play and didn't notice when he put the snail in his mouth. Later he was choking to death without anyone knowing it'. The village head called in the wet nurse, who admitted to taking the boy to the market with her and having some snails to eat.

The village head insisted that Thạch Cầu remain and relax for several days. As Thạch Cầu was taking his leave, the village head duly presented him with the three thousand piastres plus a large container of quality tea. Thạch Cầu responded, 'I only made that demand so that you and your wife would believe I was going to cure your child, and thus be less fearful. Now that your child is well I wish to refund it. I have no right to take so much'. Although both husband and wife beseeched him repeatedly and sincerely to change his mind, in the end Thạch Cầu accepted only ten piastres and two tiny packets of tea and went on his way.[1]

SEVERAL things are worth noting in this story. The frightened parents looked first to local practitioners. When that failed a Western physician was brought in, but the parents were obviously uncertain about allowing their child to go to a Western hospital, especially when no promise of success was forthcoming. Fortunately a specialized traditional practitioner in a nearby province was located and dealt with the problem decisively. There were no spiritual incantations, no metaphysical explanations. Thạch Cầu was clearly a Confucian literatus who believed in natural solutions to natural problems. He also refused to link expert aid with large financial gain. However, he knew that men like the village head would assume that a high price equated high competence. Hence the ruse involving three thousand piastres.

Although Thạch Cầu enjoyed the diagnostic challenge and determining the proper treatment, he tended to instruct others when it came to preparing remedies and caring for the patient. He used his victory for didactic purposes, not only concerning proper supervision of infants, but also to ram home a point about upright behaviour having nothing to do with wealth. Indeed, he probably saw himself in the first instance as a moralist, employing healing skills as a means to that end.

Except for the minor intrusion of a French doctor, the above story could have been recounted two hundred or even six hundred years ago. Although Thạch Cầu quickly perceived the cause of the trauma to be in the throat, he never considered operating. Nor did he regard his work as completed once the obstruction was dislodged, instead remaining to be certain there were no complications and that recovery was complete. Thạch Cầu may have been in one sense an 'ear, nose and throat specialist', but he concerned himself with the whole of the patient's organic and psychological system and, beyond that, the behaviour of the community at large.

At least three medical traditions coexisted in Vietnam prior to the impact of Western medicine. Thuốc Bắc, or 'Northern medicine', possessed the best credentials. Only those Vietnamese (or resident Chinese) capable of reading Chinese characters could presume to diagnose and prescribe. Proudly drawing its legitimacy from ancient Chinese medical classics, Northern medicine began with the belief that out of *Yin-Yang* force interactions and the eight trigrams one could construct a model of the entire universe, valid on both material and moral planes. The human body was thus a microcosmic reproduction of the vast dynamic natural forces at work in the universe. Moreover, and perhaps most importantly, the body was intimately and constantly linked to those external forces, so that good health depended in large part on tuning internal functions to the environment, as well as building defences against disruptive changes. By the same token, disease was defined as impairment of the overall balance between external and internal, physical and moral forces.

On top of that fairly straightforward dualistic model an incredibly intricate doctrine evolved, the result of both endless metaphysical speculation and empirical observations by astronomers,

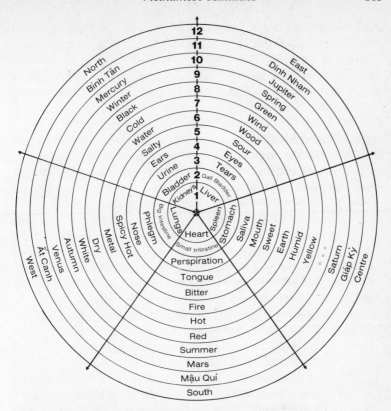

1 The Five Main Organs
2 The Five Secondary Organs
3 The Five Body Fluids
4 The Five Sensory Organs
5 The Five Flavours
6 The Five Elements

7 The Five Vital Essences
8 The Five Colours
9 The Four Seasons
10 The Five Planets
11 The Five Year Clusters
12 The Five Directions

Fig. 8.1. Sino-Vietnamese Conceptions of Man and the Universe

Adapted from: Pierre Huard and Maurice Durand, *Connaissance du Viet-Nam* (Paris and Hanoi, 1954), 64; Đỗ Đình Tuân, *Đông-Y Lừợc-Khảo* (Saigon, 1971), 87; Dường Bá Bành, *Histoire de la Médecine du Viet-Nam* (Hanoi, 1951), 76.

botanists and medical practitioners. Particularly remarkable was the preference for units of five, and the consequent system of concordances among perceived phenomena (see Fig. 8.1). On the other hand many drugs and methods of treatment clearly emerged by trial and error, only later being incorporated by Chinese metaphysicians into medical ideology. As with any comprehensive ideology there were internal inconsistencies, as well as differences over time and space. Nonetheless, the basic concepts do not seem to have changed from the early Han dynasty to the twentieth century.

How important all this intellectual paraphernalia was to individual Vietnamese practitioners of Northern medicine is hard to assess. Certainly those who wrote about medicine took it seriously, arguing that knowledge of the cyclical patterns and transformations of nature was the key to dealing with disease.[2] Paradoxically, this deductive bias helped to make every case unique in the eyes of well-read physicians, since no symptom could be divorced from the season of the year, geographical position, individual horoscope and emotional temperament of the patient.

Vietnamese practitioners of Northern medicine relied on the standard four-part Chinese clinical examination: visual inspection, auditory perception, questioning the patient, and taking his pulses. As in China, pulse-taking was the most important. Opinions varied on how many different pulse types could be identified, but any physician incapable of dealing with at least twelve was probably suspect.[3] Pulse-taking was even more crucial with female patients, since almost all Northern medicine practitioners were male and prohibited from inspecting women in detail. However, they could examine a woman's face, the second most valuable source of clinical information. Physicians took note of the colour and texture of the skin, condition of the eyes and tongue, and the patient's general demeanour in terms of fear, pain, lassitude or alertness. Following classical doctrine, they believed that different parts of the head revealed the condition of corresponding internal organs (e.g. tongue–heart, nose–lungs, ears–kidneys). Indeed, each part of the head could be sub-divided and examined for further clues. Thus, while the eye in its totality was linked to the liver, the upper eyelid was tied to the spleen, the lower eyelid to the stomach, the white of the eye to the lungs, and so on. Tongue and ears offered similar multiple windows to the body's interior.

Vietnamese texts mention many other techniques of examination, from listening to the patient cough to viewing and even tasting his urine. Significantly, asking a patient for his past medical history or questioning him in detail about symptoms often seemed

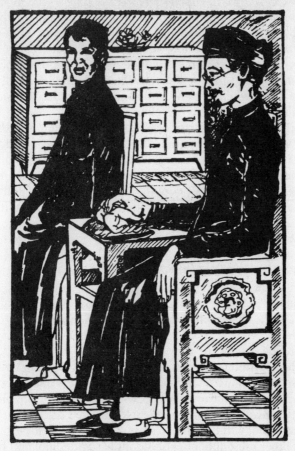

Fig. 8.2. Taking the Pulses, Vietnam, c.1940. (Đỗ Đình Tuân, *Đông-Y Lừộc-Khảo*, 2.33)

to be downgraded. This may have had something to do with prestige, a good physician being expected to know what was wrong from outward signs, not have to rely on the perceptions of an untutored patient. A practitioner asking a lot of questions was likely to be considered incompetent.

As the physician built up a symptomatic pattern he naturally moved towards diagnosis. Doctrine dictated that he first decide whether the illness was *nội thưởng*, that is to say emanating mainly from within the body due to poor physical maintenance or emotional strain, or *ngoại cảm*, the result of external forces (time of year, weather, 'humours', food, drink) disrupting the body's systemic harmony. After that he needed to determine whether the disease was still superficial in character (*biểu*), or already lodged deep in the major organs of the body (*lý*). Then 'hot' and 'cold' components had to be delineated. Finally he reviewed all symptoms to judge whether some actually disguised the ultimate sources of illness, rather than revealing them.[4]

The therapeutical doctrine of Northern medicine was even more complicated. In the first instance, particular drugs could be administered to produce sweating, expectoration, defecation, urination, vomiting, heat reduction or heat increase. Other ingredients were designed to excite or soothe particular organs. Still others might be added to offset harmful side-effects. Some drugs attacked 'trunk' causes, while others dealt with 'branch' symptoms. If one prescribed ingredients to evict 'perverse humours' (*tà khí*), it probably required one to add something to support 'correct humours' (*chính khí*) as well. Not surprisingly, concoctions became very intricate. The largest prescription I have located so far in Vietnamese publications involved twenty-four ingredients.[5] In the late 1920s, a village pharmacy shop in Quảng Nam carried 142 ingredients, while a spot check of a marketplace in the town of Vinh turned up seventy-four items.[6]

As the reprinting of fixed recipes suggests, not all practitioners possessed the knowledge or inclination to write a unique prescription for each case. They developed a repertoire of prescriptions tied to the availability of ingredients, and used them according to symptomatology. If their first choice did not appear to work, three or four other prescriptions existed for the same complaint. Indeed, compendiums of prescriptions were available in printed or manuscript form, often focusing on one disease or one sub-category of medicine.[7] Because some Northern medicine ingredients were extremely rare, treatment could become very expensive for the patient, capable of ruining an entire family financially if the disease persisted for very long.

Acupuncture and moxa treatment were also known to Vietnamese practitioners, to be used either separately or in combination with oral prescriptions. Based on the Chinese theory of meridian lines and sensitive spots connecting all organs and parts of the body, very fine needless or small clumps of smouldering mugwort were employed both to alleviate disease symptoms and to effect cures. For some reason, however, neither technique

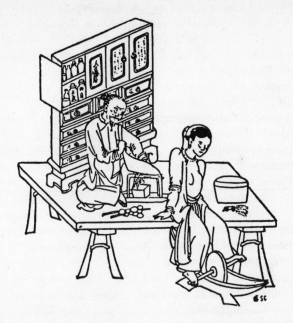

Fig. 8.3. Medical Practitioner and Assistant Preparing Ingredients, Vietnam, c.1900. (Huard and Durand, *Connaissance du Vietnam*, 171; reproduced courtesy of École Française d'Extrême-Orient.)

appears to have occasioned much interest among Vietnamese medical writers.[8] For example, Nguyễn Đình Chiểu, the famous nineteenth century writer, devoted only a few lines of his long narrative poem on medicine to acupuncture and moxa (*châm cứu*).[9] He also specifically condemned those acupuncturists who learned their trade by merely fiddling with needles, thus giving the overall 'medical calling' (*đạo y*) a bad name.[10]

The second tradition available to Vietnamese prior to the entry of Western medicine was *Thuốc Nam*, or 'Southern medicine', which relied almost exclusively on tropical plants and animals native to Vietnam. It was the poor man's medicine, generally using ingredients readily available nearby and involving a minimum of processing. Most knowledge was passed unselfconsciously from one generation to the next. Thus, everyone understood that for a common cold one could eat rice gruel laced with onion, place one's head under a blanket for a herbal steam bath, or rub a coin hard across certain of the body's sensitive points. Headaches could be treated by pinching or pricking the forehead. Preheated bamboo tubes or small glass cups were applied to the skin to suck out perverse humours. Garlic or soapberry helped someone in danger of fainting, ginger relieved stomach aches, and a broth made from tangerine rind lessened nausea. Chewing fresh tea leaves or guava buds might halt diarrhoea, apricot leaves might relieve dysentery.[11]

Generally Southern medicine was the cure of first resort. If one lacked the confidence to prescribe for oneself or a close family member, neighbours were quick to offer advice and assistance. Sometimes a particular villager developed sufficient reputation for healing to be sought out by people in adjacent villages. However, he or she seldom received more than a chicken, a stalk of bananas or some glutinous rice by way of remuneration. The real reward for success was increased local prestige and influence, undoubtedly one reason why mandarins and literati looked on such Southern healers with suspicion. Another reason was the inherently hetero-dox character of Southern medicine. Each family might keep several remedies secret from the outside world. Some villages were known to do the same, passing knowledge jealously from one generation to the next. Certain areas incorporated the medical lore of non-Vietnamese ethnic groups (highland tribes, Khmer, Cham), a practice quite offensive to those who considered the issue one of civilization versus barbarism. Nguyên Đình Chiểu, for example, demanded to know if they might go the next step into heresy and use Siamese and Lao remedies.[12]

Nevertheless, other literate Vietnamese practitioners saw fit to extoll the benefits of Southern medicine, albeit still within a basically Northern or Chinese theoretical framework. One of the most notable was a fourteenth century Buddhist monk, Tuệ Tĩnh, who compiled a series of texts on etiology, therapeutics, pharmaceuticals and proper living.[13] None of Tuệ Tĩnh's original writings survive, but eighteenth century books compiled from monastery materials and attributed to him reveal a desire on the one hand to demonstrate complete assimilation of Chinese medical concepts, and on the other to modify Chinese practice to accord with specific Vietnamese conditions. *Nam Dược Thần Hiệu* (Miraculous Effects of Southern Medicines), for example, employs a format derived from a tenth century sung dynasty text, discusses 182 diseases in thirteen categories, and offers a total of 3 872 remedies. It also describes the curative properties of 630 species of flora. In this and other texts there is particular concern to identify and promote medicinal ingredients readily available locally, for example ginger, onion, garlic, saffron and salt, as distinct from expensive Chinese imports. Eighty-two ingredients discussed in *Nam Được Thần Hiệu* possess *nôm* (Vietnamese characters) as distinct from Chinese character identifications, and a number of remedies have yet to be found in Chinese medical texts.

In popular lore Tuệ Tĩnh became known as the Saint of Southern Medicine (*Thánh Thuốc Nam*), and his most famous teaching remains, 'Use Southern medicine to treat Southern people'. Ironically, in 1385 the reigning Trần dynasty ruler is said to have donated Tuệ Tĩnh, together with nineteen other Buddhist monks, to the 'Northern' Ming dynasty by way of tribute.[14]

Even more famous was Hải Thượng Lãn Ông, born to a family of prestigious scholars and mandarins in 1720.[15] As a young man Lãn Ông distinguished himself at the capital with his talent for poetry and capacity to assimilate the Chinese classics. Nonetheless, he subsequently abandoned thoughts of a bureaucratic career and became absorbed by medicine, possibly as a consequence of searching for a cure for his own chronic ailment. After ten years poring over available texts (including those attributed to Tuệ Tĩnh) and caring for patients in the Hoàn Châu area of Nghệ An province, Lãn Ông's reputation spread more widely. People began calling him 'Saint of Medicine' (*Thanh Y*), and practitioners came from all directions to become students. Nonetheless, summoned to the capital late in life to examine the ill heir to the Trịnh seigniory, Lãn Ông was treated with suspicion by the chancellor and palace physicians alike.[16]

Meanwhile, for over two decades, Lãn Ông had been preparing a number of manuscripts. In them, he explained his philosophy of medicine, recorded thousands of popular prescriptions, and discussed a wide variety of ailments in meticulous detail.[17] One chapter, containing Lãn Ông's personal reflections on the art of healing, became a literary classic.[18] Although deeply committed to Chinese medical theories, particulary as enunciated in the *Nei-ching* (Classic of Internal Medicine), Lãn Ông's boundless curiosity and powers of observation often led him in unique directions. Most provocatively, he declared that the renowned second century classic, *Shang-han lun* (Treatise on Ailments caused by Cold), by Chang Chung-ching, was not applicable to Vietnam, both because ancient metaphysical formulations placed such diseases at the northwest point of the compass, far from the southern tropics, and because his own experience indicated that Vietnamese patients reacted unfavourably to strong 'heat-conveying' agents like ephedra or cinnamon. This assertion of Lãn Ông's continued to divide Vietnamese practitioners right up to the 1970s.[19]

Today Hải Thượng Lãn Ông is considered the father of Vietnamese medicine, not only the traditional branch, but also as authentic home-grown precursor of the meticulous clinical approach underlying modern cosmopolitan medicine. He often recorded therapeutic failures more carefully than successes, hoping that he or someone else would learn from them. Current writers also make much of Lãn Ông's ability to employ foreign concepts creatively, adapting them to particular Vietnamese conditions. That this assessment is not entirely *ex post facto* patriotic hyperbole is suggested by the endorsement of two eminent French colonial writers, Pierre Huard and Maurice Durand. They compare Lãn Ông with the sixteenth century Saxon, Janus Cornarius, who although still greatly admiring the Greek medical legacy, nevertheless demanded that 'German remedies be employed to care for Germans'.[20]

A third Vietnamese medical tradition involved dealing with harmful spirits, preferably by preventing them from entering the body at all, or, failing that, by finding a way to exorcise them and hence regain physical and mental equilibrium. Unlike Northern and Southern medical traditions, no single term identified this approach to disease and healing. The spirits went by many names, and techniques for dealing with them were innumerable. Concern began during pregnancy, when mothers wore amulets to protect the foetus, and continued into childbirth, when a symbolic notice was hung outside the home to ward off visitors for fear that someone of 'bad corporal essence' (*xấu vía*) would make the infant sick. For the first year the infant's real name was not mentioned, to lessen the chances of being noticed by demons. Until the age of twelve (eleven by Western reckoning), magical formulae were available to ward against *Con Ranh*, a demon specializing in killing children.[21]

When any family member became seriously ill, defensive prayers would probably be offered to the ancestors, and someone sent to a fortune teller to try to ascertain which particular spirit was causing the trouble, and where one might go to offer food and seek forgiveness. If that failed to work, a variety of Buddhist monks,

Taoist priests, sorcerers and mediums were available, although they might have to be brought from some distance. Talismans could be purchased, special vows made, intricate rituals undertaken. Either the patient or his close relative could proceed to cleanse himself, abstain from eating meat, and sleep at a temple or pagoda in hope of experiencing a dream which revealed the source of the problem. On the advice of a geomancer it was sometimes necessary to shift the grave of an ancestor or move one's own residence to a more favourable position.[22]

It was commonly believed that humans possessed three 'souls' (*hồn*), unlike animals with two, or plants with one. These could be attacked or lured out of the body. Death meant loss of all three souls, unconsciousness the loss of two, and various mental or physical disorders the loss of one. Although the departure of all three souls was irrevocable, one or two could be located and retrieved. Then there were 'corporal essences' (*phách; vía*), each linked to a body orifice and internal function. Men had seven, women nine. These too could be lost and regained. They possessed positive or negative force, so that a good *phách* exercised beneficial effect on others, whereas a person with bad *phách* needed to be avoided.[23]

It is important to ask—even if not possible to answer in detail here—how the three medical traditions outlined above related to each other. Both Northern and Southern medicine were primarily secular and naturalistic in character, not religious or spiritual. A stomach ache or an abcessed tooth was treated with pharmaceuticals, or perhaps acupuncture or moxabustion. If these did not work another technique would be attempted, or the patient would go to a different practitioner. There were no incantations, no ghosts, no battles of hex and anti-hex.

However, all is not what it seems. Many Northern medicine assertions had no obvious basis in physical reality, nor was it felt necessary to test them experimentally. For example, the stated value of *Yang* being nine, the square of that number somehow produced the distance that blood advances in a quarter hour, from which one determined fifty revolutions of blood throughout the body per day. The *Yin* number six was likewise employed to deduce how many times a person breathes in one day.[24] From this it was only a small step to employing astrology and horoscopy in medical diagnosis and prognosis. Some practitioners believed that the exact time when a person became ill, was injured or wounded helped to determine the prognosis. For example, a chest injury on the right-side that occured between 4 p.m. and 6 p.m. would cause one to collapse and die forty days later, if one did not drink the four-item brew available for that dire contingency. On the other hand, being injured a bit earlier or later produced entirely different results and required different treatments.[25]

Some Northern medicine practitioners in Vietnam had no reservations about including magical components in their repertoire, whether in order to make allowance for public credulity or because they acknowledged some efficacy themselves. Thus, one remedy for post-partum illness specified that a particular leaf had to be picked in utmost secrecy or it would lose its effectiveness.[26] Another in the same text, after delineating the symptoms of a bewitched person (absent-minded, empty-headed, evasive), prescribed the drinking of one bowl of warm blood from the neck of a freshly killed black dog in order to 'expel the poisons and perverse humours from the body'.[27]

It was precisely those sorts of prescriptions in an allegedly Northern medicine text that infuriated the purists. Nguyễn Đình Chiểu, for example, urged that quacks be punished severely by the state. Rather wistfully, he painted a dream of medical charlatans being denounced by outraged poor farmers and hauled before a judicial mandarin. First on trial was an uneducated simpleton who relied solely on family traditions plus a few ancient ideas learned orally and applied dogmatically, not realizing how many different permutations were explained in the medical classics. Second was the acupuncturist, mentioned earlier, who also had no comprehension of the underlying principles, and, besides, charged exorbitantly. Third came the Southern medicine practitioner who had the temerity to mix long-established Northern medicines with his questionable jungle and mountain drugs, partly to trick patients into paying higher prices. Then there was the Taoist priest, condemned for departing from Lao-tzu's legitimate teachings and promoting rank superstitions. Finally came a Buddhist monk, seemingly the worst offender, who on the one hand refused to offer practical solutions to life's problems, yet on the other accepted gifts from ill people in exchange for a vial of water mixed with 'sacred' ashes.[28]

Nonetheless, Nguyễn Đình Chiểu did not deny the existence of harmful spirits that caused illness. In fact, after referring to some ancient Chinese methods of exorcism, involving pharmaceuticals, acupuncture and appropriate ritual, he then suggested his own techniques for driving five different types of demons or ghosts from the body.[29] Perhaps the key to this apparent contradiction lay in the following passage:

Our Way has many stratagems to eliminate harmful spirits;
Demons, ghosts, monsters and fiends experience difficulty passing a Sage.
Hence taker heed in the classical medical texts,
Of words and actions that must be transmitted broadly.

In short, Nguyễn Đình Chiểu was ultimately concerned to uphold the single true Neo-Confucian faith against heterodoxy, not to claim that all diseases could be resolved by physical diagnosis and treatment. There were orthodox solutions to ghosts that obviated the need for illegitimate and disruptive competitors.

Although court and mandarinate might agree with Nguyễn Đình Chiểu's arguments in principle, they often ignored them in practice. And ordinary people seemed to forget them entirely when faced with a disease crisis. Epidemics of cholera, smallpox or plague are most instructive in this respect. A rash of deaths in or near the capital would see ranking officials scurrying in all directions to organize offerings to every possible temple or shrine, no matter how unorthodox, and frantic reliance on a variety of faith healers and spirit mediums. After the epidemic had passed, women of the court might be blamed for such deviations, but that was merely a formality. Meanwhile, the population at large tried to take matters into their own hands, organizing processions of men armed with spears, machetes, drums and firecrackers to march around villages and drive away the hoards of threatening ghosts. Thorn bushes were placed across roads, bamboo stakes daubed with lime planted on paths, and banners inscribed with demon-defying slogans hung at strategic points. At Buddhist pagodas prayers where directed to Kwannon and to Quan Đế, one of the heroic generals of the Three Kingdoms period in China. Elsewhere a priest led a group to clench a particular herb between their teeth, prostrate themselves repeatedly, and beg Heaven to save them.[30]

Each family also took its own defensive action, sticking Chinese characters on the door, daubing the walls and rafters with lime, perhaps lighting wet faggots to smoke out any disease ghost which slipped through. The name of the disease was never mentioned, as that might attract the spirit's attention.[31] When all failed and a member of the family became ill, another set of procedures was available. One of the most striking involved crafting a bamboo and paper effigy of the threatened invidual (*con nộm*), then following the directions of a sorcerer in offering it to the cholera or smallpox ghost together with some food and drink. Meanwhile, pharmaceutical mixtures were not ignored. Northern medicine texts described a range of treatments, some quite possibly efficacious. Cholera remedies, for example, often prescribed the sipping of small amounts of liquid concoctions every fifteen or thirty minutes, which at very least helped to offset dehydration.[32]

Nineteenth and early twentieth century accounts of epidemics in Vietnam suggest remarkable group effort aimed at dealing with a truly terrifying threat. Of course fear was abundant, yet there must also have been sufficient hope to occasion such wide-ranging counteractions. Even in death a person might prove helpful: a custom existed of temporary and incomplete burial, so that the corpse would be in a better position to reply to questions posed by harmful spirits in a manner that led them away from close relatives.[33] In the end, if the struggle proved fruitless and yet another relative or friend was seized, it was said that his or her 'destiny had been accomplished' (*hết số*).

Popular sayings offer some clues to Vietnamese attitudes about disease and health:[34]

Ôm tiếc thân, lành tiếc của
In sickness one grieves a wasting body, in health the loss of money.

Mê ăn uống thì nhủ dùng răng mình mà đào huyệt
Eating and drinking passionately is like using one's teeth to dig one's own grave.

Bệnh tùy khẩu nhập, hoa tùng khẩu xuất
Maladies enter through the mouth, misfortune goes out the same way.

Thầy chữa bệnh không chữa mệnh
Doctors can deal with illness, but not alter fate.

Nhiều thầy, thúi ma
Too many healers mean a stinking cadaver.

Vô đậu bất thành nhân
Those who haven't suffered smallpox are not wise in life.

Confronted with disease, Vietnamese asked the same questions as individuals the world over: 'What kind of sickness do I have?

What are my chances? What caused this sickness? Why did it happen to me (of all people)?' In seeking answers the patient was quick to consult with family elders, knowledgeable neighbours and part-time village practitioners. However, any decision to seek help beyond the village involved further questions: 'How much will the treatment cost? How long will it take? Will that stranger treat in a sympathetic manner?' The longer an illness persisted, the more likely that even a senior patient would lose control of decision-making to relatives, slipping into a well-defined 'sick' role that allowed him or her to relinquish all responsibilities, passively to accept each new treatment, and to enjoy the most devoted attention and sacrifices of the family.[35] On the other hand, prior awareness of the psychological and financial costs to the family of prolonged treatment sometimes led individuals to ignore symptoms and endure pain until a disease was well advanced.

The medical profession did not seem to enjoy high status in Vietnam, even though a few individual practitioners like Tuệ Tĩnh or Lãn Ông became quite famous. I suspect this had less to do with the quality of services offered than with the inability of practitioners to institutionalize. At no time, for example, did Vietnamese rulers allow medical practitioners to form a professional organization, to wear special clothing, or to accredit trainees. Although one might become famous by prescribing for the rich and powerful, one could also be punished summarily if an important patient failed to respond to treatment. Not surprisingly, gifted individuals preferred to concentrate on passing the civil examinations and working their way up the mandarinal ladder—leaving to failed candidates the chance to make a living in medicine (often combined with roles as local teachers and scribes).

Shortly after consolidating nationwide power in 1802, the founder of the Nguyễn dynasty, Gia Long, moved to link medicine with the state. A palace medical hierarchy was established, followed by designation of provincial medical authorities, who, however, had to devote themselves equally to caring for the royal elephants.[36] Local practitioners were permitted to establish small temples of medicine (*Y Miếu*), not unlike the more prestigious temples of literature (*Văn Miếu*). The main altar was consecrated to three legendary Chinese emperors long identified with Northern medicine: Fu Hsi, Shen Nung and Huang Ti. At some point, at least in the Hanoi temple, tablets were added to commemorate Tuệ Tĩnh and Lãn Ông.[37]

Such royal initiatives were designed to incorporate a portion of existing medical beliefs to the dominant Neo-Confucian political ideology, not to upgrade the state of the medical profession. Only King Tự Đức (r. 1847–83) went a bit further, establishing a small medical school to train palace doctors, and ordering officials to identify skilled practitioners in the provinces. Those individuals who demonstrated an ability to cure specific ailments would be given cash rewards. However, those who tried to deceive would be gaoled.[38] Faced with ever more serious attacks by the French, it is doubtful that Tự Đức's officials had much time to look for local medical practitioners, or that many of the latter stepped forward to chance either reward or punishment.

Although Western missionaries brought their own medical theories and practices to Vietnam in the seventeenth century, the impact was negligible, unlike their remarkable accomplishments in converting several hundred thousand Vietnamese to Catholicism. With the notable exception of some anatomical charts, they had nothing to offer which was superior to Vietnamese medicine of that day. A Fr. Langlois, already known for organizing a small hospital in Siam, attached himself to the court in Huế, but later fell out of favour and died in prison in 1700.[39] In 1789, a French naval surgeon, J. M. Despiau, linked up with the head of the Nguyễn clan, followed him to Huế and witnessed his enthronement as Gia Long. Despiau's subsequent activities do not seem to have been recorded, except in 1820, when he was sent by King Minh Mạng to Macao to study smallpox, and apparently brought back the technique of Jennerian vaccination.[40] However, for the next half century there was no Western doctor at the Huế court, nor any Vietnamese interest in Western medical developments. Only as the French Army recruited Vietnamese soldiers after 1860 did one small segment of the population experience Western medicine, surgery in particular.

In 1902, Governor General Paul Doumer created a School of Indigenous Auxiliary Doctors in Hanoi. The first director was Dr Yersin, internationally famous for discovering the plague bacillus at Canton in 1894. Three years later a Medical Assistance Bureau was established, supervising operations of eighty facilities throughout Indochina. The largest part of these resources was directed towards the resident French population, but it was also in the immediate interests of the colonial authorities to try to contain outbreaks of smallpox, cholera and plague. This they were increasingly able to accomplish, one of the reasons for a steady increase in population after the turn of the century. Nonetheless, by 1930 only 240 auxiliary doctors and pharmacists had graduated from the Hanoi School, approximately one per 67 000 people.[41] Since most graduates clustered in the cities of Hanoi, Haiphong and Saigon, very few Vietnamese villagers ever saw a practitioner of 'Western medicine' (*Tây Y*) unless it was the French health inspector making his rounds once every year or two.

Vietnamese primary school teachers had more impact. Armed with government-approved hygiene manuals about teeth brushing, clean clothes, basic anatomy and contagious diseases, they usually linked better health with the development of a strong citizenry and ultimately an independent nation. Although little or no attempt was made in these textbooks to explain germ theory, endemic disease or community preventive medicine, an alert, enterprising teacher could learn about such things and more, by purchasing a few books and subscribing to journals of the day. As early as 1917 a Hanoi monthly was offering brief histories of modern astronomy, physics and biochemistry. Pasteur's life and work was extolled. Tuberculosis, a serious problem in Vietnam, received special attention. The functioning of the human brain was described, and a long essay on psychology serialized.[42] Beginning in 1925 a number of Western medical compendiums were published in Vietnamese. Books and pamphlets on sexual hygiene, pregnancy, childbirth and venereal disease also appeared for the first time, occasioning angry outbursts from Confucian traditionalists. In 1930 a popular fortnightly journal, *Phụ Nữ Tân Văn* (Women's News), began running a column on medical topics by a prominent Western-trained physician. Soon the journal was criticizing the colonial authorities for failing to mount serious campaigns against malaria, tuberculosis, cholera, syphilis, rabies and leprosy. When these criticisms apparently fell on deaf ears, some writers suggested that only overthrow of the imperialist system could clear the way for effective public health programmes.[43]

Traditional medical practitioners were no less capable of using the printing press. Most impressive was the fat Vietnamese language compendium put out annually by Haw Par, the famous Chinese Tiger-Balm medicine king. By 1931 this combined almanac, manual and patent medicine advertisement was 370 pages long, and 100 000 copies were being printed.[44] It may have been at this time that Northern medicine and Southern medicine came routinely to be subsumed under the term 'Eastern medicine' (*Đông Y*), obviously a reaction to pressure from Western medicine proponents. Also, to be 'Eastern' in the 1920s and 1930s meant defending spiritual values against the crass, materialistic West. Those who did not wish to buy into that argument simply adopted the popular term 'our medicine' (*Thuốc ta*). Although young Vietnamese intellectuals steadfastly condemned popular superstitions, for example fortune telling, trances and demonology, they seldom attacked dispensers of indigenous medicine.[45] Indeed, when the colonial authorities moved in 1938 to restrict traditional practitioners, some left-wing intellectuals protested vehemently, among other things pointing out how specious were French arguments of protecting public health when they continued to promote opium smoking.[45] Unlike China in the 1920s and 1930s, Vietnam experienced no full-fledged debate over the relative merits of traditional and modern medicine.[47]

Meanwhile, however, the small contingent of Western-trained Vietnamese doctors gained confidence and experience. Their stronghold was the Hôpital Indigène du Protectorat in Hanoi, connected with the medical school and containing a hundred beds.[48] Although none were permitted to teach, Dr. Hồ Đắc Di became the first accredited Vietnamese surgeon there in 1935, and Dr Tôn Thất Tùng the first accredited intern in 1938. The medical challenges were considerable, as most Vietnamese continued to avoid Western hospitals or clinics except as a last resort, when their condition was likely to be grave. Nevertheless, the Protectorate Hospital often had two patients to a bed and more lying on the floor. Starving vagrants were carried in by the police, examined by students, given some medicine and broth, but often died after a few days.[49]

Unclaimed corpses went to the Department of Anatomy for dissection. In some ways this was the core of Western medical education. Vietnamese students were acutely aware of the traditional medical taboo against both dissection and major surgery. Confucian doctrine warned that one's body, even in death, belonged to one's parents and was not to be carved up. Buddhist doctrine ruled out practice on animals. Perhaps more important, cutting flesh was beneath the dignity of a gentleman, and could be dangerous to the practitioner's own health. However, none of those points serve to explain why, over the centuries, no one had bothered to correct received anatomical charts by simply observing bodies mangled by accidents, warfare or execution. Of course, there was a bias against tampering with ancient wisdom, yet that had not prevented Hải Thượng Lãn Ông from rejecting *Shang-han* doctrine. I suspect that the deductive preference for diagnosing and treating patients holistically led even the most curious traditional practitioners away from inductive analysis of individual parts.

In any event, some Hanoi medical students clearly relished the cultural iconoclasm inherent in dissection. Apparently teacher supervision was lax. One former student recalls brandishing leg bones like swords, throwing clumps of fat at each other, even putting a severed penis in the purse of a female friend.[50] More seriously, those aiming to be surgeons used their free time to dissect meticulously scores of additional cadavers. Dr Tôn Thất Tùng dissected more than 200 cadaver livers between 1935 and 1939, developing a technique for exposing them completely in fifteen minutes. Together with Professor Meyer May he then operated successfully to remove a liver cancer, only to be stunned when their report was rejected by the Paris Academy. He then shifted his attention to the study of severe parasitical infestations, doing autopsies to map the complex movements of ascarids in particular. In 1941 he designed a procedure to remove dead ascarids blocking the entrance to the gall bladder, an operation which subsequently became routine throughout the world. The more he researched parasites, however, the more Dr Tùng realized that the underlying cause was poverty, and the necessary solutions beyond his powers as a surgeon.[51]

During World War II, when it was impossible to obtain Western pharmaceuticals from Europe, the Indochina colonial authorities sponsored an urgent search for substitutes, eventually claiming some four hundred innovations. Vietnamese pharmacists, led by Hồ Đắc An, succeeded in producing locally a number of modern medicines, including histidine, cholesterol, benzoic acid and feramine. Traditional practitioners were also called in to present their wares for scientific scrutiny. Highest priority was assigned to identifying, producing and distributing remedies for amoebic dysentery and intestinal parasites.[52] Because some Northern medicinal ingredients from China were almost as scarce as Western ingredients, Southern medicine enjoyed a strong revival. Faced with shortages, Đỗ Phong Thuần, a well-known Northern medicine practitioner, recalled that, 'We woke up, remembered plants in our own gardens and forests, and used those'.[53]

Attention to local ingredients and remedies continued for followers of the Democratic Republic of Vietnam (DRV) after they were driven from the cities and towns in 1945–46 by the returning French forces. Indeed, DRV leaders made a virtue of necessity, extolling Eastern medicine as a precious historical legacy. They drew the line at 'superstitious' customs, without, however, mounting any campaigns of eradication. Meanwhile, urban areas under French control returned to dependence on pharmaceutical imports.

A number of Western-trained medical personnel associated themselves with the DRV at its inception. The first scientific book published under the new regime was *Acute Pancreatic Inflammation and Surgery*, with the author, Dr Tôn Thất Tùng, readily selling his own bicycle to cover printing costs. Retreating from Hanoi in late 1946, the staff of the former Protectorate Hospital made up the core of a mobile operating unit and medical school. When operating in the open, scores of highland minority people clustered to watch, even climbing the surrounding trees. They regarded Dr Tùng as a sorcerer with powers second only to the 'chicken ghost'. To facilitate quick movement of patients under enemy attack, a Spanish Civil War technique of placing plaster casts over operated areas of the body was adopted, the main disadvantage being stench. In 1949, Dr Đặng Văn Ngữ travelled from Japan to the northwest mountain liberated zone carrying both the knowledge and fungi spores to manufacture penicillin and streptomycin. Soon small teams were being dispatched to battle zones to produce antibiotics on the spot.[54] Meanwhile, French commanders tried to prevent sulfonamides and quinine from reaching the DRV forces.[55] A particular brand of sulfonamide injection, brand-named Dagenan, came to be highly prized in DRV-controlled zones. Indeed, for a while it was common to label a well-rounded, all-purpose revolutionary activist as a 'Dagenan cadre'.[56]

Despite such developments in Western medicine, the vast majority of Vietnamese continued to rely on traditional remedies. However, changes were evident. Some Eastern medicine practitioners chose to incorporate Western pharmaceuticals and techniques. Most notable was quinine, originally taken up for malaria, but then employed less discriminately against 'cold' fevers.[57] Some urban Vietnamese combined Nivaquine, aspirin and perhaps a vitamin pill as a tonic.[58] Powerful Western drugs designed to treat syphilis, containing mercury, arsenic and bismuth, were acquired by traditional practitioners to use for the same purpose. Western-trained practitioners complained at the number of overdosed patients brought to their hospital wards to die. Sulfonamide came to be employed in combination with a *mélange* of Northern medicine incredients. Copper sulfate and zinc sulfate were adopted for eye ailments.[59]

Most remarkable by the 1940s was the widespread enthusiasm for needle injections. It would be interesting to know exactly when and why this Western technique became so popular. In the first decade of the twentieth century Vietnamese were still reported by French administrators to be unenthusiastic about lining up for smallpox vaccinations. Yet, between August 1937 and August 1938, faced with a rampant cholera epidemic, 9 650 000 people, or about one-half the population, accepted inoculation.[60] From there perhaps it was natural to seek out injections when already stricken by a disease, not to mention taking a variety of intramuscular tonics. Whether some practitioners endowed injections with magic properties is unknown. In any event, into the gap between Eastern and Western medicine stepped a special breed of health practitioners, often called 'medical assistants' (*y tá*), who sold shots directly to the consumer. The increasing availability of antibiotics in the 1950s strengthened their position. In fact, since Western-trained doctors and village nurses now came to be judged according to the number of shots they administered, it was routine to inject vitamins or camphor if nothing else was needed. Camphor produced some fever, seen by patients to be a hot or *yang* effect in the traditional sense.[61]

Partition of Vietnam in 1954 inevitably produced two very different health systems. In the South, the government extolled Western medicine and tried repeatedly to restrict the role and status of traditional practitioners. In the North, building on practical experience obtained during the anti-French Resistance, Hồ Chí Minh urged all medical cadres to study means of 'harmonizing' Eastern and Western remedies. For the first time in Vietnamese history the government granted institutional legitimacy to Eastern medicine practitioners, while however pressing them to eschew 'superstition'. Meanwhile, the advent of the Second Indochina War forced ordinary citizens in both regions to fall back on local initiatives and remedies. Popular attitudes became more complex than ever. To cite an extreme case, a sophisticated Saigon woman might patronize a Western-trained plastic surgeon one day, visit a herbalist the next day, and perhaps hedge her bet by calling in a sorcerer or medium the third day.

Although Vietnam now has a single health system, and the government intends to develop an 'identifiably Vietnamese medical science',[62] no one claims that individuals faced with a health crisis respond in a unified, coherent manner. Ironically, that seems to bother Vietnamese health officials more than it does Western observers, who have come to question unilinear or monolithic approaches to disease and healing.

1. Recounted in Đỗ Đình Tuân, *Đông-Y Lược Khảo* (Saigon, Hoa Lú, 1971), 1:173–5. The story probably dates from about World War I, as we know from French sources that Dr des Barres arrived in Indochina in 1902.

2. See, for example, the late nineteenth century work by Nguyễn Đình Chiểu, *Ngủ Tiều Vấn Đáp Y Thuật* (Saigon, Tân Việt, 1952), 49–76.

3. Đỗ Phong Thuần, *Đông Y Học Thực Nghiệm* (Saigon, Trí Đăng, 1970), 29–35, offers readers a 208-line poem describing 27 different pulses.

4. Đỗ Đình Tuân, op. cit., 1:105–19.

5. Thích Tâm An, *Muốn Làm Người Dũng Sĩ* (Saigon, 1969), 75–7. The prescription is for someone beaten or squashed close to death. One wonders how all the ingredients could be located in time. Apparently some 'basic' prescriptions in China contained as many as one hundred drugs.

6. Albert Sallet, *Le médecin annamite et la préparation des remèdes* (Paris, Imp. Nationale, 1931), 26–7.

7. Thus, Trần Hàm Tấn, 'Notes bibliographiques sur la pharmacopée sino-vietnamienne', *Dân Việt Nam* (Hanoi) no. 2 (Dec. 1948), 30–6, lists eight pharmacological texts dealing with smallpox, ten with childhood diseases, and four with female disorders.

8. Only one entry in the 58-item bibliography of Dương Bá Bành, *Histoire de la médecine du Viet-Nam* (Hanoi, École Française d'Extrême-Orient, 1951[?]), 5–12, deals specifically with acupuncture.

9. Nguyễn Đình Chiểu, 151–2.

10. Ibid., 378–81.

11. Lê Trần Đức, *Tuệ Tỉnh và Nền Y Dược Cổ Truyền Việt Nam* (Hanoi, Y Học, 1975), 32.

12. Nguyễn Đình Chiểu, 381–4.

13. Lê Trần Đức, 'Tue Tinh and the Beginnings of National Medicine', in Hoàng Bảo Châu et al., *Traditional Medicine*, Vietnamese Studies no. 50 (Hanoi, Foreign Language Publishing House, 1980[?]), 130–42. Trần Hàm Tấn, 29–36, contains 13 texts attributed in some way to Tuệ Tỉnh.

14. Lê Trần Đức, *Tuệ Tinh và Nền Y Dược*, 12.

15. His original name was Lê Hữu Trác. Lê Trần Đức, *Thân Thế va Sù Nghiệp Y Học của Hài Thượng Lãn Ông* (2nd rev. ed., Hanoi, Y Học, 1970); Le Khac Thien, 'Hai Thuong Lan Ong, Great Master of Traditional Medicine', in Hoàng Bảo Châu, op. cit. 143–59.

16. Hải Thượng Lãn Ông, 'At the Palace of the Trinh Lords', in Hoàng Bảo Châu, op. cit., 163–72. He implies that his prescription was ignored. In any event, the patient died shortly thereafter.

17. His encyclopedic *Hải Thượng Y Tong Tam Linh* (Treatise on Medical Knowledge by Hai Thuong) contained 28 volumes, almost all of which survived in

an 1866 printed version. Pierre Huard and Maurice Durand, 'Lan Ong et la médicine sino-vietnamienne', *Bulletin de la Société des Études Indochinoises* (Saigon), Nouvelle Série, 28, 3 (1953), 221–65.

18. It is titled 'Châu Ngọc Cách Ngôn' (Maxims of Pearl and Jade), and published *quốc ngữ* versions are available from Hanoi (1971) and Saigon (1972).

19. For example, Đỗ Phong Thuần, op. cit., 8, cites Lãn Ông to substantiate his decision to exclude all discussion of *shang-han* (in Vietnamese, *thường hàn*) illnesses, whereas Đỗ Đình Tuân, op. cit., 2:177–267, devotes ninety pages to the topic.

20. Huard and Durand, op. cit., 21. The same authors, in *Connaissance du Viet-Nam* (Paris and Hanoi, École Française d'Extrême-Orient, 1954), 60, also compare Lãn Ông in this respect with Nagata Tokuhon, the seventeenth century Japanese physician.

21. Léopold Cadière, *Croyances et pratiques religieuses des Viêtnamiens* (Saigon, École Française d'Extrême-Orient, 1955), 2:198–209; Đào Duy Anh, *Việt Nam Văn Hóa Sử' Cường* (Saigon, Bốn Phường, 1951), 182–6, 192–3.

22. Đào Duy Anh, op. cit., 304–12.

23. See Cadière, op. cit., 3:180–95, for a more intricate discussion.

24. Pierre Huard and Ming Wong, *Chinese Medicine* (London, Weidenfeld and Nicolson, 1968), 64. The authors also mention similar numerological assertions in the West, for example those of Agrippa von Nettesheim (1486–1533).

25. Thích Tâm An, op. cit., 5–10.

26. Dan Tuong (comp.), *293 Bài Thuốc Gia Truyền Đông Y* (Saigon, 1971), remedy no. 96.

27. Ibid., remedy no. 24.

28. Nguyễn Đình Chiểu, op. cit., 369–93.

29. Ibid., 287–9.

30. Cadière, op. cit., 3:195–243; Albert Sallet, 'Les esprits malfaisants dan les affections épidémiques au Binh-Thuan', *Bulletin des amis de vieux Hué* 13, 1 (1926), 81–8. Cf. Colin Brown, 'The Influenza Pandemic of 1918 in Indonesia', below, for descriptions of analogous behaviour elsewhere.

31. Đào Duy Anh, op. cit., 192; Bùi Hiển, 'Ma Đậu', in *Nằm Vạ* (Hanoi, Đời Nay, 1958), 17–26.

32. Dan Tuong, op. cit., remedies 38–40.

33. Cadière, op. cit., 4:212–16. Especially at risk were siblings born on a day, month or year (plus or minus twelve) coincidental with the deceased.

34. Sallet, op. cit., 134–48.

35. Tran Minh Tung, 'Health and Disease: The Indochinese Perspective', in *Working with Indochinese Refugees* (Chicago, Travelers Aid, 1978[?]), 45–6.

36. Đường Bá Bành, op. cit. 47. Similar administrative initiatives are recorded in the late fifteenth century annals of the Lê dynasty.

37. Huard and Wong, op. cit., 102.

38. *Đai Nam Thực Lục Chính Biên* (Hanoi, Khoa Học Xã Hội, 1973–76), 28:301; 33:279, 33:327. I am very grateful to Professor Nguyễn Thế Anh for pointing out these efforts by Tự Đức.

39. Đường Bá Bành, op. cit., 62.

40. Đường Bá Bành, op. cit., 63; Huard and Wong, op. cit., 135.

41. Fifty-eight of these graduates were European. Phan Huy Dan, *Quelques suggestions sur la réorganisation sanitaire au Vietnam* (Paris, R. Foulon, 1949), 25–9.

42. *Nam Phong Tạp Chí* (Hanoi), articles appearing between July 1917 and December 1921.

43. David G. Marr, *Vietnamese Tradition on Trial* (Berkeley, University of California Press, 1981), 78–82, 212–14, 339–40.

44. Lủổng Y Vi-Te Sanh, *Nhị Thiên Dủổng* (Saigon, 1931).

45. One exception is Trong Lang, 'Vỏi các Ông Lang', *Hanoi Tân Văn*, nos. 57–73 (March-July 1941).

46. *Dại Chúng* (Saigon), nos. 2 (19 Nov. 1938), 5 (16 Dec. 1938), and 9 (21 Jan. 1939).

47. Ralph C. Crozier, *Traditional Medicine in Modern China: Science, Nationalism, and the Tensions of Cultural Change* (Cambridge, Harvard University Press, 1968), 58–148.

48. In 1936 the name was changed to Yersin Hospital, then later to Phủ Doan Hospital, and finally, in 1958, to Vietnam-German Democratic Republic Friendship Hospital.

49. Tôn Thất Tùng, *Dủổng vào Khoa Học của Tôi* (Hanoi, Thanh Niên, 1978), 16–23; Nguyễn Tuấn Phát, *Một Vài Cảm Nghỉ* (Saigon, Khai Trí, 1969[?]).

50. Nguyễn Tuấn Phát, op. cit., 103.

51. Tôn Thất Tùng, op. cit., 27–41.

52. A. Gibot and R.F. Auriol, 'Le problème des médicaments en Indochine de 1940 à 1945', *Produits Pharmaceutiques* 2, 3 (March 1947), 109–19.

53. Dỗ Phong Thuần, op. cit., 85.

54. Tôn Thất Tùng, 43–62; P.V., '80th Anniversary of the Hanoi Faculty of Medicine', *Vietnam Courier* (Hanoi) 19, 1 (1983), 19–20.

55. Phan Huy Dan, op. cit., 52.

56. Interview with members of the SRV Ministry of Health visiting Canberra, 27 May 1984.

57. Dỗ Phong Thuần, op. cit., 70, 80–81, endorses quinine for malaria, but also lists a Northern medicine alternative if quinine is unavailable or causes discomfort. He criticizes quinine's use for other illness.

58. Nguyễn Tuấn Phát, op. cit., 17–21.

59. Dủổng Bá Bành, op. cit., 65, 67–9.

60. Phan Huy Dan, op. cit., 37.

61. Chester A. Bain, 'The Persistence of Tradition in Modern Vietnamese Medicine', *Southeast Asia* (Carbondale, Ill.) 3 (Winter 1974), 617.

62. Hoàng Bảo Châu, op. cit., 11–13.

IV   THE BIOLOGY AND POLITICS OF DEATH

9 Death and Disease in Nineteenth Century Batavia

SUSAN ABEYASEKERE

'THE unwholesome air of Batavia . . . is the death of more Europeans than any other place upon the Globe of the same extent.'[1] Thus Captain Cook in 1770 summed up the prevailing view about the capital of the Dutch East Indies.[2] During the nineteenth century, visitors' opinions were gradually modified until Europeans ceased to describe Batavia in such terms. Had Batavia therefore become a healthy city in the course of the century? Certainly for Europeans the picture had changed: their death rates fell dramatically, until the only health problem which provoked comment was the occasional cholera epidemic, from which they were unable to shield themselves completely. But for the vast majority of the urban population, Batavia remained a remarkably unhealthy place. What had altered in the health picture of the nineteenth century was not medical care, since both preventive and curative medicine could offer little of use, but rather the environment of the Europeans. They had escaped the deadly confines of the old town in favour of the more salubrious suburbs and they benefited most from the first hesitant government excursions into public health, while the Chinese and Indonesians continued to suffer from environmentally related diseases.

Lacking reliable urban birth and death figures, we have to look elsewhere for evidence of general health levels.[3] The population of Batavia grew slowly in the nineteenth century—more slowly than the Java-wide growth rate[4] and far less rapidly than in the first decades of the twentieth century. Between 1815 and 1900 it seems that Batavia's population increased by a little over two and a half times (from about 47 000 to 115 000), while between 1900 and 1930 alone it almost quadrupled.[5] In the absence of migration or birth statistics it is difficult to assess the significance of the level of health for population growth, but an analysis of Batavia's growth

189

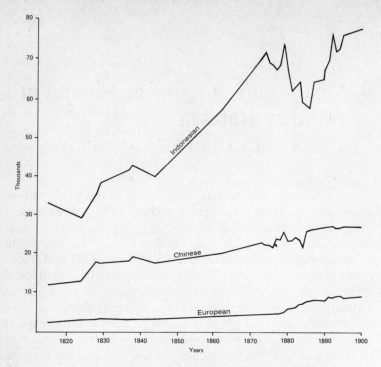

Fig. 9.1. Population of Batavia, by Ethnic Group, 1815–1900

Sources: Raffles, 1:Table 1, 2:246; C. S. W. van Hogendorp, 'Algemeen Jaarlijksch Verslag van den Staat der Residentie Batavia over 1824', Collectie Van Hogendorp nr. 83, Algemeen Rijksarchief, Den Haag; Bleeker, 'Bijdragen', 449–51, 456; 'Statistische gegevens'; *KV*, 1875–90, 1892–97, 1902.

by ethnic group shows dips and plateaus in the growth of Chinese and Indonesian groups which generally coincided with reports of major epidemics (Fig. 9.1). Cholera epidemics were first recorded for Batavia in 1821 and 1851–53; then from the 1860s cholera and fever epidemics occurred sporadically until the end of the century and beyond. Although we lack reliable statistics for numbers affected by these epidemics,[6] official reports reveal something of the suffering: e.g., in the cholera epidemic of 1864, 4 474 cases of the disease were registered in the town, of which 37% were fatal. At that time the population of Batavia was about 82 000.[7]

Apart from the dramatic impact of epidemics, a number of debilitating illnesses were endemic in Batavia—notably malaria and dysentery. No doubt their underlying influence contributed to

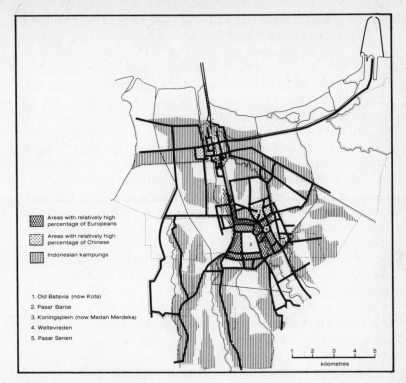

Fig. 9.2. Ethnic Distribution of the Population of Batavia, c. 1885

Source: Map 'Batavia en Omstreken', drawn by J. Vos (Batavia, Albrecht, 1887).

the slow growth of the population. However, in order to understand the effect of these illnesses, it is more realistic to examine
individual ethnic groups and areas of the city, as generalizations
conceal significant variations.

The Sociology and Geography of Disease

Batavia was inhabited by three main ethnic groups—Europeans,
Chinese and Indonesians. In 1878, for example, Indonesians com-
prised by far the largest group (70%) of the society, with the
Chinese reaching almost a quarter of the total and the Europeans
only 4.5%.[8]

In the nineteenth century there were distinct Chinese and European areas of residence in Batavia (Fig. 9.2). The Europeans

had recognized that the old walled town of Batavia, first built by the Dutch East India Company at the mouth of the River Ciliwung in 1619 and criss-crossed by canals in the Dutch fashion, was a most unhealthy place to live. Overcrowded, its canals often stagnant because the water flowed more sluggishly every year, and frequently flooded, the place had become so notorious among Europeans that they left it in droves to settle in the new and higher suburbs further south; those who worked at the offices and warehouses near the port travelled in by carriage. Governor-General Daendels' decision in the early nineteenth century to break down the walls of the town and move the administration to Weltevreden, a few miles inland, merely formalized a *fait accompli*. In the nineteenth century virtually no Europeans lived in the *benedenstad*—the lower town or Batavia proper. This gave them enormous health advantages. Although they did not understand the causes of malaria, observation had taught them that it was dangerous to spend the night in the old town—precisely the hours when the malaria mosquitoes were active. Batavia swarmed with *Anopheles* mosquitoes of several kinds; the larvae bred in the brackish, still water of the swamps and fishponds that lined the northern coast. As silt carried down by the Ciliwung River steadily extended the marshy coastline, breeding places multiplied.[9]

In Weltevreden the land was better drained and the Europeans inhabited bungalows with well-ventilated rooms surrounded by gardens which, in the case of the wealthy, amounted to veritable parks. Europeans took care to filter their drinking water and boil it, and they had ample food. There is every reason to expect, therefore, that they are avoided the worst of the environmentally related illnesses which afflicted the poorer inhabitants of the lower town.

What little evidence is available about the death rate among Europeans in the nineteenth century confirms improvement over the decades. Bleeker reported a steep decline in mortality from 227.7 per thousand Europeans in Batavia in 1819 to 53 per thousand in 1844.[10] By 1903–11 Ouwehand could report an average per year of just 28.9 deaths per thousand Europeans.[11] When postmortem examination by doctor became compulsory for Europeans in 1907, it was possible to comment more accurately on causes of death. Over the period 1908–11, it appeared that the fatal illnesses among Europeans were, in descending order of importance, cholera, tuberculosis, typhoid, malaria and dysentery.[12] Because the nature of infectious diseases was not understood until the late nineteenth century, most Europeans were still unable to insulate themselves entirely from the impact of epidemics. In 1864, for example, it was reported that 240 Europeans died during a cholera epidemic, a sizeable proportion of the approximately 4 000 Europeans living in the city at the time, and about 14% of all reported cholera deaths.[13]

Like the Europeans, the Chinese were also to be found mainly in an identifiable area of Batavia, although as the century progressed the Chinatowns proliferated to include not only the 'Chinese camp' just outside the former walled town (the area now known as Glodok) but also Chinese settlements around Pasar Baroe and Pasar Senen, the other commercial centres (Fig. 9.2). According to Bleeker's figures of 1844, the majority of the Chinese were to be found in the lower-lying parts of town.[14] Their living quarters were invariably crowded and subject to flooding, and had poor access to clean drinking water. Of the old Chinese camp, Bleeker wrote that most of the 1 069 closely packed houses there had only dirt floors, and when floods occurred the water sometimes stood three to four feet deep inside. In 1887, an inhabitant of this area complained to one of the Malay-language newspapers that a Chinese stall-holder created a nuisance by letting his ducks loose every day in a ditch whose water local people used for bathing and washing rice and clothes.[15]

Unfortunately the only death rates reported for the Chinese in the nineteenth century are those given in 1844 by Bleeker, whose figures must certainly represent under-reporting: he calculated an average death rate for Chinese in Batavia between 1833 and 1838 of 60.5 per thousand. This compared with an average death rate for Europeans during the same years of 78.8 per thousand, which is likely to have been more accurate.[16] The next reference to death rates for Chinese does not come until Ouwehand's report for the years 1903–11, showing the Chinese with an average death rate of 45 per thousand—considerably higher than the Europeans' rate of 28.9 and less than the Indonesians' rate of 64.3.[17] I have not been able to locate data about diseases suffered by the Chinese in Batavia; it seems likely that they succumbed to the same environmentally related illnesses as the Indonesians, although it was noted by some doctors that typhoid was more often a cause of death among Chinese than among Indonesians.[18]

It is not possible to identify the Indonesians with any one locality in Batavia, since their *kampung* (unplanned residential areas) sprang up all over town, and in every ward except the Chinese camp they predominated; they did after all comprise more than two-thirds of the total urban population. Rather than any geographical generalization, the health record of the Indonesian community is best explained by the fact that they were the poorest group in the town. Whereas the Chinese derived an income chiefly from commerce and the Europeans from higher-level business and bureaucracy, the Indonesians' role was as menials—servants and coolies—and as providers of poorly paid services such as street-vending and laundry. More than other groups, therefore, they were likely to suffer from poor nutrition and housing and their attendant diseases. Evidence suggests there was considerable variation in their living conditions and susceptibility to particular diseases, often according to the area of town in which they lived. In general their housing, built of wood, woven bamboo and thatch among the gardens of the *kampung*, was more airy than that of the Chinese, and often they were able to provide at least some fresh food for themselves in the form of fruit, vegetables and poultry. However, their houses were insanitary and frequently built in swampy areas—the parts of the town deemed less desirable for settlement by the more well-to-do Chinese and Europeans. In the outer *kampung*, the Indonesians were subject to accidents of a more rural than urban nature which were gleefully reported by the European newspapers: falls from fruit-trees were commonplace, and occasionally an Indonesian peacefully defecating at night over a river or canal was attacked by a lurking crocodile.[19]

Indonesians who lived in the more elevated areas of town to the south enjoyed better health than those in the lower part, which was subject to flooding and pervaded by malaria mosquitoes. Even in the 'upper town' however, the death rate among Indonesians reported by Ouwehand for 1903–8 was 48 per thousand: in the 'lower town' it was as high as 98. During the cholera epidemic years 1910–11, the figures were 73 and 148 respectively.[20] As pointed out above, Indonesians had far higher death rates than Chinese and Europeans in the period 1903–11. Ouwehand's investigations of the registers of Muslim cemeteries for 1910–11 revealed that about one-third died of fever (probably malaria). He also reported that a survey of enlargement of the spleen (a good and simple indication of malaria) produced more favourable results the further south one went—declining from a maximum in one area where 90% of those examined had enlarged spleens.[21]

The research of van Gorkom showed a shockingly high death rate of Indonesians in some parts of the town; up to 394.7 per thousand in the sub-district of Djembatan Lima Koelon, a very crowded older part of the 'lower town', during the cholera epidemic of 1911–12.[22] Only a high rate of immigration could keep up the population of such areas, which would otherwise have died out in a few years.

In the old town there were certain notorious pockets of disease—the *pondok* or doss-houses where in 1912 an estimated 12—20 000 coolies lived in unbelievably crowded and insanitary conditions.[23] When epidemics struck, they generally appeared first and with greatest devastation in these *pondok*, since many coolies were wharf-labourers who contracted infections brought in by ship, and diseases were rapidly communicated to fellow-*pondok* dwellers by means of polluted water-supplies and poor sanitation.

Infant mortality rates in nineteenth century Batavia were probably very high, as they were when investigated in the early twentieth century. The Muslim cemetery registers mentioned above showed that of the 14 000 deaths recorded there in 18 months during 1910–11, about a quarter occurred under the age of one year.[24] In 1935–37, de Haas found that among Indonesians nearly 60%, and among Chinese nearly 50%, of total mortality was due to deaths of children below age five.[25] Poor environmental conditions hit children hardest. Since it is likely that the Indonesian population contained proportionately more children than the other two ethnic groups, the higher crude death rate among Indonesians could have been caused in large part by infant mortality. Unfortunately the lack of data about age groups makes it impossible to give age-specific mortality rates for the nineteenth century.

Public Health

If much of the poor health of Batavia's inhabitants could be traced to the environment, what was done in the nineteenth century to tackle that cause? Governments were indeed aware of the need for public works programmes (to improve drainage in particular), yet it was still not politically acceptable among the Dutch for governments to intervene too far, or to spend too much in a colony which was mainly intended to yield a profit. However, the fact that Batavia was the seat of government and contained the highest concentration of Europeans in the Dutch East Indies meant that the authorities felt more obliged to take action there. Corvée and convict labour was used to dig drainage canals. Such works had been undertaken ever since Batavia was founded by the Dutch—it was after all originally a canal town—and recurred in spurts in the nineteenth century. Digging canals could itself be fatal for many workers and for people on nearby land, as such activity often stimulated the spread of malaria. Significantly the authorities found it hard to recruit workers for excavation jobs, so notorious were the health problems.[26]

New drainage canals were built in the 1820s and 1870s, especially after the big floods of the latter decade. On the other hand, many of the canals that criss-crossed the old town were filled in, to avoid the health dangers of stagnant water which had followed the silting up of the river. Similarly, some swamps around the town were drained to prevent the 'miasmas' which European thinkers blamed for fevers. Although in the late eighteenth century the Company had taken measures to forbid burial within the city walls in order to prevent contamination of wells[27], the government took little effective action to ensure that people had safe water supplies. A constant source of complaints in the newspapers of the second half of the nineteenth century was the filthy state of the canals, used as a receptacle for every kind of waste. In the 'lower town' ordinary people were obliged to resort to canals for much of their water, with predictable consequences. During droughts, inhabitants of the lower town had great trouble finding drinking water. Even after artesian wells were sunk in some places in the late nineteenth century, the problem was not solved. For instance, in 1888 the *Bataviaash Nieuwsblad* (21 July) reported that since artesian water hydrants in two *kampung* of the lower town were not working, inhabitants had to buy drinking water brought in from outside, at a cost of three cents for two tins full—at a time when coolies, who were the main dwellers in such areas, earned twenty cents to one guilder a day.[28]

Public health was obviously not considered a major government concern. No attempt was made to deal with sewage, apart from certain regulations (apparently ignored) against emptying rubbish into waterways. The continuing existence of *pondok* proved the failure of government to tackle housing as a source of disease. After the Health Act of 1882 was passed, an Inspector was appointed to police health standards in public places, but one man for the whole of Java could make little impression on the problem. Some efforts were made to improve water supplies by sinking artesian wells, but these were mainly located in 'European' areas. The government excused itself to some extent on the grounds that a large proportion of the area of Batavia was privately owned, and it was considered the responsibility of landlords to improve conditions on their estates.[29]

In the medical arena, the government acknowledged some responsibility, and in the nineteenth century important innovations were made—with little overall impact. A breakthrough which occurred at the beginning of the century was the government's first venture into public preventive medicine in the form of smallpox inoculation. Before the great advances in bacteriological research in the late nineteenth century, smallpox was the only infectious disease for which doctors could offer effective preventive measures. Following the introduction of smallpox vaccine into Java in 1804, the authorities took control of promoting widespread vaccination. They showed considerable ingenuity in training and employing Indonesian vaccinators, including women and Muslim leaders, which helped overcome prejudice against the new technique. By the 1820s thousands of people were being vaccinated each year in the Batavia residency.[30] Undoubtedly this had some effect on mortality, especially among children, who were the main victims of the disease.[31] Smallpox was not wiped out during the nineteenth century in Batavia: a constant stream of immigrants from country areas where inoculation was less common kept the disease alive, but fewer cases were reported than elsewhere in Java, where epidemics sometimes erupted.

Under the Dutch East India Company, medical policy had been concerned only with Company servants—apart from the establishment of the so-called Chinese Hospital, which was financed by taxes on the Chinese community.[32] In the nineteenth century the major medical preoccupation of the government was still with servants of the state, and in particular with the military. The biggest hospital in Batavia, as elsewhere, was still the military hospital. However, as Batavia was a major centre of European settlement, its civilian health service was better than that of most towns. The government provided some civilian medical care, including two or three doctors, two midwives and an apothecary (all European) as well as Indonesian vaccinators and 'native doctors' (*dokter-djawa*). By the second half of the century Batavia had two private doctors as well, who were paid by the government to give some free medical help in order to relieve the burden on its own staff.[33]

In the nineteenth century the authorities undertook the training of Indonesians to help provide medical care. The first move was the recruitment of Indonesian smallpox vaccinators. By 1851 this blossomed into the opening of the so-called *dokter-djawa* school attached to the hospital at Weltevreden. Although it was originally intended to train paramedics with a short course in the Malay language and then send the trainees back to their place of origin, this procedure was later deemed unsatisfactory because the paramedics, having no access to medical literature, were unable to sustain and improve their medical knowledge in isolated regions. From 1875 onwards, a full-scale European-style medical course was introduced and in 1898 the institution became STOVIA (School Tot Opleiding van Inlandsche Artsen—School for Training Indies Doctors), which became famous for nurturing Indonesian nationalist leaders. As far as Batavia was concerned, although it was the centre of training it benefited little from the services of 'native doctors', who were still posted back to their place of origin on completion of training. Looking at the list of graduates from the school,[34] it is significant that only six out of 377 graduates from 1854 to 1900 originated in Batavia, probably because few Batavian Indonesians reached the education level required for entrance.

A more discouraging story could be told about the training of Indonesian midwives. As early as 1817 the Government paid the European midwife in Batavia to instruct Indonesian women as midwives.[35] Later a section was attached to the Weltevreden hospital for the training of women from all over the archipelago, in the same way as had been done for the 'native doctors'; but the school was abolished in 1857 because it was proclaimed 'unsuitable'; there was no real demand by Indonesians for its graduates, it was claimed. Thenceforth the training of midwives was entrusted to individual European doctors.[36] Again, no women from Batavia trained as midwives.

The fact that there were few Western-trained doctors and midwives in Batavia was largely academic; their services were too foreign and expensive for most of the population. Although the poorest could obtain some free services, most European doctors preferred private practice, where a consultation in the 1880s cost two and a half guilders.[37] Similarly, the hospitals where Western medical service was provided for the poor were not popular. The hospitals intended for non-Europeans were the Stadsverband (first-aid post) and the Chinese Hospital, both in the lower town. They treated only a fraction of the sick: about 3–4 000 a year in the Stadsverband and 5–600 in the Chinese Hospital, which from 1827 was supported by Government funds.[38] There were obvious reasons for the failure of hospitals to attract Indonesians, apart from the unfamiliarity of Western medical care. Throughout the century, complaints of over-crowding, poor and unsuitable food, rough and careless nursing and cursory treatment by doctors were recorded.[39] Towards the end of the century, the medical historian Schoute stated, the Stadsverband at Glodok 'was an institution where only convicts, prostitutes and vagabonds were brought— and then with force; no one ever went there voluntarily'.[40] Hospitals were regarded as a last resort for the gravely ill, which naturally perpetuated their reputation for burying rather than curing people.

Medical Systems

What, then, did European medicine have to offer the population of Batavia in the nineteenth century? Apart from smallpox prevention, little was known by Western doctors about the main diseases of Batavia until the late nineteenth century, when first the connection between hygiene and health was understood and then the causes of malaria and cholera were discovered. Even then, the results of those scientific advances did not seriously affect the practice of medicine until the twentieth century. Though the highly respectable and standard medical text of the 1880s, Dr C. L. van der Burg's *De geneesheer in Nederlandsch-Indië* (The Physician in Netherlands India),[41] has some sensible advice to offer about cleanliness and moderation in eating and drinking (ideas stemming, one suspects, as much from Dutch Protestantism as from science), its suggestions for dealing with the major diseases of the time are often almost worthless.

During the first half of the nineteenth century, great debate raged among Europeans about whether cholera was infectious and if so, how. When the first great cholera epidemic threatened Batavia in 1820, the government doctor advised that strict quarantine measures should not be attempted because they would panic people; anyway, he said, the illness was spread by the air.[42] During the 1851 cholera outbreak, official medical advice was to burn fires in the *kampung* 'to cleanse the air', and to clean the bodies and clothes of cholera victims 'in the normal way'[43], which probably meant in river water. By the 1880s, van der Burg was sure that cholera was infectious, but admitted that he knew of no sure preventive or cure. He proceeded, however, to give recipes for cholera drinks based on laudanum, of the kind which were available on demand to Batavia's inhabitants during epidemics in the late nineteenth century. On the other hand, official medical opinion held that beri-beri, which was a serious problem among convicts and soldiers, was an infection—only later was it shown to result from vitamin deficiency.

Van der Burg's work reveals that people were still utterly confused about the causes of malaria; he does not even recommend the use of mosquito-nets as a preventive measure. However, in the second half of the nineteenth century Europeans were becoming aware of the uses of quinine. Van der Burg and even newspapers recommended quinine treatment in case of fever.[44] Indeed, in the late nineteenth century cinchona was grown extensively on plantations in West Java, but quinine was not freely available or cheap enough for most people, and its medical limitations were still not understood.[45]

With low demonstrable effectiveness added to high cost and unfamiliarity, it is not surprising that Western medicine made little inroad into the lives of most citizens of Batavia. But the medical menu was much more diverse than the government acknowledged: it offered both professional services and folk or commercial remedies over a span of medical systems—Western, Indonesian and Chinese. Relatively highly paid, formally trained medical professionals included some Arabic *hakim*, Malay and Javanese *dukun* (healers) and Chinese doctors, in addition to European physicians and surgeons. Such people had high status within their own ethnic communities and even beyond. Statistics on European doctors in Batavia have already been mentioned; although the numbers of other personnel are uncertain, some indication can be gained from official reports that the residency of Batavia (a region with roughly ten times the population of the town) had 1 074 Indonesian *dukun* and 89 Chinese doctors in 1885.[46] Most of the Chinese would have been located in town, since few of their compatriots lived in rural areas.

Many Western doctors felt able to learn from Asian medicine, partly perhaps because their own background put them in sympathy with Asian views on 'humours' (hot, cold, wet and dry and so on)[47] but also no doubt because, aware of the deficiencies of their own science and cut off from the expertise and medical supplies of their own homeland, they hoped that they could learn to use local ingredients. A series of students followed in the footsteps of the famous Rumphius in investigating the medicinal properties of Indonesian plants. Bleeker, author of a lengthy study in 1843–45 of the fauna and flora of Batavia, believed, like other writers of the time, that local remedies were efficacious. For instance, he remarked that the peel of the mangostan was considered locally to be a cure for some forms of chronic dysentery, and mentioned that he often used it in the hospital at Weltevreden.[48]

For their Asian counterparts, Western doctors in Batavia had rather less respect:

Native servants affected by intermittent fevers were visited by old women from the *kampung* (so-called *dukun*). The only help which these women rendered was the making of many mysterious gestures and the smearing or rather spitting upon of some part of the body (e.g. toes, back, etc.) with red *sirih* (betel-nut) juice, freshly chewed. The patients had unlimited faith in this form of treatment.[49]

Such comments as this one from Bleeker came at a time when Western doctors had scarcely ceased using leeches for frequent bleeding of malaria patients. Here it is worth bearing in mind a distinction recently pointed out by David Mitchell in his study of fold medicine in Sumba:[50] medicine is both a science—the skills of altering the natural course of illness—and an art—helping people to cope with the experience of illness. In nineteenth century Batavia the science of medicine was not very advanced among any of the available systems, and it was doubtless galling for European doctors to find that the art of medicine was much more successfully practised by their rivals.

It is quite difficult in any medical system to draw the line between professionals and others. In Batavia the term *dukun* in particular seemed to cover an enormous range of medical activities. In a recent study of traditional healers, Boedhihartono lists eleven specialist *dukun*, including *dukun bayi* (birth attendant), *dukun pijet* (massage healer), *dukun jamu* (herbalist), and *dukun ramal* (fortune-teller).[51] Some of these people could perhaps be classified as paramedics, like midwives and 'native doctors'. Other

practices are definitely more concerned with the art of medicine
rather than its science: in Western eyes such practitioners would
be equated with the 'quacks' who frequented European society. In
another part of the medical spectrum were people who merely sold
prepared medicines: these ranged from European apothecaries to
Chinese shop-sellers with their imported dried merchandise and
Javanese pedlars, usually female, of *jamu* (herbal medicines).[52]

It is worth noting that as one progresses across the spectrum in
all three medical systems, from paramedics and pedlars to highly
paid and trained specialists, the number of women practitioners
decreases. It seems that their status also declined during the
century. For instance, there are accounts of famous Chinese
women doctors in Batavia in the eighteenth century, but not in the
nineteenth;[53] the down-grading of the training of Indonesian midwives as compared with the up-grading of 'native doctors' is
significant; and by the end of the nineteenth century European
male doctors went out of their way to deride the female authors of
household medical handbooks such as that by Njonja E. van
Gent-Detelle.[54]

Batavians' Responses to Disease

While most people probably stayed largely within either a
Western or an Asian medical system, others were eclectic. Most
foreign immigrants were males, who formed liaisons with or married local Eurasians, Indonesian or Indonesian-Chinese women,
who naturally brought their own culture into nominally 'European' or 'Chinese' households.[55] Thus there are many reports of
non-Indonesian families turning to medical treatments outside
their own culture. European doctors complained in 1818 that in
the Chinese Hospital, where they were supposed to be supervising
care,

Chinese and other quacks and so-called *dukun* who also have free
access to this house, make profits and rob the sick of their money with the
deceitful promise of a speedy recovery or by selling all kinds of things,
which they call remedies; thereby they urge the patients to ignore or
reject the prescriptions and medicines given them by the Town Doctor or
Physician.[56]

Medical books by European (usually Eurasian) women happily
mixed Western and Asian home remedies (thus accounting for

some of the scorn of European doctors). Europeans were fond of being massaged by the expert hands of the *dukun pijet*. Van der Burg noted that the Chinese liked to consult European physicians— but they also consulted Chinese doctors and Indonesian *dukun* and often used Chinese medicines as well as the prescriptions of the European doctor.[57] Poor Indonesians probably had less choice. They relied on cheap preventive medicines as well as cures— buying *jamu* and growing their own herbs.[58]

Despite the range of medical choices open to Batavia's citizens, there is no evidence that any was efficacious in dealing with the problems of urban ill-health experienced in the nineteenth century. As malaria-bearing mosquitoes continued to breed unchecked in the brackish marshes in and around the city, and as Batavia's population grew, it seems likely that malaria claimed increasing numbers of victims.[59] Improved communications also resulted in the rapid spread of infections: the new scourge was cholera. The numbers of people struck down by both malaria and cholera in Batavia indicate a medical problem beyond the control of the preventive and curative systems of the time.

How then did people cope? In some cases not very well at all; cholera in particular was likely to cause panic. Exceptional individuals worked heroically against fearful odds. Roorda van Eysinga wrote of the 1821 epidemic:

There were days when in Batavia 160 people were carried off by [cholera]; seized by strong cramps, they gave up the ghost in a few moments . . . I had the good fortune not to be infected, and to see many of my patients recover; but I was so weary that I could hardly keep going. It was very difficult, in an intensely hot climate, to treat patients who, if they belonged to the lower class, mostly lived in little brick rooms. These rooms had to be kept closed to prevent any draught. Then the patients had to be bathed with warm water, and the terrible condition of the victims whom I instructed to be rubbed with arrack (which I did myself when help was lacking) made the treatment one of those unbearable employments which should rightly be described as *hellish*.[60]

The novelist Daum gives a picture of the demoralizing effect on Batavia's Europeans of one of the epidemics of the 1880s:

Cholera raged furiously. Everyone did his best to disguise it and not stir up fear, but one could not ignore the fact that the natives were carrying away their corpses by the dozen, and that from early morning until darkness fell, their melancholy *Allah ill' Allah* echoed along the roads.[61]

Even Daum's main character, the dashing Connie, is mortally afraid: she drinks champagne heavily as a preventive and has a medicine chest full of patent remedies.

Although the Chinese and Indonesians had no such eloquent recorders of their reactions to epidemics, contemporary newspapers do give occasional glimpses. It appears that people sometimes panicked and abandoned the victims of disease, although to judge from the scarcity of such reports, this was unusual. In 1883 a European paper claimed that three Indonesian cholera victims, one of them a woman, had been found in a shed by the river: 'Their lips and hands were already blue. According to our information, the people of the *kampung* behind . . . put them out when they showed signs of illness and left them to their fate'.[62] More commonly, people resorted to religion as a protection. As individuals, Indonesians placed great reliance in the powers of 'holy water'.

There were also community rituals to ward off disease. As *Sinar Terang* reported on 21 August 1888:

It is now cholera season, so the people of *kampung* Noordwijk Wetan hold a *selamatan* (ritual) to keep illness out of their *kampung*. Many *kampung* people gather together with *hajis* to read prayers while walking around the entire *kampung*—40 or 50 people, including the superintendent of the ward and his deputy. In front of the open door of a house is placed an earthenware pitcher full of water with seven *peser* (half cents) for the prayers: when the group comes to a house with a pitcher they pray and take the money.

Similarly, *Pembrita Betawi*, on 12 July 1901, reported that in the Chinese Camp and Pasar Senen the Chinese called in the *barongsay* (dragon) players at times of cholera epidemic:

When cholera threatens the city of Batavia, the *barongsay* players make some profit, for every night the creature roams about the Chinatown being rewarded with gifts—some give a pair of candles but most give a packet containing money. It is said that these *barongsay* players can earn up to ten guilders a night. If they come to a house where there has recently been a death in the family, the players are invited to enter and to dance around the yard with the *barongsay*, for which they are given a parcel full of coins. Some superstitious Chinese families invite the *barongsay* to perform in their house every night, because they believe the cholera demon fears the *barongsay*.

As a most dramatic and quick-acting disease, cholera elicited extreme reactions. Other slower-working but equally deadly illnesses were probably accepted more fatalistically, as easier to fit into the common pattern of high mortality in those days.

Batavia in Context

Comparisons between Batavia and other north Javanese ports are difficult due to the lack of urban mortality statistics in the nineteenth century. However, the slower rate of growth of Batavia is striking when compared with Surabaya, its closest rival. Whereas Raffles reported Surabaya in 1815 as having a population of 24 574, compared with 47 083 for Batavia,[63] by 1895 Surabaya, with 124 529 people, outstripped Batavia's 114 566.[64] One likely cause of Batavia's slower growth was the less crowded hinterland, which probably created less pressure for migration to town, but Batavia's natural growth rate may also have been depressed by greater unhealthiness. It is significant that from 1873 to 1894 the death rate of the residency of Batavia was consistently reported as higher than that of Surabaya; indeed the death rate frequently exceeded the birth rate.[65] We can consider these statistics in conjunction with some more detailed studies made in the early twentieth century. These reveal first of all that in 1911/12 urban Batavia had a far higher death rate than West Java as a whole[66] and secondly, that in 1903–11 urban Batavia's mortality averaged 57.8 per thousand compared with 36 for Surabaya.[67] There seems to be some evidence, therefore, for the belief that the city of Batavia was unusually unhealthy, compared both with rural areas and with the most similar town, Surabaya.

Comparison with European cities bears out the modern argument that to talk of tropical disease is misleading, since what are now regarded as exotic tropical disorders, such as malaria and cholera, were once widespread in the West, too.[68] Cholera ravaged European towns in the nineteenth century, and in the first half of that period Dutch towns experienced malaria epidemics.[69] Descriptions of living conditions in European towns in 1800–50 parallel those in Batavia: e.g., a Dutch source refers to the poor of Gouda in 1842 drinking untreated water from the canals into which the drains emptied.[70] The main medical difference between Batavia and European towns seems to be that in the second half of the century European governments introduced effective public health measures on a wide scale, and nutrition improved as a result of rising wages and cheaper and more adequate food supplies. In both British and Dutch cities sanitation, housing and the environment generally improved, and the death rate declined accordingly.[71] Van Gorkom reported that in 1894 the death rate in the large cities of Holland fell below that in the countryside for the first time in the century.[72]

As usual, governments were slow to transfer to the colonies lessons learned at home. Cholera, which as a new disease had acted as a catalyst for reform in Europe in the nineteenth century, brought very little change in health policy in the Indies. The Dutch Health Acts of 1865, which 'opened a new era of medical and health care',[73] were only dimly reflected in the Indies' Health Act of 1882. Batavia experienced less benefit from a newly awakened health awareness in Holland than Indian cities did from British campaigners like Chadwick. There was nothing in nineteenth century Batavia to compare with the sanitation crusades of British administrators in towns such as Allahabad.[74] Although no comparative statistics are available for the nineteenth century, both Ouwehand and van Gorkom found that Batavia's death rate in the first decade of the twentieth century not only exceeded that of other Javanese towns but also compared unfavourably with that of other large Asian cities—even Calcutta.[75] Clearly the massive drop in European mortality made no impression on the overall picture.

In nineteenth century Batavia, attempts to improve living conditions for non-Europeans were virtually non-existent, while care was taken to provide well-laid-out suburbs for the colonial elite, and artesian wells were sunk mainly in 'their' areas of town. A similar social short-sightedness characterized most regimes in the nineteenth century; what differentiated Batavia from many other cities was that there one's chances in the stakes for life and death were increasingly determined by one's position in the racial hierarchy created by the colonial rulers.

I wish to thank Patrick Miller for his assistance with the preparation of graphics.

1. *Captain Cook's Journal, 1768–71* (1893; reprint Adelaide, Libraries Board of South Australia, 1968), 364.

2. On the issue of the early unhealthiness of Batavia, see Leonard Blusse, 'An Insane Administration and an Unsanitary Town: the Dutch East India Company and Batavia (1619–1799)', in R. Ross and G. T. Telkamp (eds), *Colonial Cities* (The Hague, Nijhoff, 1984).

3. It is impossible to determine with any certainty what the death rate was for Batavia before the twentieth century. Even firm population figures for Batavia are hard to find until regular official data for towns were issued in 1880 (*Koloniaal*

Verslag 1880, Bijlage A; hereafter cited as *KV* plus year). Registration of births and deaths was not compulsory until the twentieth century. The authorities did begin recording general birth and death rates among Indonesians in Batavia in 1873, but these were reported only at the residency level, which does not allow conclusions to be drawn for the population of the town, which was about one-tenth the size of the residency.

4. Admittedly, the question of Java's population growth in the nineteenth century is a hotly disputed one. Widjojo Nitisastro, *Population Trends in Indonesia* (Ithaca, Cornell University Press, 1970), 5–6, presents the often-quoted figures that show Java increasing from almost 5 million in 1815 to almost 29 million in 1900, and then proceeds to throw doubt on their reliability, especially for the first half of the century. See also Peter Boomgaard, 'Morbidity and Mortality in Java, 1820–1880', and Peter Gardiner and Mayling Oey, 'Morbidity and Mortality in Java, 1880–1940', above.

5. Statistical sources are T. S. Raffles, *The History of Java* (1817; reprint Kuala Lumpur, Oxford University Press, 1965), 1: Table 1; *KV*, 1902; and *Volkstelling Nederlands-Indië 1930*, 1:132. This constitutes an annual growth rate of 1% from 1815 to 1900 and 4% from 1900 to 1930.

6. Available figures underrepresent the number of probable cholera cases: mild attacks could be confused with simple diarrhoea. As for actual deaths, it was well known that local officials preferred to understate the victims in the area under their jurisdiction, since a high level did not reflect well on themselves. Malaria was often confusingly subsumed in a wider class of 'fevers'. Cf. Boomgaard, op. cit.

7. Cholera figures from *KV*, 1864, 79. Lacking an urban population figure for 1864, I have estimated it from the incomplete statistics given in 'Statistische gegevens, Stad en voorsteden Batavia met betrekking tot te heffen belastingen 1860–62'. Residentie Archieven, Batavia, no. 35, Arsip Nasional, Jakarta.

8. *KV*, 1880, Bijlage A.

9. M. L. van Breemen, 'De Verbreiding van malaria te Weltevreden en Batavia', *Geneeskundige Tijdschrift voor Nederlandsch-Indië* (hereafter cited as *GTNI*) 58 (1918), 633–5. Blusse, op. cit., links the silting up of the Ciliwung River to the clearing of the hinterland for sugar cultivation in the eighteenth century. See Boomgaard, op. cit., on the relevant species of *Anopheles*.

10. P. Bleeker, 'Bijdragen tot de Geneeskundige Topographie van Batavia. IV. Bevolking', *Tijdschrift voor Nederlandsch-Indië* 8, 2 (1846), 472. Swaving calculated a further decline, after a cholera peak of 73.9 per thousand Europeans in 1853, to 50.3 in 1860; see W. J. van Gorkom, *Ongezond Batavia, vroeger en nu* (Batavia, Javasche Boekhandel, 1913), 43.

11. C. D. Ouwehand, 'Mortaliteit te Batavia', *GTNI* 52 (1912), 298.

12. Van Gorkom, op. cit., 53. No analysis of differences among Europeans by sex or age is made in this reference.

13. *Java-Bode*, 21 September 1864; *KV*, 1864, 79. It is likely that deaths from cholera were better reported for Europeans than for other ethnic groups, thus leading to an overstatement of the proportion of Europeans among the dead.

14. Bleeker, op. cit., 495–6.

15. *Pembrita Betawi*, 13 April 1887.

16. Bleeker, op. cit., 459. Bleeker's mortality statistics, based on local reports, were probably most reliable for Europeans and least for Indonesians, for whom he cites an unbelievably low death rate of 40.3 per thousand between 1833 and 1838 (ibid., 457–8). This must be due to under-reporting.

17. Ouwehand, op. cit., 298.

18. E.g., ibid., 308.; J. E. Dinger, A. Marseille and J. W. Tesch, 'Onderzoek naar de epidemiologie der febris typhoidea in de studie-wijk voor hygiene te Batavia', *GTNI* 79 (1939), 2714.

19. E.g., *Java-Bode*, 29 March 1856.
20. Ouwehand, op. cit., 297–8.
21. Ibid., 300–6.
22. Van Gorkom, op. cit., 66–7.
23. Ouwehand, op. cit,. 302.
24. Ibid., 303.
25. J. H. de Haas, 'Sterfte naar leeftijdsgroepen in Batavia, in het bijzonder op den kinderleeftijd', *GTNI* 79, 2 (1939), 713.
26. There were continual complaints about the difficulty of finding labour to dig the new harbour at Tanjung Priok and the canal connecting it to Batavia; see *Maandverslagen omtrent de werkzaamheden aan den bouw der Havenwerken van Batavia* (Batavia, 1877–85). D. Schoute, 'De Geneeskunde in Nederlandsch-Indië gedurende de negentiende eeuw', *GTNI* 74 (1934), 886, reports a similar story in 1800–1802 when the Government was making defence and flood works around the town. 1 200–2 400 men were put to work, but 'the rapid death' frightened people so much that scarcely 800 remained. One third of the officers involved died of fever. Cf. Boomgaard, op. cit., on the wider implications of 'man-made' malaria.
27. F. de Haan, *Oud Batavia* (Batavia, G. Kolff & Co., 1922), 2:344.
28. *KV*, 1890, 246.
29. According to official figures (*Regeeringsalmanak*, 1885, Bijlage B), in 1884 18 870 people lived on private estates within Batavia town. This constituted about one-fifth of the total population of the town.
30. Schoute, op. cit., 74 (1934), 1277–83.
31. M. D. Teenstra, *De vruchten mijner werkzaamheden gedurende mijner reize over de Kaap de Goede Hoop naar Java en terug . . .* (Groningen, H. Eeckhoff, 1829), 292, reported that although an estimated one-tenth of all children below fifteen years still died of smallpox in Java, inoculation was having good results; cf. Boomgaard, op. cit.
32. Schoute, op. cit., 74 (1934), 1018.
33. *KV*, 1873.
34. *Ontwikkeling van het geneeskundig onderwijs te Weltevreden, 1851/1926* (Weltevreden, G. Kolff & Co., 1926).
35. Schoute, op. cit., 74 (1934), 1165.
36. Ibid., 75 (1935), 669–70.
37. C. L. van der Burg, *De geneesheer in Nederlandsch-Indië* (Batavia, Ernst & Co., 1883), 1:370.
38. Schoute, op. cit., 74 (1934), 1728.
39. Ibid., passim.
40. Ibid., 75 (1935), 1469.
41. Van der Burg, op. cit.
42. Schoute, op. cit., 74 (1934), 1431.
43. Ibid., 75 (1935), 1051.
44. *Java-Bode*, 26 July 1881; van der Burg, op. cit., 2:84–5.
45. Cf. Boomgaard, op. cit.
46. *KV*, 1887, Bijlage A.
47. Charles Leslie, 'Introduction', in Leslie (ed.), *Asian Medical Systems: a Comparative Study* (Berkeley, University of California Press, 1976), 4.
48. P. Bleeker, 'Bijdrage tot de medische topographie van Batavia', *Tijdschrift voor Nederlandsch-Indië* 5–7 (1843–45). The reference to mangostan is in ibid., 6, 2 (1844), 123.
49. Ibid., 6, 1 (1844), 474–5. This same use of chewed *sirih* was noted by van der Burg, op. cit., 1:68.
50. David Mitchell, 'Folk Medicine in Sumba: A Critical Evaluation', in D. Mitchell (ed.), *Indonesian Medical Traditions* (Monash University, 1982), 2–3.

51. Boedhihartono, 'Current State and Future Prospects of Traditional Healers in Indonesia', in ibid., 23–4.

52. In 1860 there were reported to be thirty Chinese apothecaries in Batavia; 'Algemeen Verslag der Residentie Batavia, 1861', Bijlage no. 13, Arsip Nasional, Jakarta.

53. Claudine Salmon, 'Le role des femmes dans l'emigration Chinoise en Insulinde', *Archipel*, no. 16 (1978), 164. It should be noted that the so-called Chinese women mentioned were actually of Indonesian or part-Indonesian origin, making it unclear what variety of medicine they practised.

54. E.g., van der Burg, op. cit., 1:356–8; cf. van Gent-Detelle, *Boekoe obatobat voor Orang Toea dan anak-anak* (Djocdja, 1880).

55. Susan Abeyasekere, 'Women as Cultural Intermediaries in Nineteenth Century Batavia', in Lenore Manderson (ed.), *Women's Work and Women's Role: Economics and Everyday Life in Indonesia, Malaysia and Singapore* (Canberra, Centre for Development Studies, 1983), 15–30.

56. Schoute, op. cit., 74 (1934), 1170.

57. Van der Burg, op. cit., 1:36.

58. Bleeker, 'Bijdragen tot de medische topographie', 6, 2 (1844), 467–70, noted that various medicinal herbs were grown in *kampung* gardens in Batavia.

59. This conclusion can be drawn from the official statistics (in *KV*) on patients treated by European doctors; cf. Boomgaard, op. cit.

60. P. P. Roorda van Eysinga, *Verschillende reizen en lotgevallen* (Amsterdam, Roorda van Eysinga, 1830–32), 3:146–7.

61. P. A. Daum, *Hoe hij raad van Indië werd* ('s-Gravenhage, J.C. Opmeer, 1888), 112.

62. *Java-Bode*, 1 August 1883.

63. Raffles, op. cit., 2:276–7 and 1:Table 1.

64. *KV*, 1897, Bijlage A.

65. Ibid., 1873–94, Bijlage A.

66. Van Gorkom, op. cit., 61.

67. Ouwehand, op. cit., 298.

68. R. N. Chaudhuri, 'Tropical Medicine—Past, Present and Future', *British Medical Journal*, 21 August 1954, 423.

69. I. J. Brugmans, *Stapvoets voorwaarts. Sociale geschiedenis van Nederland in de negentiende eeuw* (Bussum, Fibula-Van Dishoek, 1970), 75.

70. Ibid., 35. Similar evidence of pollution of the drinking water of the poor in British towns is to be found in F. B. Smith, *The People's Health, 1830–1910* (Canberra, Australian National University Press, 1979), 215–20.

71. A. Querido, *The Development of Socio-Medical Care in the Netherlands* (London, Routledge & Kegan Paul, 1968); Brugmans, op. cit.; G. Rosen, 'Disease, Debility and Death', in H. J. Dyos and M. Wolff (eds), *The Victorian City: Images and Realities* (London, Routledge & Kegan Paul, 1973).

72. Van Gorkom, op. cit., 58–9.

73. Querido, op. cit., 31.

74. J. B. Harrison, 'Allahabad: a Sanitary History', in K. Ballhatchet and J. Harrison (eds), *The City in South Asia: Pre-modern and Modern* (London, Curzon Press, 1980).

75. Van Gorkom, op. cit., 62–64; Ouwehand, op. cit., 297–8.

10 Plague in Java

TERENCE H. HULL

PLAGUE is caused by the bacillus *Pasteurella pestis*.[1] Rodents, and particularly rats, act as hosts to the organism, and while the disease is often fatal to the carrier, it is believed that some species of rat, or perhaps individual members of the species, have developed an immunity to infection, and carry the bacilli in their bloodstreams with no ill effects. Periodically, the bacilli spread to other species which are not immune and the new rodent hosts quickly die. The rapid spread to other rats occurs via fleas, which leave the corpse of early victims in search of food. Sometimes the carrier flea alights on a human rather than another rat, and the disease changes from an epizootic to an epidemic, as large numbers of people contract the infection.[2] Before 1940 the outlook for plague victims was not good. Most sufferers, often over 90%, died within days. The majority developed lumps called 'buboes' which were filled with virulent pus, and suffered high fever, toxaemia and extreme weakness. Within a few days their veins became distended, leading to haemorrhages which give the body a dark pallor, hence the term 'Black Death'. A minority of victims, usually fewer than 10%, manifested infections which centred on the lung (pulmonary plague) or throughout the bloodstream (septicaemic plague), and for them death was more certain and quick. Additionally, people with pulmonary plague could infect others directly, because the bacilli were ejected in droplets as they coughed, but otherwise the disease was only spread through the intervention of a vector such as a flea.

Plague in Indonesian History

It is generally believed that plague did not affect the population of Indonesia prior to 1910,[3] when a cargo ship carrying rice from Burma introduced infected rats and fleas into Surabaya. This

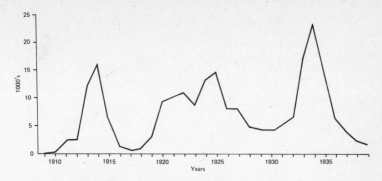

Fig. 10.1. Plague Deaths in Java, 1910–39

probably occurred in October, when the Government was building up food stocks in preparation for anticipated food shortages before the harvest. In November 1910, cases of human plague were identified in Turen, Malang,[4] and by the end of that year seventeen people were reported to have died from the disease. Over the next thirty years the epidemic spread along the volcanic spine of Java, keeping mainly to upland areas, moving slowly from east to west.[5] Official records show over 215 000 deaths between 1911 and 1939, but the actual numbers are undoubtedly somewhat higher (Fig. 10.1). The disease, though distinctive, was not always reported.

By European standards, the demographic impact of plague in Java was unremarkable. It did not constitute a major cause of death in the island as a whole, and even in the districts where the epidemic hit hardest it was erratic, taking victims seemingly at random and leaving the bulk of the population unharmed. While most residencies experienced some form of epidemic, only five had over 10 000 deaths during the thirty years before World War II.[6] The discovery of a practical vaccine in the mid-1930s seemed to spell the end of plague in Indonesia, and the development of antibiotics in the 1940s ensured that even those who contracted the disease could be saved if treatment was started early enough. Thus it is understandable that plague has tended to be ignored in considerations of the medical history of Indonesia. It is a disease of the past, largely overshadowed by more common and persistent ailments which have claimed victims in the millions.

Nonetheless, the history of plague in Java is of broader relevance than the simple analysis of relative epidemiological impact

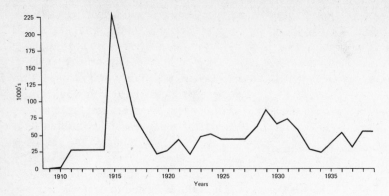

Fig. 10.2. House Improvements in Java, 1910–39

might indicate. Quite out of proportion to its eventual demographic implications, the outbreak of plague in East Java called forth the mobilization of financial and organizational resources unprecedented in the public health services of the colony. Governmental interventions affected Indonesians in major ways, often over long periods of time. Travel was interrupted, tens of thousands of people were put into isolation camps, property was confiscated, homes burned, and, in the eyes of many thousands of families, the bodies of their relatives were outrageously defiled through post-mortem spleen puncture to confirm plague as a cause of death.[7] Over one and a half million houses were refurbished by the government to make them rat proof, many more were inspected for rats' nests by the plague service, and the entire practice of house construction in Java was modified by regulations imposed by the government and through the retraining of village builders (Fig. 10.2). Ironically, whatever beneficial effects such measures may have had in the long run, it is difficult to demonstrate conclusively that they helped to save lives as the epidemic made its westward progress. Plague and the anti-plague campaign, then, may have been of greater significance for the changes they brought to the health and housing systems of Indonesia than for their direct impact on the mortality levels of the native population.

Sources of Data

From the first outbreak in 1910, plague was the object of great concern to the colonial bureaucracy and the small but growing medical profession. Systems of routine record keeping were immediately instituted to aid epidemiological study, and a variety of laboratory and field studies were undertaken to study the habits of the bacilli, rats, fleas and other parasites. Results were reported in the medical journal of the Netherlands Indies and in papers for conferences. Because of the worldwide concern with plague in the first three decades of the century, early workers on plague in Java sought guidance from the international research community to give direction to their planning, and they reported the results of their efforts in English as well as Dutch.

By coincidence, the introduction of plague in Indonesia occurred as a new journal was being launched to deal with matters of public health. The *Mededeelingen van den Burgerlijken Geneeskundigen Dienst in Nederlandsch-Indië* (*MBGDN*; Reports of the Civil Medical Service of the Netherlands Indies) brought out its first issue in 1912, with the entire contents being devoted to analysis of the plague epidemic in Malang. Over the next few years articles frequently appeared discussing the biology of rats or the frequency of fleas on trapped rodents, or the geographic progress of the disease and its relation to temperature, humidity, rainfall and other seasonal factors. In the 1930s (after the journal's name had been changed in 1925 to *Mededeelingen van den Dienst der Volksgezondheid* [*MDVG*; Reports of the Public Health Service]), data on deaths and cases were published as part of the Annual Reports of the Plague Eradication Campaign (*Verslag Betreffende de Pestbestrijding op Java*) or the Public Health Service. Occasionally reports of experiments with vaccination were published, sometimes with summary data on cases of deaths for selected regions. The *MDVG* is the major source for a quantitative analysis of the epidemic.[8]

The First Wave: 1910-1914

The seventeen people who died in Turen in 1910 had come from only two villages. They had probably caught the disease from the fleas of a rat that had contracted the disease in Burma or en route to Surabaya in a cargo ship. Later researchers demonstrated that the fleas could have lived in the warehouse for several days on gunny-sacks after abandoning the corpse of their infected rat-host.[9] Then the starving fleas probably jumped onto another rat which had managed to get into the rice warehouse, and from this source an epizootic of plague among rats in Surabaya was started. Rats may have then travelled on goods wagons out to rural stations where rice was distributed to people needing supplementary grain in the period preceeding the harvest. At this point the disease spread from rats to humans and the epidemic was under way.[10]

In the first months of the outbreak researchers were most concerned with answering the question of why the outbreak started in a rural area rather than the town of Surabaya, where the epizootic must have broken out. Swellengrebel and others conducted various experiments with rats and fleas to shed some light on this problem. They measured the distance rats could travel, the height fleas could jump, various characteristics of the dying rat, and the behaviour of the starving flea. The theory which emerged as plausible, though clearly unprovable, was that the rats of Surabaya were more likely to live under the brick-walled houses in shallow burrows. When they died, their fleas had difficulty travelling up into houses, both because of the distances involved, and because ants on the ground were natural predators. Village house-rats, on the other hand, lived in thatched roofs, or on rafters hidden by mat ceilings. When they died their fleas could jump down to humans living below. Furthermore, fleas are more mobile, and have a longer lifespan in cool areas. Thus they were more likely to infect humans in the upland villages than in the hot coastal cities. This was a special form of the 'rat–flea–human' hypothesis, and according to van Thiel 'Indonesia became the first tropical country where "the hypothesis" was accepted in its full consequences and where measures were taken accordingly'.[11] In practical terms this meant interrupting the line of transmission by removing rats and/or fleas from contact with humans by rat-proofing houses, trapping rats and killing fleas and other parasites. However, at this stage they were unsure as to whether the flea was the only vector, or whether other parasites might also be infective.

As the research continued, the plague was spreading. From Turen it moved to Karanglo, and by March 1911 cases were reported in nearly all of the districts of Malang and in Kediri and Surabaya. By the end of the year over 2 000 people had died. In 1912, a similar number of people were affected. It probably appeared to many officials that the epidemic could be either confined to a small area of East Java or with appropriate measures even eradicated before serious increases in the number of deaths.

The European officials took the disease very seriously—haunted perhaps by the spectre of the Black Death which had ravaged their own flat land in the past—but Javanese villagers could have had little concept of the illness or its lethal potential. How then must they have felt when the government, in February 1912, set up road blocks on the major thoroughfares in the affected areas and insisted on fumigating all clothing and goods with carbon disulphide (CS_2) gas before travellers could proceed? Swellengrebel[12] reported that in the month between 14 February and 15 March 1913 over 56 000 travellers were disinfected and their clothes thoroughly searched for parasites, which were sent to the laboratory for analysis. Nearly 3 000 parasites were found, of which only three were rat fleas, and only two of these were of a type implicated in the transmission of plague. The rest were common lice (*Pediculus hominis*) or bedbugs (*Cimex rotundus*).

Despite this demonstration that Javanese were largely free of rat fleas, the government redoubled its efforts to control the spread of infection by fumigation, to kill all the possible vectors, and by rat-proofing dwellings. One prominent researcher in East Java at this time was Dr O. L. E. de Raadt. As the Assistant Inspector of the Civil Medical Service and manager of the anti-plague campaign in Malang he was an indefatigable scientist, designing elaborate experiments to test the physical prowess of rats and fleas. In June 1913 he wrote a paper which revealed a particularly important attitude in the light of later events. Titled 'Can the Plague be Spread by Head-Lice?', the paper reported on a series of trials whereby lice 'obtained by combing the luxuriant hair of a female plague patient' were crushed and injected into five rodents. All five died within a few days. 'This proves', wrote de Raadt, 'that head-lice which have sucked the blood of plague patients have absorbed the plague virus and must consequently be considered capable of transmitting the disease.'[13] Humans, then, rather than being the random, helpless victims of a disease carried by rat fleas, were thus implicated as hosts themselves, and the various parasites common on the human body were taken to be dangerous vectors which had to be controlled to prevent rampant infection.

The number of plague deaths and places affected rose dramatically during 1913, and cases were found in Surakarta and Madura that were thought to have been carried there by travellers or in goods vans. As the end of the year approached, it was clear that the epidemic was going to achieve a five-fold increase in victims and that some more systematic measures would have to be taken to control the disease. Throughout 1914 the programme of fumigation, house improvement, isolation of victims and evacuation of villages was implemented under the direction of the Civil Medical Service, the local government authorities and the Technical Service, the latter being largely in charge of public works. Serious disagreements over tactics arose. Dr P. C. Flu argued for fumigation of village houses and disinfection of clothing, on the grounds that isolation and evacuation of the population were very unpopular and that villagers generally went back to the villages at night to care for their gardens and guard their property. Proponents of evacuation (including Otten) countered that fumigation was too expensive, and much disliked by householders, who were thus tempted to hide the fact of plague deaths in order to avoid the procedure. Both groups complained that the Technical Service's programme of refurbishing houses was too slow to be acceptable to villagers, and in any case the improvements often did not reach the necessary standard to prevent infestation by rats.

On 29 December 1914 a resolution was issued by the Chief-Inspector and Head of the Civil Medical Service ordering the then Inspector, Assistant Head of the Service, to take control of all matters concerning the plague in the plague districts, and to move to Malang to establish the headquarters of a special Plague Service. Dr W. J. van Gorkom took up this post on 2 January 1915. Three weeks later the Governor-General signed an ordinance giving authority for the new service to manage all aspects of the anti-plague campaign except quarantine (which was covered by a separate ordinance). The Head moved quickly to establish a new administrative structure for the service. In September 1914 the Chief-Inspector had defined the duties of the medical staff as coming partially under the control of territorial leaders, but now the Head of the Plague Service established the autonomy of the Service in the plague districts by overriding that notional control. Management, he declared, 'has been put in the first instance in the hands of medical men',[14] and it may be inferred from this that he identified the faults of the previous system as being the result of the disorganization or ignorance of lay authorities. The Head of the Technical Service requested a leave of absence in January, and soon after was dismissed, thus leaving the way open for the complete integration of all activities under the medical authorities. 'There is only one single service', declared van Gorkom,

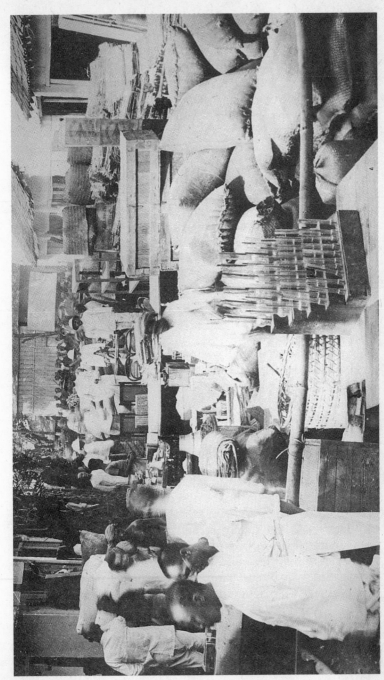

Fig. 10.3. Inspection of houses and household effects during the plague-fight in Java (reproduced courtesy of the Koninklijk Instituut voor de Tropen).

' . . . there can be never any question of independence' of any of the subdivisions.[15] Moreover, though the various ordinances under which medical affairs were organized mentioned a variety of measures to be taken on the basis of 'technical advice', van Gorkom denied that this implied any autonomy of action by technical specialists. Rather, 'everything necessary in that respect shall be done in concurrence with a medical man'.[16] The new Plague Service thus marked the triumph of those who advocated strong vertical chains of command under the leadership of medical specialists. Non-medical activities were clearly subordinate to medical authority, and were regarded as being fully integrated components of the Service. Justifying all these reforms was the threat of plague. Strong immediate action was needed, it was argued, because of the horrendous consequences of the spread of the disease, and only the medical profession understood the disease well enough to determine the appropriate strategy. By this time nearly 15 000 Javanese had died in the epidemic, and the government turned to doctors to prevent catastrophe.

Remission: 1915–1919

The newly reorganized Plague Service continued the practices of the previous campaign but focused all planning and execution on issues that were taken to be of particular importance in the epidemiology of the disease. Isolation of family members of victims was now formally recommended to prevent the spread of the disease by lice or other parasites. Suspected cases were to be notified to the authorities immediately, and if the victim had already died (as was the case in the majority of reports)[17] the funeral was to be delayed to allow a surgeon or *mantri* (health worker) time to perform the spleen puncture to confirm the diagnosis of plague. Verified cases were to be buried quickly thereafter, and the family members removed to a temporary shelter some distance from the village. Their clothing was to be thoroughly disinfected, and they were to wash themselves with disinfectant soap. While fumigation of houses with carbon disulphide gas under tarpaulin was common before 1915, Otten demonstrated that the procedure was not justified because rats moved back in the dwellings soon after the canvas covers were removed. In any case the procedure was both cumbersome and costly. Thus priority was shifted to making structures rat proof, by replacing thatch roofs with tiles, and building rafters designed to prevent rats from building nests unnoticed. A general clean-up was also advocated to remove rubbish that might otherwise serve as nesting places. These improvements were to be examined by a medical specialist who could attest that they met medical, in addition to engineering, standards.

Plague *mantri* were trained and sent to villages to serve as contacts between doctors and the people. They were to live in the villages, so the local population would learn to trust them and willingly report any suspected cases of plague immediately. Because it was known that the population were generally wary of the plague officials—after all, they imposed some very harsh measures—the *mantri* and the surgeons were instructed to 'carry some medicaments and some wound-dressing requisites, to be distributed amongst the population on application'. This, it was hoped, would 'popularize' the Service. The medicines were mainly simple creams and syrups, and, interestingly, the fieldworkers were instructed *not* to give plague serum[18] as a prophylactic unless it was specifically requested, 'because of the aversion of the population against injections'.[19]

Van Gorkom was optimistic in May 1915 that the measures were producing the desired effect. The number of cases being reported was declining, even as the method of identifying cases was improving. By the end of the year the number of deaths reported for East Java was only a third of the previous year's total. Overall figures were not down by as large a factor, because a new outbreak of the disease in Surakarta had claimed 1 406 lives. As a result, the Surakarta residency was added to the Plague Service area in March 1915. Over the next two years the total number of deaths continued to fall, though new outbreaks were reported in Rembang, Semarang and Yogyakarta. It must have seemed that the measures taken by the Service were effective and that the epidemic could be controlled through the application of proper epidemiological procedures. Unlike India (where 4.2 million people died between 1909 and 1918), it appeared that Java would be spared the horrors of a major catastrophe, because of the thorough understanding of the rat–flea–human line of transmission and the development of an effective public health campaign to address the problem scientifically.

The Second Wave: Central Java 1919–1928

Despite the major efforts being made to improve houses in villages, the numbers of deaths began to climb after 1917, because the disease began to affect more villages in Central Java, where the Plague Service was not well established. Thus, even as tens of thousands of houses were being repaired in Malang and Madiun, thousands of people were dying in Kedu. Otten[20] referred to the 'explosive' character of the outbreaks in Central Java in 1919, and a map showing the dates at which subdistricts recorded their first cases reveals the steady spread of the epidemic from the slopes of Mt Ungaran near Semarang, south to the slopes of Mt Sendoro and Mt Sumbing and then east to Merbabu and Merapi, completely encircling each of these volcanoes within a year. This put the Service under considerable pressure. It was not possible to train staff fast enough or mobilize resources completely enough to cover the rapidly expanding territory of the epidemic. The strategy of isolation–evacuation–refurbishing was both difficult to coordinated and very expensive. Thus researchers were encouraged to develop less costly means of dealing with the epidemic.

Vaccination appeared to be one promising avenue. Efforts were directed at the development of a live plague vaccine that would offer immunity over an extended period of time but would not cause serious side-effects. Unfortunately, one of the scientists, a man named Borger, contracted an infection while working in the laboratory and died soon after. Flu reported that because of this incident 'the attempts . . . to get a vaccine against plague were stopped' in the Netherlands Indies.[21] In fact, work continued in the early twenties, and a field test of Haffkine's vaccine from India and a 'Java Strain' was conducted in Central Java by Otten in 1920–21. The results were not encouraging, since an immediate immunity of only 50% was obtained, and this declined over time.[22] It appeared that for the time being, at least, the Service should continue to concentrate on house refurbishing and inspection.

Refinement of the 'Rat–Flea–Human' Hypothesis

Many of the measures undertaken in the early years of the epidemic were based on the assumption that fleas were unaffected in their role as vectors of disease between rodent and human victims. Researchers in Malang reading the reports from India were intrigued by the problem of explaining exactly how the flea passed bacilli into the human bloodstream. The British in India contended that the fleas contaminated the blood with their excrement while they were feeding. Swellengrebel was sceptical, and in 1913 reported that 'Mr. Otten and myself repeatedly observed large quantities of these fleas sucking blood, but we never could detect a flea defecating'.[23] In consequence they concluded that 'rat-fleas in Java are able to introduce plague-bacilli into the body of their host without defecating', and, instead, transmission must be through the fleas' proboscis, but 'whether from the salivary glands or from the mid-gut by regurgitation, is a problem as yet unsolved'.[24] Even more of a problem was the question of why the flea would regurgitate blood into the victim. Unlike the *Anopheles* mosquito, which passes malaria plasmodium mixed in the anti-coagulant fluid injected in the victim's bloodstream prior to feeding, the flea does not use such procedures. A paper published in England by Bacot and Martin in 1914, in a special supplement on plague in the *Journal of Hygiene,* provided the explanation. Fleas were not just neutral transmitters of the disease, but were themselves victims of the plague bacilli, which formed colonies blocking the gizzard, proventriculus and stomach. As the flea bit a rat or human and began sucking their blood, this blockage prevented ingestion into the stomach. Instead, the starving insect quickly tired, and the elastic recoil of the proventricular valve and the oesophagus forced blood back into the bloodstream, carrying some of the bacilli which had been blocking the flea's digestive track. Moreover, infected fleas were found to have very short lifespans under high temperatures, thus helping to explain why the disease seemed to be more common in cooler upland areas. But most important, Bacot and Martin established that while many other parasites such as lice might become infected with plague, their physiology was such that they did not experience blockage and thus were not normally *infective.* The flea most likely to act as vector was found to be the *Xenopsylla cheopis*, which was also most commonly found on house rats.[25]

These discoveries had clear policy implications, but as Hirst remarks, 'reorientation of ideas did not take place for many years'.[26] There are a number of reasons why this should have been the case in Java. First, the policy makers were themselves committed researchers who were busy defending their own theories of transmission at the time the Bacot and Martin paper appeared. De

Raadt, Swellengrebel and Otten had a considerable investment both emotionally and financially in their own laboratories. Second, as colonial administrators they were acutely conscious of competition with the British colonial administration and regarded most of the plague research from India with scepticism. The fact that Bacot and Martin worked in the Lister Institute in London may have prevented their work being well regarded or widely recognized in Java. Finally, though it is hard to establish through documents, a form of psychological inertia may have sustained belief in general theories of transmission long after a specific vector had been identified, since the involvement of lice, bedbugs, and fleas other than *X. cheopis* implied the sort of human responsibility for disease which many Dutch officials conveniently attributed to the Javanese.

Gradually the Plague Service modified its techniques in line with financial realities, scientific discoveries and the geographic challenges posed by the epidemic. As it moved westward, the disease affected villages located in increasingly difficult terrain. The massive efforts at evacuation, fumigation and roadblocks characteristic of East Java ten years earlier were not found as often in Central Java in the twenties. Instead, a focused policy of house improvement and inspection became routine, and in annual reports graphs abounded showing plague deaths in each subdistrict, with arrows pointing out the starting and completion dates of house improvement. Invariably, and not surprisingly, the improvements were completed about the same time as the deaths fell to zero. However, in a remarkably large number of cases, the house improvement programme did not start until *after* the deaths had reached a peak and were declining. Nonetheless, the Service claimed that the data showed clearly that 'the disease disappeared as if by magic from the infected subdistricts as soon as the improvement of housing conditions was taken in hand'.[27]

In 1925 a Division of Public Health Education was established in Java as part of the Hygiene Campaign. In co-operation with the Rockefeller Foundation, the government set up field stations, and in 1933 opened a school for the training of hygiene *mantri*, who were to assist villagers to improve their health conditions by adopting sanitary procedures for cooking, washing, sleeping and eating. The manual used by the *mantri* stressed the need for pit latrines, tile roofs, fresh air and clean hands.[28] As part of their training, the *mantri* spent equal time in classrooms and villages over a two-year period. They were the prototypes of the modern primary health-care worker.

Coincidentally, the hygiene programme was getting under way as the Plague Service was entering its second decade, and both focused on housing as the primary issue in health care. There was a major difference in approach, though. While the Plague Service stressed *intervention* and a high degree of medical supervision of activities, J. L. Hydrick, the Rockefeller-sponsored doctor, advocated education aimed at promotion of community awareness and self-sufficiency.[29] The plague campaign in East Java had been a singular incursion by a public health programme into villages, but by the late twenties plague workers were only one of a number of health specialists making regular visits to discuss house improvement.[30] In all likelihood this facilitated modifications in the way the Service handled its own tasks. In 1915 van Gorkom had contended that the Service would have to restrict its modifications of houses to rat-proofing, because of 'the character of the dwellings' improvement as an emergency measure against a special danger'.[31] By 1928 improvement of housing was being accorded a higher priority by the government for reasons other than plague, and thus the Service maintained its programme in Central Java and Surakarta in 1928–30, even after the numbers of cases had fallen substantially (see Fig. 10.3).

Ironically, years later it was contended that the reduction in plague deaths due to house improvement was offset by an increase in deaths due to malaria. Removal of the kitchen from the main house and improvement of ventilation meant that more mosquitoes were attracted inside, including those carrying the malaria plasmodia.[32]

The Third Wave: West Java, 1930–1934

There had been some cases of plague in West Java in 1920 and 1921 when the Central Java epidemic was at its peak, but they were confined to a small area in Batavia. From 1923 on, the number of cases grew, first in Cirebon and later in the Priangan, but until 1931 the annual number of plague deaths in the province was kept under 2 000 per year. In 1932 the total reached 4 366, and in 1933 over 15 000 people died, mainly in the Priangan. 'The causes' of the outbreak, according to the Plague Service Annual Report for 1933, 'are not of a peculiar nature; in the natural course of events

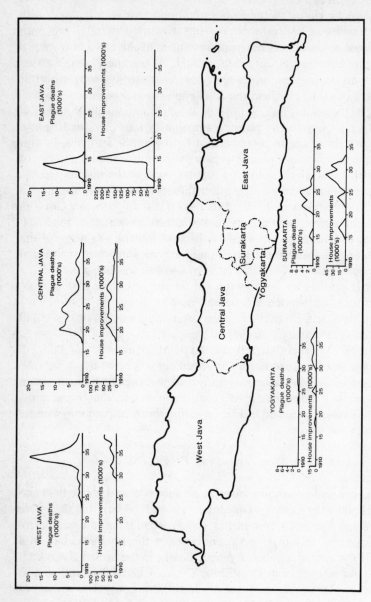

Fig. 10.4. Plague Deaths and House Improvements in Java, by District, 1910–39

one would expect sooner or later a rapid and violent dispersal of the disease, from the moment the plague penetrated the Priangan where the dense population and the mountain climate favour spreading'.[33] However, twenty years of experience in dealing with plague in East and Central Java apparently did not prepare the Plague Service for the events in the Priangan regency, where more people died in the three years 1933–35 than were affected in the entire province of East Java, 1910–39.

The events in West Java are neatly summarized in the graphs of Figure 10.3 and the data in Tables 10.1 and 10.2 (see Appendix). As the most serious outbreak of the Java epidemic was gathering momentum, the programme for house improvements was being cut back. The budget of 1 650 000 guilders in 1932 fell to 844 000 in 1933, but in terms of realized expenditures the position was even worse. From a 1929 peak of 1.8 million guilders, the economic depression pressed government expenditure on house improvement down to 1.5 in 1930, then to 1.4, 1.0, 0.8 and finally to 0.65 in 1934. Despite the fact that the most important element of the programme was being severely cut back in the face of the most serious outbreak of plague to date, H. J. Rosier, then head of the campaign, reported in 1934 that 'the success of house-improvement was sufficient everywhere, as usual'.[34] This apparently sanguine remark was offset by the report that in the 'Priangan a good many economic objections against the house-improvement were made'.[35]

The problems of the Service were not only economic. In 1933 serious incidents in Garut and Tegal-Brebes indicated the strong aversion of the population to the spleen-puncture procedure which had become the cornerstone of the intelligence operation's attempts to determine plague deaths. In one case an official was murdered.[36] In the same year 101 people in Garut were reported as having refused the procedure, while 888 clandestine burials were discovered. In response, and despite the serious economic times, the Service determined that the intelligence department charged with seeking out cases would have to be increased in the Priangan, to deal with the rapidly increasing number of cases and the difficulties encountered in dealing with opposition from families.

Breakthrough: 1934–39

In October 1934 Dr Otten, who was at this time Director of the Pasteur Institute in Bandung, reported that he had successfully developed a live-plague vaccine which was substantially more effective than the Haffkine and Java strains which he had used in 1920–21 in Central Java. Initial tests showed a 90% immunity and almost no side-effects. Permission was given for a preparatory test vaccination experiment to be conducted in Bandung regency in November and December 1934, and these tests confirmed his initial results. Given the serious nature of the ongoing outbreak in the Priangan, however, before the final results of the Bandung experiments were known, the government approved a mass inoculation campaign to start in January 1935. The course of the epidemic was reversed virtually immediately. Over two million people were vaccinated during the year. Whenever a re-emergence of the disease occurred, the population of affected villages was revaccinated. In September 1937 mass revaccination was carried out in Bandung to prevent an anticipated seasonal rise in the number of cases. In four years, 2.9 million people were vaccinated at least once and 6.5 million revaccinations were administered. Otten claimed that this was done 'without any harmful consequence to health and life of the population'.[37] His pride at this remarkable turn of events was piqued by the failure of others to recognize its significance. He complained bitterly when the internationally sponsored Conference on Rural Hygiene 'was unable to endorse' his conviction that the vaccine constituted a major contribution to world public health, but put this down to the general attitude of the League of Nations, which 'in matters of medical hygiene . . . behaves as it does in politics: it strives only for compromise'.[38]

In 1938 and 1939, as the number of plague deaths in West Java fell from 1 447 to 1 123 and the epidemic was thought to have been brought under control, the fragile tissue of international political compromises collapsed. First the Netherlands and later Indonesia were invaded and subjected to radical changes of government. In the thirty years which had passed since the first victim of the Java plague epidemic died in Turen, the colony had undergone many changes in public health policy. The three waves of the epidemic were successively concentrated in each of the three major provinces in turn, and each wave was characterized by a change of Plague Service strategy. East Java experienced a battery of interventions predicated on the assumption that the disease was spread by many vectors. Central Java's epidemic covered a broad area, and the campaign concentrated on house improvement. The West Java outbreak was the most severe, and unfortunately coincided with the Great Depression, which saw reductions in the health budget. The housing improvement programme recovered somewhat in the late 1930s, but by that time the success of the Otten vaccine in controlling the disease had been established, and the attempt to improve village construction techniques was continued as much for general public health reasons as for the control of the plague.

Epilogue

The *MDVG* ceased publication during the Japanese occupation, and was replaced by other scientific journals after the establishment of the Republic. In 1940 the number of plague cases reported by the Public Health Service was only 312; fewer than for any year since 1910. Pollitzer cites records showing an increase in cases to 550 in 1941 and a fall to 339 in 1942,[39] but Velimirovic cites B. Wirodipoero in contending that these are slight underestimates.[40] The latter records an upturn in cases in 1943, a decline to zero in 1945 and a major outbreak in 1946–49, with over 7 500 deaths in 1948.

After 1950 the reconstituted anti-plague service had new weapons in its armoury to fight rats and fleas. The discovery of DDT and dieldrin made it possible to concentrate on killing the host and vector rather than merely keeping them out of the house.[41] Moreover, the development of antibiotics (especially Tetracyclin) greatly improved the prognosis for victims who could be given medical treatment quickly. The service used these innovations as well as the time-honoured procedures for case identification, rat-proofing and isolation to deal with outbreaks in Surakarta and Boyolali in the early 1950s.

Two researchers from WHO, Baltazard and Bahmanyar, took the opportunity afforded by the Surakarta outbreak to have another look at the epidemiology of plague in Java. They found, contrary to de Raadt and others, that the source host for the plague was not the house rat, but a field rat, *Rattus exulans ephippium*. This species is highly resistant but very receptive to the *P. pestis*, and as such is the only species of rat in Java able to maintain the infection without ill effects to itself. It is a vagabond, visiting villages sporadically when hunger and an increase in numbers encourage it to leave the fields. Then it transfers the disease through fleas to house rats, and an outbreak of human plague is possible. This finding explains why plague in Java tended to be brief in any given area, yet inexorable in its spread. The conclusion Baltazard and Bahmanyar drew from these findings is that 'almost all the measures now applied might usefully be discontinued. The Plague Control Service could then concentrate on an eradication campaign in order to accelerate the already inevitable disappearance of the disease'.[42] Unanswered is the question of what would have happened in Java had the Service in Malang in 1911 concentrated on rats in the fields rather than in the houses.

Plague was not a major disease in Java from a demographic standpoint, but it did leave its mark on the public health system in a number of ways. It provided the ideal opportunity for doctors to establish hegemony over a programme that involved the co-ordination of a variety of specializations. The horror of the disease justified a number of intrusive procedures which violated both the civil and property rights of the families and neighbours of plague victims. Over time the Service developed routine procedures for dealing with suspected plague victims that offended the personal and religious sensibilities of surviving family members, despite the lack of clear medical justification for the practices. In the process, an entire generation of Javanese medically trained professionals was socialized into a particularly unfortunate relationship with their village compatriots. Like their Dutch teachers, they were aloof and quick to apply interventions with little consideration of patients' sensibilities.

Finally, it is interesting to speculate that the course of the house improvement campaign, which gave relatively greater benefits to East than West Java, may also be responsible for the fact that in 1971 the proportion of houses regarded as of lowest quality was 6.5% in the former and 16.5% in the latter, and, similarly, infant mortality was much lower in the east than in the west. It would be ironic, indeed, if the greatest demographic impact of van Gorkom's programme was not the prevention of plague deaths in the three decades from 1910, but rather its contribution to infant survival in the three decades of Indonesian independence. Ironic, perhaps, but on the basis of the available evidence, not impossible.

Susan Abeyasekere, Anton Lucas and Anthony Reid provided me with helpful comments on a draft of this paper. Marian Obenchain did most of the data processing and Pat Mooney typed all the many versions of the paper. I am grateful to all of them for their help.

  1. A recent alternative naming is *Yersinia pseudotuberculosis sub pestis*.

2. An epizootic is the rapid spread of disease among animals. An epidemic refers specifically to infections of humans.

3. See, however, Barbara Lovric, 'Bali: Myth, Magic and Morbidity', above, on the evidence for early plague in Bali.

4. N. H. Swellengrebel, 'Record of Observations on the Bionomics of Rats and on Other Subjects, Bearing on the Epidemiology of Plague in Eastern Java', *Mededeelingen van den Burgerlijken Geneeskundigen Dienst in Nederlandsch-Indië* (cited hereafter as *MBGDN*) 2 (1913), 89.

5. A small outbreak of human plague in Makassar between 1922 and 1930, peaking in 1924, was the only recorded incidence of the disease in the Outer Islands. In all, 115 cases of bubonic plague were found. Because of the limited nature of this episode, the epidemic can largely be regarded as confined to Java. N. van der Walle, 'De ratten en rattenvlooien van Makassar: enkele opmerkingen naar aanleiding van de voorgekomen pestgevallen', *Mededeelingen van den Dienst in Nederlandsch-Indië* 21, 4 (1932), 273.

6. The Annual Report for 1934 (184–6) shows that in the worst year of the epidemic only seven subdistricts had a plague death rate as high as 20 per thousand population and eighteen had rates between 19 and 20 per thousand. While these rates significantly raised the overall death rates in the villages concerned, they did not even approach the rates of England for 1348–49, which are estimated at between 300 and 450 per thousand; J. Hatcher, *Plague, Population and the English Economy 1348–1530* (London, Macmillan Press, 1977), 25.

7. According to the Annual Reports of 1933–39, spleen puncture was performed not just in cases of suspected plague but, in districts where any cases had occurred, at all attended deaths. Thus in 1933, though only 17 000 plague deaths were recorded, 60 347 punctures were performed and 1 668 refusals recorded out of 80 710 attended deaths. 'Verslag betreffende de pestbestrijding op Java over het jaar 1933' (Annual Report 1933), *Mededeelingen van den Dienst der Volksgezondheid in Nederlandsch-Indië* (hereafter cited as *MDVG*) 24, Supplement (1935), 279. The puncture was regarded by Rosier as 'the method par excellence for the determination of plague', but lately WHO has recommended puncture of the liver, lungs and heart, since it is too difficult to reach the spleen; M. Bahmanyar and D. C. Cavanaugh, *Plague Manual* (Geneva, World Health Organization, 1976), 8.

8. It is not, unfortunately, an easy source to use. Definitions seem to have changed frequently and of course the boundary and administrative structural changes between 1910 and 1940 make the construction of comparative series difficult. We have also found a number of errors in later reports which attempted to recapitulate earlier data. The modern spelling of place names is used throughout this paper regardless of whether the place so named still exists as an administrative unit (e.g., Priangan instead of Preanger).

9. P. C. Flu, 'Some Epidemiological Observations on Plague', *MBGDN* 3 (1921), 250–87.

10. Ibid., 271.

11. P. H. van Thiel, 'History of the Control of Endemic Diseases in the Netherlands Overseas Territories', *Annales des Sociétés Belges de Médicine Tropicale* 51, 4–5 (1971), 447.

12. Swellengrebel, op. cit., 70.

13. O. L. E. de Raadt, 'Can the Plague be Spread by Head Lice?', *MBGDN* 4 (1916), 40.

14. W. J. van Gorkom, 'Plague Service. Report over the First Quarter 1915', *MBGDN* 5 (1918).

15. Ibid., 8.

16. Ibid.

17. As van Gorkom exclaimed: 'Alas! the number of deaths reported is still exceeding largely that of the cases of illness' (ibid., 11).

18. The Haffkine plague serum was a horse serum developed in India, but it had low effectiveness and produced serious side effects, including the possibly fatal danger of serum reaction.

19. W. J. van Gorkom, 'General Introduction for the Execution of Measures for Combating the Plague in Java', *MBGDN* 5 (1918), 81. By contrast, modern Indonesians actively request injections (*suntikan*) for even minor ailments and tend to distrust other treatments.

20. L. Otten, 'De pestbestrijding op Java 1911–1935', *Feestbundel 1936, Genees-kundig Tijdschrift van Nederlandsch-Indië* (Batavia, Kolff & Co., 1936), 95.

21. P. C. Flu, 'Experiments Immunisation against Plague', *MBGDN* 3 (1919), 25.

22. Annual Report 1933, 217; H. J. Rosier, 'Verslag betreffende de pestbe-strijding op Java over het jaar 1934' (Annual Report 1934), *MDVG* 25, 2 (1936), 148; also L. Otten, 'De pest op Java, 1911–1923', *MBGDN* 2 (1924), 225ff.

23. Swellengrebel, op. cit., 10–11.

24. Ibid., 11.

25. L. F. Hirst, *The Conquest of Plague* (Oxford, Clarendon Press, 1953), 184–7.

26. Ibid., 186.

27. Annual Report 1933, 271.

28. J. L. Hydrick, *Intensive Rural Hygiene Work and Public Health Education of the Public Health Service of Netherlands India* (Batavia, Public Health Service, 1937).

29. Ibid., 2, 3, 5.

30. Note also that the malaria campaign stressed home improvement. H. J. Rosier, 'Verslag betreffende de pestbestrijding op Java over het jaar 1937' (Annual Report 1937), *MDVG* 27, Supplement II (1938), 117.

31. Van Gorkom, op. cit., 63.

32. I. Snapper, 'Medical Contributions From the Netherlands Indies', in Pieter, Honig and Frans Verdoorn (eds), *Science and Scientists in the Netherlands Indies* (New York, Board for the Netherlands Indies, Surinam and Curacao, 1945), 309–20.

33. Annual Report 1933, 269.

34. Rosier, Annual Report 1934, 209.

35. Ibid.

36. Annual Report 1933, 271.

37. L. Otten, 'A Live Plague Vaccine and the Results', *MDVG* 31, 1 (1941), 109.

38. L. Otten, 'Immunization against Plague with Dead and Live Vaccine', *MDVG* 27, 1–2 (1938), 122.

39. R. Pollitzer, *Plague* (Geneva, World Health Organization, 1954).

40. B. Velimirovic, 'Plague in South-East Asia: A Brief Historical Summary and Present Geographical Distribution', *Transactions of the Royal Society of Tropical Medicine and Hygiene* 66, 3 (1972), 479–504.

41. Bahmanyar and Cavanaugh, op. cit., 55–59.

42. M. Baltazard and M. Bahmanyar, 'Recherches sur la peste à Java', *Bulletin of the World Health Organization* 23 (1960), 245; also Velimirovic, op. cit., 483–4.

Appendix
TABLE 10.1
PLAGUE DEATHS IN JAVA, BY DISTRICTS, 1910-39[a]

Region	1910–14	1915–19	1920–24	Plague Deaths 1925–29	1930–34	1935–39	Total
Banten	0	0	0	0	0	0	0
Batavia	0	0	18	0	12	101	131
Priangan	0	0	0	1 142	41 927	19 315	62 384
Buitenzorg	0	0	0	0	123	62	185
Cirebon	0	0	520	4 812	1 234	509	7 075
WEST JAVA	0	0	538	5 954	43 296	19 987	69 775
Pekalongan	0	0	1 613	5 482	6 776	4 496	18 367
Semarang	0	639	7 449	1 018	17	0	9 123
Banyumas	0	0	2 146	5 244	23	559	7 972
Kedu	0	2 825	23 446	9 985	3 317	1 317	40 890
Rembang/Jepara	0	0	2	0	0	0	2
CENTRAL JAVA	0	3 464	34 656	21 729	10 133	6 372	76 354

TABLE 10.1 continued

Region	1910–14	1915–19	1920–24	Plague Deaths 1925–29	1930–34	1935–39	Total
YOGYAKARTA	0	17	667	2 104	1 584	163	4 535
SURAKARTA	7	2 034	14 758	8 269	20	14	25 102
Bojonegoro	0	0	0	0	0	0	0
Surabaya	1 461	994	496	127	0	0	3 078
Madura	121	29	0	1	0	0	151
Malang/Pasuruan	19 680	2 735	205	402	47	84	23 153
Besuki	0	0	0	0	0	0	0
Madiun	2 541	229	4	1	0	0	2 775
Kediri	7 780	2 032	167	118	0	0	10 097
EAST JAVA	31 583	6 019	872	649	47	84	39 254
JAVA–MADURA	31 590	11 534	51 491	38 705	55 080	26 620	215 020

(a) Reported deaths underestimate the true numbers because of failure to detect cases, refusal of families to report cases, and misdiagnosis. However, given the distinctive nature of the disease, it is expected such factors would account for only a small proportion of deaths.

Source: MDVG, various years.

TABLE 10.2

HOUSE IMPROVEMENTS SPONSORED BY THE PLAGUE SERVICE IN JAVA, BY DISTRICT, 1911–39[a]

Region	1911–14	1915–19	1920–24	1925–29	1930–34	1935–39	Total
				Houses Improved			
Banten	0	0	0	0	ND	ND	ND
Batavia	0	0	0	0	ND	1 510	ND
Priangan	0	0	0	0	ND	115 367	ND
Buitenzorg	0	0	0	0	ND	ND	ND
Cirebon	0	0	0	0	ND	10 892	ND
WEST JAVA	0	0	0	0	70 814	167 236	238 050
Pekalongan	0	0	ND	ND	ND	17 803	ND
Semarang	0	17 200	ND	ND	ND	ND	ND
Banyumas	0	0	ND	ND	ND	5 503	ND
Kedu	0	4 849	ND	ND	ND	ND	ND
Rembang/Jepara	0	0	ND	ND	ND	ND	ND
CENTRAL JAVA	0	22 049	157 765	148 816	91 004	40 341	459 975
YOGYAKARTA	0	6 692	0	9 033	27 819	24 569	68 113

Table 10.2 continued

Region	1911–14	1915–19	1920–24	Houses Improved 1925–29	1930–34	1935–39	Total
SURAKARTA	0	37 261	29 962	118 002	60 212	0	245 437
Bojonegoro	0	0	ND	0	0	ND	ND
Surabaya	0	15 485	ND	0	0	ND	ND
Madura	0	4 498	ND	0	0	ND	ND
Malang/Pasuruan	31 548	132 205	ND	0	0	ND	ND
Besuki	0	0	ND	0	0	ND	ND
Madiun	75 399	97 322	ND	0	0	ND	ND
Kediri	280	200 956	ND	0	0	ND	ND
EAST JAVA	107 227	450 466	182	0	0	816	558 691
JAVA–MADURA	107 227	516 468	187 909	278 851	249 849	232 962	1 570 266

(a) Data in the Annual Reports for 1933–39 wrongly classify house improvements for 1911–19 as having occurred in Central rather than East Java.
Source: MDVG, various years.

11 The Influenza Pandemic of 1918 in Indonesia

COLIN BROWN

THE influenza pandemic of 1918 was probably the greatest single natural disaster ever to hit this earth. According to one source the pandemic was 'the most destructive in history; in fact it ranks with the plague of Justinian and the Black Death as one of the severest holocausts of disease ever encountered'.[1] No one knows precisely how many people died either from the flu itself or from associated illnesses such as pneumonia, but a round figure of 20 million seems likely. The country worst hit was India, where some 12.5 million deaths were recorded.

In Indonesia, it seems probable that at least 1.5 million people died; by way of comparison, the plague killed just over 215 000 people between 1911 and 1939.[2] Despite this, the episode has attracted remarkably little scholarly attention. With commendable speed, in the same month that the epidemic was at its peak, the colonial authorities set up a Commission of Inquiry with a brief to:

investigate the nature of the disease, the cause of same, the manner in which it came, the area it covered, the mortality which occured and the experiences regarding preventative measures and treatment, compiled during this epidemic.[3]

The Commission's report, published in 1920, is heavily technical in flavour, devoting much attention to the clinical and biological elements of the epidemic, and recording comparatively little of what it meant to the population of the Indies. No writers have subsequently taken on the task of describing more fully the impact of the pandemic on Indies society. This essay is an attempt to fill this gap.

Generally speaking, the influenza observed in the Indies had the same general characteristics as that reported elsewhere.[4] The onset of illness was rapid, and usually without prior warning. A high fever set in, lasting from about three to five days. Common symptoms included a dry hacking cough, violent headaches and articular lumbar and muscular pains. The disease was of sufficient virulence to cause death within a few days of the appearance of these symptoms. However, at least as important in causing death was the capacity of the disease to exacerbate existing illnesses or render the patient more vulnerable to other ones. Pneumonia was frequently brought on by the disease, as were malaria, haemorrhages (especially of the nose and lungs), dysentery and tuberculosis. These complications were often induced by the patient's returning to work immediately after the initial fever had died down, but before full recovery had been effected. It was the number of complications associated with the disease, and their intensity, which set the 1918 pandemic apart from earlier ones.

Origins and Spread

The pandemic emerged from the battlefields of western Europe in the northern summer of 1918, the last summer of World War I.[5] The origins of the disease are not known with certainty; it seems probable that it was imported from the United States with American troops, then beginning to flood into Europe to join in the war, though there may also have been independent foci in Russia and Siberia, and China. But, from the explosion-point in western Europe, the disease spread rapidly. It reached Bombay in June, thence to the Straits Settlements; it was first reported in Indonesia at Pankattan, on the east coast of Sumatra, later in the same month.[6] By the end of July, major outbreaks of the disease had been noted in several parts of Java, and in Kalimantan. In this initial attack, though, the disease seems to have penetrated no further east than Java: Bali, Sulawesi and the islands to the east were untouched. And although high levels of morbidity were recorded, mortality was generally quite low. A second wave of the disease, arriving in October, was much more widespread, however. This time, very few parts of the archipelago were unaffected, the eastern islands in particular being very badly hit. It was this second wave which brought most deaths.

Fairly detailed figures on mortality, down to the regency (*kabu-*

paten) level, are available for Java and Madura—the standard reservations have to be entered as to their absolute accuracy, but they are probably of good indicative value. Perhaps the best way of measuring the impact of the disease is to look not simply at the mortality rates for 1918, but rather at the extent to which these rates exceed previously established norms. I have taken, as a simple indicator of this, the ratio of the 1918 rate to the average rate over the six immediately preceding years, 1912–17.[7] If this ratio is unity, then the flu had no significant impact; the greater the ratio is above unity, the greater the impact. And of course, if the ratio is less than unity, the implication would be that fewer deaths were occuring than previously, despite the flu.

On the eighty-one regencies in Java and Madura, the un-weighted mean of the ratios was just over 1.9. There were fifteen regencies in which the ratio exceeded this mean by more than one standard deviation (see Table 11.1). Of these, no fewer than twelve were located in East Java, being concentrated in particular in the region south from Surabaya to Kediri and Madiun, and east to the Oost Hoek. There is little by way of a clear pattern linking these regions: some are rich and others poor, some densely populated and some not, some close to major population centres and other relatively isolated. Their East Java location is almost the only firm link.

At the other end of the scale, in twelve regencies the ratio was more than one standard deviation below the mean. And the interesting point here is that most of them—nine—were in west Java. Again, apart from provincial location, there is little by way of geographical or economic pattern linking them. Three regencies (Sumedang, Bandung and Garut) recorded ratios less than unity, which, if at all accurate, would indicate that health conditions there in 1918 were somehow better than they had been in preceding years, despite the flu.

Explaining why this differential pattern of mortality should have occurred is difficult. Broadly speaking, the mild first wave of the disease hit the western part of Java first, then faded out fairly rapidly as it spread eastwards through the island. Those areas hit hard by the first wave were often not badly affected by the second. The correlation between these two events is not a perfect one. But it would appear that exposure to the first wave gave people a measure of protection or immunity from the second.

Information on mortality levels in regions outside Java is much

TABLE 11.1

INDEX OF FLU-RELATED MORTALITY RATES, BY REGENCY, JAVA AND MADURA, 1918

Region	More than one S.D. [a] above the mean	Up to one S.D. above the mean	Up to one S.D. below the mean	More than one S.D. below the mean
WEST JAVA			Indramayu Tangerang Cirebon Batavia Krawang Buitenzorg Cianjur Cilacap Sukabumi	Sumedang Bandung Garut Tasikmalaya Lebak Mr. Cornelis Majalengka Pandeglang Serang
CENTRAL JAVA	Boyolali Salatiga Temanggung	Grobogan Batang Purworejo Banjarnegara Sragen Klaten Blora	Brebes Tegal Purbalingga Kudus Pati Pekalongan Yogyakarta	

Region	More than one S.D.(a) above the mean	Up to one S.D. above the mean	Up to one S.D. below the mean	More than one S.D. below the mean
		Kulon Progo Wonosobo Solo Kebumen Banyumas Demak Jepara Gunung Kidul	Pemalang Purwokerto Magelang Rembang Semarang	Sampang Pamekasan Bangkalan
EAST JAVA	Blitar Panarukan Trenggalek Madiun Pasuruan Bondowoso Banyuwangi Lamongan Tulungagung Ngawi Ponorogo Sumenep	Kediri Magetan Malang Jember Surabaya Gresik	Sidoarjo Tuban Bangil Probolinggo Mojokerto Pacitan Kraksaan Jombang Berbek Lumajang	

(a) Standard Deviation

harder to come by and more difficult to evaluate. Nonetheless, it does seem that the further east the second wave spread, the more deaths it caused, in line with the pattern noted in Java. In Sulawesi, Maluku and Timor, for instance, the *Koloniaal Verslag* of 1918 noted high death rates, though it did not specify just what the rates were.[8] In southeast Sulawesi, a Catholic missionary on tour in the interior reported deaths 'everywhere'; in one village 177 people had died out of a population of 900, in a period of just three weeks.[9] In Tana Toraja, 10% of the population is reported to have died because of the flu.[10] The Resident of Bali and Lombok recorded that deaths on the island of Lombok amounted to just over 36 000, or 5.9% of the entire population of the island.[11]

Differential Impact

Although we do have some information of the impact of the disease at the regency level, we really know very little about the differential impact of the disease: which groups in the community suffered most. All we have are some scattered fragments of information about particular groups, which might perhaps give some idea of the pattern of attack.

Amongst Europeans—for whom the data are most complete—the most common single cause of death during 1918 was disease of the respiratory organs, accounting for just over 12% of the deaths.[12] Flu came second, causing 11.7% of the deaths, followed by diseases of the alimentary organs (7.8%). It should be remembered, though, that contracting flu rendered people vulnerable to other ailments which otherwise might not have been deadly. Thus the figure for deaths directly attributed to flu almost certainly greatly underestimates the real impact of the disease.

Reflecting the general tendency for flu-related deaths in Java to be more common in the east, more Europeans died in Surabaya than in Jakarta and Semarang combined. However the most striking factor about these data is not the number of deaths, but the number of people who did not die: mortality rates were extremely low, compared with those for the Indonesian community. Whereas about 1.8% of Indonesians on Java died, the comparable figure for Europeans was probably about one-tenth of that.

With respect to the Indonesian population, less is known with any degree of precision. As might have been expected, institutions which brought relatively large numbers of people into close contact with one another were often foci for attack, especially if those institutions were open ones, permitting a fairly free movement of people in and out. Perhaps the most obvious examples of such institutions were schools and orphanages. The newspapers of the time carried a large number of articles recording the impact of the flu on these institutions. Absenteeism was reported to have been high, and in many places schools were closed as a result.[13]

Amongst the military, morbidity rates were high, though mortality rates were not. The army establishment in 1918 stood at 41 159 officers and men. Of these, 3 174 (just under 8%) were treated for flu; of these sufferers, 121 (nearly 4%) died.[14] Thus of the total army establishment, only about 0.3% died. Presumably the main reasons for this low mortality rate include the better medical and nursing care available to members of the military, better food and housing, and the generally stronger physical condition of soldiers compared with the civilian population. It is also the case, of course, that there were no women or children in the military. Unfortunately, the available data do not allow firm conclusions to be drawn about whether women or children had mortality rates higher or lower than those of adult males, although it will be argued below that for children the rates were probably higher than for those adults.

Members of that other great uniformed and regimented institution, the prison system, fared less well. The *Koloniaal Verslag* for 1918 noted, with admirable frankness, that 'As a result of the Spanish flu, health conditions prevailing among prisoners leave much to be desired'.[15] But conditions in individual gaols varied considerably. In Garut, for instance, the authorities managed to keep the gaol strictly isolated from contact with the outside world, with the result that it remained completely free of the disease.[16] However, the large Central Gaol in Batavia could not be kept isolated. Indeed, it suffered a severe attack during the first wave of the epidemic in July–August. But this first attack turned out to be advantageous to the inmates, for while the morbidity rate was high, the mortality rate was low; and exposure to the first wave seems to have accorded many of the gaol inmates and staff an immunity to the second, otherwise more deadly, wave.[17] In other, smaller, prisons, though, death rates were much higher.[18]

It might have been expected that contract labourers on plantations and in the mines would have suffered the same fate as prisoners. Such probably was the case, though the information available is slight and scattered. On the relatively isolated island of Bangka, for instance, although about one in four workers fell ill, the mortality rate was quite low: only thirty-one deaths were recorded, out of a total workforce of 10 000 (0.3%).[19] Low mortality rates were also recorded for tin mines at other relatively isolated locations such as Lingga and Karimun, in Riau.[20] But in Tanjung Pinang, also part of the province of Riau, but much more heavily populated and open to the movement of people and goods, death rates were much higher. Out of 4 052 contract labourers, 438 were reported to have died—nearly 11%.[21] High death rates were also found among plantation workers on the tea estates of West Java, causing production levels to drop off significantly, and in Lampung and West Kalimantan.[22]

Contemporary analyses of the global pandemic tended to pinpoint people of ordinary working age as the ones most likely to be stricken and to die.[23] In this respect, it was argued, the 1918 epidemic differed from earlier epidemics, most notably that of 1889–90. However, some more recent research has suggested that this view is incorrect, that in fact most deaths occurred among the very young and the very old, just as in other flu epidemics.[24] Unfortunately, the data are not available to make a firm judgement on this issue with respect to Indonesia.

In particular, there are no reliable data on the age structure of the population at large at the time of the pandemic. The first serious attempt at a national census did not take place until November 1920. And even here, while a reasonably detailed picture of the age structure of the European population of the Indies was produced, in the case of the Indonesian population the only division made was between those aged under fifteen, and those aged fifteen and over.[25] In the absence of any better contemporary data, it is impossible to draw any meaningful conclusions about which age groups were hardest hit by the illness.

One thing, however, can be said. Of the people who died from influenza, there is some evidence that the bulk were outside the normal working age group—mid-teens to mid-fifties. Thus, in a study undertaken by van Steenis of the 777 flu-related deaths recorded in the Magelang sub-district of Central Java between 1 October and 31 December 1918, 46% were of children aged under ten years, and a further 14% were of people aged sixty or more.[26] Thus over half the total number of deaths were of people unlikely to have been in the full-time work force. How far it is reasonable to extrapolate from this study is not clear. However it is the most exhaustive study of its type found thus far, and does correlate with more anecdotal evidence that a large proportion of flu-related deaths occurred among children.[27]

Treatment of the Disease

When it came to the medical treatment of sufferers, neither European-trained doctors nor local *dukun* (healers) could offer much real help. There was no known cure for the flu. It was not until 1933 that a virus capable of inducing flu, initially in ferrets, was discovered, thereby opening the way for work to proceed in the development of antigens capable of combating the illness.[28] The most that any one could do in 1918 was to treat the symptoms of the disease, not the disease itself.

The Civil Medical Service (BGD), only recently established as an entity separate from the Army Medical Service, took the general view that the main factors permitting the rapid and extensive spread of the disease among Indonesians were poor hygiene and poor diet, together with the failure of sufferers to allow themselves sufficient time to recuperate from the disease before resuming normal employment. Thus it saw improvements in these areas as being the most effective response to the disease, at least in the long run. As for medicines, it had to admit that none was known to be effective.[29] Aspirin and quinine were often prescribed to treat the fever and the headaches, but they had no wider effect. It was not until early 1919 that emergency regulations were drawn up providing, among other things, for a programme to educate people about the disease (particularly with respect to its connection with hygiene), for free distribution of medicines to the needy, and for making simple masks available to people in infected areas.[30]

The obvious incapacity of the BGD to take much positive action against influenza drew critical responses from several quarters. One of the most rigorous and detailed was mounted in the Volksraad (People's Council) by Dr Abdul Rivai. Rivai argued that the BGD, by its failure to take effective action, was permitting a mortality rate in Java which would be totally unacceptable in Europe. The Service, he charged was following an inhumane policy of *laissez mourir*—allowing people to die. 'I will fight against [this policy]', he said, 'I shall fight against it. I'll be like a bulldog holding fast to the throat of the Medical Service.'[31] But this attack was not followed up by other members of the Volksraad. The head of the BGD, de Vogel, neatly turned it aside by producing a response every bit as detailed as Rivai's original submission, and the matter dropped from view.

Several doctors and other medical staff were to lose their lives as a result of the epidemic, though the Commission of Inquiry's report noted that many of them seemed quickly to have acquired an immunity to it.[32] But others seem to have used the occasion to pursue personal gain. At least one doctor, G. G. J. Rademaker of Surabaya, took out an advertisement in his local paper announcing that due to the 'mysterious illness then prevailing' he had been forced to double his fees.[33] On the other hand in Solo the proprietor of a local *toko obat*—a shop selling patent medicines— announced that that for the duration of the epidemic he would supply medicines free of charge to anyone asking for them.[34]

Most Indonesians, of course, did not have access to Western doctors or medicines of any type. As the leadership of the Sarekat Islam in Surabaya noted, 'because of their poverty, Indonesians do not have adequate medical assistance at their disposal'. As a result, it continued, somewhat ominously but nonetheless obviously correctly, 'they are likely to provide most of the victims of the epidemic. Indonesians must therefore rely on their own medicines'.[35] Another Indonesian, the Regent of Pasuruan, R. T. Soejono, went further, arguing that Indonesians would not even accept Western medicines when they were offered to them for nothing. This, he said, was

partly because the people saw such help as charity, and partly because they were afraid that they would be asked for it all back again, further evidence that they have no faith in the government.[36]

A reporter for the *Locomotief* put the Indonesian aversion to the use of Dutch remedies in a rather less generous light. The high death rate in Purworejo, he said, was the fault of the Indonesians, not of the doctors: they chose to ignore the advice given to them by doctors and to rely instead on *dukun*, 'who recommend the preparation of some foul potion or other to drive out the evil spirits, but which often causes the (illness) to become worse'.[37] For a variety of reasons, then, most Indonesians sought help through indigenous remedies rather than Western medicines.

Indonesian treatments, like their European counterparts, were directed primarily at the relief of the symptoms of the disease, rather than at the disease itself. The most common Indonesian interpretation of these symptoms was that they resulted from some form of *masuk angin*—a fairly broad term covering a range of chills and fevers. One local paper offered its readers a choice of three remedies: the juice of a *labu* (kind of pumpkin) with a pinch of salt; a poultice consisting of lime juice, ginger and red onions, reduced to a paste and mixed with locally made (i.e., not distilled) vinegar; and a drink made from an extract of cloves, the number of cloves being equal to the age of the patient in years.[38] Another remedy which sounds rather more lethal—though whether to patient or fever I am not sure—consisted of the root of the *lempuyangan* tree, peeled and mashed, then mixed with red peppers and eaten. The mixture, my informant assured me, was 'very hot', and caused profuse sweating.

These remedies were based on the notion that the cause of the illness was something physical, which could be treated with medicines of some kind. For some Indonesians, though, the causes of the illness were not physical, but spiritual, and thus required spiritual responses. In many places *selametan* (ritual meals) were eaten or processions held. In Parakan, Central Java, for instance, it was reported that during a procession through the Muslim section of the town,

no fewer than 12 goats were slaughtered and their heads and legs buried at the road junctions, with the aim of warding off the danger of disease, which Parakan has avoided so far.[39]

It was not successful.

The Patih of Bangkalan in Madura showed, possibly unwittingly, a good grasp of one of the factors assisting the spread of the disease when he called on local religious leaders to pray for rain.[40] The unusually long dry season in 1918 which preceded the second wave of the epidemic had led to an upsurge in respiratory diseases: coughing and sneezing were obvious and easy ways for the disease to spread. And it should be noted here, in fairness to the Patih, that Bangkalan reported a very low level of mortality that year, less than the mean for Java.

Others, though, took a rather more esoteric view of the causes
of the crisis, and thus of the best means of fighting it. One person
interviewed maintained that the epidemic was a result of the
workings of *hukum kodrat* (natural law). His own parents, he said,
had foreseen the coming of the pandemic. They had said that if
people failed to carry out their religious duties properly, if they
committed adultery and other immoral acts, if they ate to excess
(or if they ate forbidden food such as dog meat), then they would
be punished under natural law. There would be a long dry season,
a shortage of food, and then a wave of illness of epidemic proportions in which many would die. And all this, my informant said,
with perhaps more than a touch of triumph in his voice, had come
to pass! The only appropriate way of reacting to the epidemic, in
these terms, was to get down to the root cause of it, to purify one's
way of life, and to live according to natural law.

Finally, of course, some saw in the pandemic the forces of
darkness. One newspaper reported that in Kulon Progo, on the
western edge of Yogyakarta, people were saying that the origins of
the disease lay in black magic. So the fight against it consisted of
seeking out the people in the village who were performing hyp-
notism and other forms of black magic, and driving them out.
'Only then', the paper said, 'would peace and good health
return.'[41]

Social and Economic Impact

Given the swiftness with which the epidemic struck, and the
high levels of morbidity and mortality it brought, it is hardly
surprising that it caused major social and economic disturbances.
The *Koloniaal Verslag* noted that everyday life was badly disrupted in many places.[42] Shops, offices and schools were closed,
and markets deserted. Perhaps the most harrowing reports are
those emanating from the eastern islands. Thus the Commission of
Inquiry noted the conditions prevailing in one location in Ambon,

where, for some time, only 8 of the 800 inhabitants were able to do
their work. The others . . . were absolutely abandoned to their fate, and
in the absence of any help they remained without food, drink and
medicine. A similar condition of misery prevailed in numerous other
places. Houses were closed, the streets were deserted; inside the houses
the children cried for want of food and drink, and no-one could help . . .
This tragic state of affairs caused by the influenza was also reported from

many places in the Moluccas [Maluku], Bali and Lombok and other places.[43]

On the island of Sumbawa it was reported that buffalo and horses were dying of hunger because local herdsmen, being stricken with the flu, were unable to take them out in search of good pasture, which was in short supply during the driest part of the year.[44]

In many places, there was insufficient manpower available to ensure the proper burial of victims. One newspaper report on conditions on the island of Buton, off the southern tip of southeast Sulawesi, said that corpses had been seen lying beside the road, and then dragged away by dogs; when death occurred indoors, the reporter went on,

the survivors, too weak themselves to drag the body away, simply removed a plank from the floorboards and allowed the corpse to fall down through the gap.[45]

This is a sensational story, to be sure, but there seems little doubt that performing proper burials was a real problem in many hard-hit areas. One person in Purworejo recounted the shock he experienced as a young teenager on seeing a burial procession pass by his house. It is difficult to say which affected him most: the fact that there were only four people in the procession, one supporting each corner of the bier, or the fact that two of the burial party were women. Either way, he felt that established customs were being seriously violated.

There are several reports of an upsurge in violence during the epidemic. In Surakarta, for instance, it was reported that there had been an increase in the number of robberies in several *kampung*; this was seen as being caused by, or at least permitted by, the fact that due to the epidemic there were insufficient healthy men available to mount the normal night watch.[46] A journalist writing from Madura also reported an increase in the number of robberies and murders carried out.[47]

Far more serious is the suggestion that the epidemic was partially responsible for setting off the large-scale anti-Chinese riots in the Central Javanese town of Kudus in November. A contemporary Chinese writer, Tan Boen Kim, in his account of the events, devotes considerable attention to the impact of influenza on the town.[48] He notes that although some Chinese fell victim to the disease, and a few Europeans, Javanese accounted for the great majority of deaths it caused. This he attributed primarily to the Javanese lack of knowledge of, and attention to, hygiene and cleanliness, especially in rural areas 'where many people are filthy dirty and do not care what or where they eat'.[49] In order to try to ward off the epidemic, leaders of the Chinese community organized a series of processions in which religious statues (*taopekkong*) were paraded about the town. During the fourth procession, Javanese bystanders clashed with the Chinese; a mêlée ensued which rapidly turned into a riot. Though the influenza was by no means the sole cause of the riot, it does seem to have 'played some part in arousing the feelings of the people'.[50]

This riot seems to be the only evidence of a direct connection between influenza and political unrest in the Indies in the last few months of 1918. One might speculate that the epidemic would have disturbed the social equilibrium of the communities it struck, and have thus facilitated the agitation being undertaken by nationalist groups, especially the ISDV (Social Democrats) and the Sarekat Islam. However there seems to be no evidence to confirm such an hypothesis, either in contemporary reports of these events, or subsequent analyses of them.[51]

In more general terms, my interviews with epidemic survivors suggest that the general feeling of the time was one of uncertainty mixed with fear. As one writer said bluntly, 'the people were at their wit's end'.[52] The causes of the disease were unknown; it was capable, apparently, of striking people at random; death rates were known to be high; and the onslaught could take place within a frighteningly short period of time. Many people reacted in a fairly normal way when faced with such a crisis: they returned to their home villages to wait it out. One person told me of walking from his boarding school back to his village, a distance of some twenty kilometres, carrying his sick brother on his back. He survived, and so did his brother. But shortly after his return home, several of his neighbours, previously uninfected, came down with the flu, and some of them died. It is likely that the disease was brought into the village by my informant—on his back. In fact this was probably a common way for the disease to be transmitted, and spread into many remote areas. The instinctive reaction when faced with a crisis—to *pulang kampung*, to return to one's home village—provided an excellent means of spreading the disease.

On the other hand, it should also be noted that committees

sprang up in many places with the aim of providing assistance to victims of the epidemic. Often, moving forces behind these committees were local notables: in Surakarta they included Pangeran Paku Alam, Pangeran Soeriodiningrat and the Captain of the Chinese.[53] Such exalted membership presumably made fundraising that much easier. Just how much of an impact their activities had is hard to say, though it would almost certainly have been limited to urban areas.

In economic terms, given the overwhelmingly agricultural nature of the Indonesian workforce, it might be expected that the high levels of morbidity and mortality associated with the flu would have had some concrete impact on agricultural production. The withdrawal of large quantities of labour from the agricultural workplace should have meant a decline in areas cropped and harvested. Such a phenomenon was observed, for instance, in India, where the area sown to crops in 1919 was down 4% on the 1917 figure.[54] In fact this was apparently not the case in Indonesia, at least in Java and Madura. Indeed, the areas under smallholder food crops in 1919 were generally higher than they had been in 1917, thereby continuing the upward trend established in the years immediately preceding. If these data are correct—and there is no good reason to doubt their relative accuracy—some explanation is needed. There are a number of possibilites.

First, the marginal productivity of labour could have been zero; if this were so, then a reduction in their labour force would have had no impact on production levels. This proposition is very difficult to verify, but it seems most unlikely.

Second, the rural labour force might have been supplemented by drawing in workers from other sectors of the economy. There is in fact some evidence for this. The *Soerabaiasch Handelsblad* noted that the epidemic had brought about a labour shortage in Semarang as men who had previously engaged others (*wakil*) to perform their labouring duties in their home villages found they could not engage such people. As a result they had to do the work themselves, and were thus unavailable for work in Semarang.[55] Further, Creutzberg notes that:

The government services, especially the Department of the Interior and the Department of Agriculture, Industries and Commerce, were enlisted, devoting all their energies to preventing the catastrophic effects of a famine.[56]

The *Koloniaal Verslag* for 1919, too, noted that normal administrative functions of the government 'were hampered by the granting of assistance for the cultivation of *sawah* and *pekarangan* and for the harvesting of the fields'.[57]

Third, we need to consider the composition of that part of the population affected by the epidemic. It has already been noted that there is some slight evidence to suggest that the bulk of the deaths caused by the flu occurred among people outside the normal working age group. If this is indeed the case, then the effect of the epidemic on agricultural production would have been much less than the sheer number of deaths would suggest.

This still leaves the question of morbidity. Even if deaths among working-age people were not very high, morbidity levels almost certainly were, and sick people are not generally capable of putting in a full day's work. Yet it was a characteristic of the flu that recovery was relatively quick for sufferers who did not die of the disease. For most, the period of illness probably did not exceed ten days or a fortnight; then they could resume normal employment. In terms of agricultural work, what this probably meant was that the work cycle was delayed, put back a few weeks, rather than broken. The wet-rice cycle is illustrative. Coming as it did in November-December, the second wave of the epidemic struck at a time when most rice farmers, at least in Java and Madura, would have been preparing to plant the 1918–19 crop. What seems to have happened is that the epidemic forced farmers to postpone this work while the flu raged. We do not have data on rice plantings by month, so it is not possible to check out this hypothesis in this way. However we do have monthly data on areas harvested, and these do seem to provide some confirmation. For the six years 1913–18, more sawah rice was harvested in May than in any other month—usually between 25% and 30% of the total wet-rice crop.[58] But in 1919, more rice was harvested in June than in May. In 1920 there was still some distortion to the pattern, although the May harvest was now equal to that in June. By 1921, though, the cycle seems to have worked its way back to the pre-1919 norm. This disturbance to the cycle supports the notion that wet-rice plantings at the end of 1918 were postponed by, on average, one month.

This postponement had an impact, too, on dry season crops. This is to be expected—the lengthening of the wet-rice cycle must have cut into the cycle of dry season crops. The data show that the areas under rice and maize did not vary from established patterns;

but the areas devoted to secondary crops, such as cassava, soya beans and peanuts, declined in comparison with previous years.[59] This is consistent with the hypothesis that, faced with a shortage of labour due to the ravages of the flu, farmers chose to cultivate the more valuable dry season crops and to sacrifice those which were less valuable.

There is a little evidence available on other aspects of the economic impact of the epidemic. The illness or death of the main money-earner in a household would be expected to cause financial problems and, in many cases, increased reliance on credit institutions. It might, therefore, reasonably be expected that such institutions would show an increased level of activities towards the end of 1918 and perhaps also in the early months of 1919. In the case of the Government Pawnshop Service, both the number of loans made and their value were considerably higher in 1918 than they had been in earlier years.[60] Village grain banks (*lumbung desa*) seem also to have done more business at the time of the epidemic than in the immediately preceding or succeeding years. During the financial year October 1918 to September 1919, 1.5 million people in Java borrowed rice from the *lumbung*. As the *Koloniaal Verslag* notes, assuming a household size of five people, this means that something like one fifth of Java's entire population was borrowing from a *lumbung* at this time.[61] The year 1918 also saw village banks making loans to more people than in previous and subsequent years.[62]

Such evidence is, of course, fragmentary. It needs to be kept firmly in mind that the influenza epidemic was not the only factor affecting the borrowing habits of the people at this time. In none of the cases cited above does the *Koloniaal Verslag* offer any particular reasons for the increased levels of activity in 1918 except with respect to the *lumbung*; it noted here that food shortages had contributed to the increased demands being made on them.[63] One other branch of the government, though, did explicitly note a linkage between the economic well-being of the people and the epidemic. This branch, perhaps rather surprisingly, was that regulating the production of salt. The years immediately preceding 1918 had seen a steady rise in the per capita consumption of salt in Java and Madura, from 2.94 kg. in 1914 to 3.10 kg. in 1917. In 1918, it fell back to 3.08 kg.; it recovered slightly in 1919 to 3.09, but it was not back on to the trend established earlier until 1920 when it reached 3.29 kg.[64]

The 1919 *Koloniaal Verslag* noted:

> the halting of the rising level [of consumption of salt produced on behalf of the government] in Java and Madura is in the main attributable to the influenza epidemic which was then raging . . . Sales in November 1918 were very much down on those of November 1917, in some places by 30 per cent.[65]

Of the slight increase in consumption in 1919, the following year's *Verslag* said that the increase—0.9%—'must be regarded as satisfactory, seeing that the adverse effects of the influenza epidemic of late 1918 are still being felt'.[66] Finally, noting the quite steep rise in consumption in 1920, the *Verslag* of 1921 said that this was 'in part due to the improved medical condition of the people'.[67] The linkage between the flu and salt consumption—more correctly, the purchase of salt from government stocks—is hardly clear. However, it might be suggested that the loss of income attributable to the epidemic reduced the capacity of the people to buy salt, and probably also to buy salted fish, the latter representing a significant proportion of government salt sales. The *Verslag* for 1919 does note that there was an upsurge in the illegal production of salt, an activity made easier by the long dry season in preceding months. Presumably financial strictures would have made such production even more attractive than it might otherwise have been.

Aftermath

As quickly as it had come, the epidemic disappeared. By the end of January 1919 it was all but over, though localized after-shocks continued to be reported during the rest of the year. And the traces of it began quickly to fade. The agricultural cycle evened out, borrowings from banks and pawnshops returned to earlier levels, schools, shops and offices re-opened for business. Only three consequences of any substance remained.

First, in 1921 the colonial authorities, after much debate enacted an Influenza Ordinance.[68] One of the reasons why details of deaths from influenza are known so imprecisely is that it was not a disease prescribed in the Epidemic Diseases Ordinance of 1911.[69] There was thus no requirement for doctors to report detection of outbreaks of the disease, nor any limitation on the movement of people into and out of infected areas. The BGD had none of the legal powers for coping with the flu that it did have with respect, for instance, to cholera. The new ordinance gave it, and certainly other specified government officers, such powers. Doctors were required to report to the civil authorities any outbreak of flu which caused an unusually high death rate. The authorities were then empowered, in consultation with the medical service, to enact precautionary regulations governing the holding of public gatherings, the closing of schools, and the establishment of temporary aid centres providing food, medical care, and, when necessary funerals. The latter services were to be provided free to those unable to afford them themselves. Violation of any regulations so enacted could bring a gaol term not exceeding six days or a fine of up to fifty guilders. The Ordinance also provided for the establishment of a complex system for controlling the movement of shipping, especially passenger shipping, through infected areas. This section was of particular importance given the crucial role played by shipping in spreading the disease through the eastern islands. This importance was implicitly recognized in the penalties applicable for violation of these restrictions: gaol for up to one year, or a fine not exceeding 10 000 guilders.

The second legacy of the epidemic, less concrete but long lasting, is the incorporation of the events into local folklore. In many places memories of these tragic events are still very much alive. I first heard stories about influenza in Purworejo. The epidemic was consistently described as having two major characteristics. First, it struck people down with great swiftness. One of the adages most often heard in this context is '*pagi sakit, sore meninggal*; *sore sakit, pagi meninggal*'—'sick in the morning, dead by evening; sick in the evening, dead by morning'. Clinically this is something of an exaggeration, though death within three days of the onset of illness 'was not rare'.[70] Second, the disease is remembered as being particularly severe in its impact, in terms of both morbidity and mortality. Almost everyone said they knew someone, or knew of someone, who had suffered from the disease; many knew people who had died. Few people were left totally untouched. I heard essentially similar stories in several other parts of Java. Terance Bigalke informs me that he had heard much the same stories in Tana Toraja, in Sulawesi, in the 1970s.

A third result of the epidemic, though hard to measure with accuracy, was demographic. In his major study of the Indonesian population, Widjojo Nitisastro noted that it was 'quite probable that the influenza epidemic . . . had a great impact on Indonesia's population'.[71] He shows that between 1917 and 1920, of the seventeen residencies in Java and Madura (including Yogyakarta and Surakarta), population declined in eight, including four of the six residencies of East Java. This is consistent with the observation made earlier that flu-related mortality rates in Java were highest in the east. But it is difficult to draw firm conclusions from these data, since influenza was obviously not the only factor affecting population growth rates. Madura, for instance, had a relatively high level of out-migration, and Besuki a high level of in-migration, both of which probably had a longer-term influence on their respective population growths than did the flu. It is unfortunate that the Census of 1920 was not very detailed or reliable and yielded little data that could have been used in trying to measure the demographic impact of the flu. Some more precise data, even if only tentative, on the age structure of the Indonesian population, for instance, might have helped to solve the question of age-specific death rates. In the absence of such data, it is difficult to do more than speculate.

I wish to thank Radin Fernando for his assistance in collecting much of the data upon which this paper is based, and Claire Smith, Charlotta Blomberg and Laura Forsyth for speedily and efficiently typing a messy manuscript.

1. *Encyclopaedia Britannica*, 14th edition, 12:242.

2. I. Snapper, 'Medical Contributions from the Netherlands Indies', in Peter Honig and Frans Verdoorn (eds), *Science and Scientists in the Netherlands Indies* (New York, Board for the Netherlands Indies, Surinam and Curacao, 1945), 316; cf. Terence H. Hull, 'Plague in Java', above.

3. 'Report on the Influenza-Epidemic in Netherlands-India 1918', *Mededeelingen van den Burgerlijke Geneeskundigen Dienst in Nederlandsch-Indië* 10 (1920), 78. Hereafter cited as 'Report'. Among the Committee's members were Mas Sardjito, later to become Prof. Dr Sardjito, Rektor of Universitas Gadjah Mada, and the singularly appropriately named Dr P.C. Flu.

4. This paragraph is based on 'Report', 117–33.

5. F. M. Burnet and Ellen Clark, *Influenza* (Melbourne, Monographs from the Walter and Eliza Hall Institute of Research in Pathology and Medicine, no. 4, 1942), 69ff.

6. 'Report', 141.

7. The data are drawn from *Mededeelingen van den Geneeskundigen Dienst in Nederlandsch-Indië* 4 (1923), 399–401. See Table 1.

8. *Koloniaal Verslag*, 1919, cols 71–6 and 80 (hereafter cited as *KV*, plus year).

9. 'De Spaansche Griep op Zuid-Oost Celebes', *Indië* 2 (1918–19), 830.

10. Terance W. Bigalke, 'A Social History of "Tana Toraja" 1870–1965' (Ph.D. dissertation, University of Wisconsin-Madison, 1981), 254.

11. Cited in Alfons van der Kraan, *Lombok: Conquest, Colonization and Underdevelopment, 1870–1940* (Singapore, Heinemann for the Asian Studies Association of Australia, 1980), 134.

12. The data in this paragraph and the following one are from *KV*, 1919, Bijlage Q, Table X.

13. *Locomotief*, 19 October 1918 and 8 November 1918; *Darmo Kondo* 20, November 1918 (reported in *Inlandsche Pers Overzicht* [hereafter cited as *IPO*], 1918, 47:4).

14. *KV*, 1920, cols 131–3.

15. *KV*, 1919, col. 109.

16. 'Report', 143.

17. Ibid, 135.

18. Cf. *Locomotief*, 5 November 1918, carrying a report of deaths in the gaol in Bojonegoro.

19. *KV*, 1919, cols 65–6.

20. Ibid., col. 64.

21. Ibid., col. 64.

22. *Locomotief*, 26 October 1918; *Kaoem Moeda*, 12 November 1918 (*IPO*, 1918, 46:9); *KV*, 1919, cols 115–16.

23. E.g., Burnet, op, cit., citing *Report on the Pandemic of Influenza, 1918–1919*, Ministry of Health, Reports on Public Health and Medical Subjects, no. 4 (London, HMSO, 1920).

24. E.g., Edwin D. Kilbourne (ed.), *The Influenza Viruses and Influenza* (New York, Academic Press, 1975), 485–6.

25. *Uitkomsten der in de maand November 1920 dehouden Volkstelling* (Batavia, Ruygrok, 1922), 2:120–1.

26. P. B. van Steenis, 'Enkele epidemiologische opmerkingen aangaande de Griep in de afdeeling Magelang 1918', *Geneeskundig Tijdschrift voor Nederlandsch Indië* (1919), 909–10.

27. C. W. Nortier, 'De Spaansche griep te Modjowarno', *Maandblad der Samenwerkende Zendings-Corporaties* (1919), 51–2.

28. Burnet, op. cit., 1.

29. *Locomotief*, 28 October 1918; *KV*, 1919, col. 50. See also 'Report', 137.

30. *KV*, 1920, col. 64.

31. *Handelingen van den Volksraad*, 14de Vergadering, 25 November 1918, 305.

32. 'Report', 155.

33. *Medan Boediman*, 6 November 1918 (*IPO*, 1918, 46:3).

34. *Djawi Hisworo*, 27 November 1918 (*IPO*, 1918, 46:4).

35. *Oetoesan Hindia*, 12 November 1918 (*IPO*, 1918, 46:21).

36. Ibid., 30 November 1918 (*IPO*, 1918, 48:27).

37. *Locomotief*, 9 November 1918.

38. *Bromotani*, 3 November 1918 (*IPO*, 1918, 45:5).

39. *Neratja*, 4 December 1918 (*IPO*, 1918, 49:4).

40. Ibid.

41. *Koemandang Djawi*, 30 December 1918 (*IPO*, 1919, 1:1). See also 'De Spaansche Griep op Zuid-Oost Celebes', 831.

42. *KV*, 1919, col. 175.

43. 'Report', 145.

44. *KV*, 1919, col. 237.

45. *Oetoesan Hindia*, 14 January 1919 (*IPO*, 1919, 3:23).

46. *Djawi Kondo*, 8 February 1919 (*IPO*, 1919, 6:6).

47. *Neratja*, 2 December 1918 (*IPO*, 1918, 49:1).

48. Tan Boen Kim, *Peroesoehan di Koedoes* (Batavia, Goan Hong, 1920), esp. chapter 4, 'Penjakit Influenza', 63–75.

49. Ibid., 74.

50. Lance Castles, *Religion, Politics and Economic Behaviour: The Kudus Cigarette Industry*, Cultural Reports Series no. 15 (New Haven, Yale University Southeast Asia Studies, 1967), 63.

51. A full search of the Archives has not been carried out. However, there is no

mention of such a connection reported in the *IPO*; in the reports submitted by colonial officials, collected by the Arsip Nasional and published as *Sarekat Islam Lokal*, or the *Memori Serah Jabatan* for West, Central and East Java and the Princely States of Yogyakarta and Surakarta, or by Kwantes and published in *De Ontwikkeling van de Nationalistische Beweging in Nederlandsch-Indië*, Vol. 1, 1917-mid 1923 (Groningen, Tjeenk Willink, 1975); or in the *Encyclopaedie van Nederlandsch-Indië*, 3:700–702. Also silent are R.T. McVey, *The Rise of Indonesian Communism* (Ithaca, Cornell University, 1965); Timur Jaylani, 'The Sarekat Islam Movement: Its Contribution to Indonesian Nationalism' (M.A. thesis, McGill University, 1959); and Deliar Noer, *The Modernist Muslim Movements in Indonesia, 1900–1942* (Singapore, Oxford University Press, 1973). More research could be undertaken; but it seems reasonable to assume that there is unlikely to be anything of major significance overlooked.

52. 'De Spaansche Griep', 830.
53. *Locomotief*, 30 November 1918.
54. Cf. T. W. Schultz, *Transforming Agriculture* (New Haven, Yale University Press, 1964), 68.
55. *Soerabaiasch Handelsblad*, 21 August 1921. I am indebted to John Ingleson for this reference.
56. P. Creutzberg, *Het Economisch Beleid in Nederlandsch-Indië*, Part II (Groningen, Tjeenk Willink, 1974), xxvi.
57. *KV*, 1919, col. 50.
58. *KV*, 1920, Bijlage W, Table I.
59. Ibid., Bijlage W, Tables II–VI.
60. *KV*, 1917, col. 163; *KV*, 1918, col. 157; *KV*, 1919, col. 199; *KV*, 1920, col. 241.
61. *KV*, 1918, col. 144; *KV*, 1920, col 188.
62. *KV*, 1918, col. 99; *KV*, 1919, col. 144; *KV*, 1920, col. 189.
63. *KV*, 1919, col. 144.
64. *KV*, 1915, col. 263; *KV*, 1917, col. 276; *KV*, 1918, col. 270; *KV*, 1919, col. 306; *KV*, 1920, col. 337; *KV*, 1921, col. 287.
65. *KV*, 1919, col. 307.
66. *KV*, 1920, col. 337.
67. *KV*, 1921, col. 289.
68. *Staatsblad van Nederlandsch Indië*, 1920, no. 793.
69. Ibid., 1911, no. 299; cf. Peter Gardiner and Mayling Oey, 'Morbidity and Mortality in Java, 1880–1940', above.
70. 'Report', 127.
71. Widjojo Nitisastro, *Population Trends in Indonesia* (Ithaca, Cornell University Press, 1970), 67–8.

12 Blame, Responsibility and Remedial Action: Death, Disease and the Infant in Early Twentieth Century Malaya[1]

LENORE MANDERSON

THE statistics of early twentieth century Malaya point to a recurrent tragedy of some dimension. Of every four infants, at least one would die in its first year of life; only two of every three would reach adulthood. Yet the records, both colonial and indigenous, are largely silent on the impact of these deaths on the bereaved: in part a consequence of a greater interest in political and particularly courtly life than in the everyday life of ordinary people; in part as a result of the especially private bereavement that follows infant death.[2] To colonial administrators, however, the numbers alone indicated the extent of the problem, and the battle to reduce the infant mortality rate was to be a major aspect of public health work in the decades that followed.

Defining the Problem: Patterns of Infant Death to 1910

To the turn of the century, infant mortality rates attracted little comment. They were, predictably, high, but adult mortality rates, including those following outbreaks of malaria and the more enigmatic beri-beri, gained most official comment and practical response. In the first decade of the twentieth century, the infant mortality rate received some scrutiny, particularly in light of the suggestion that the majority of the deaths were due to largely remediable conditions.[3]

At the turn of the century, the infant mortality rate for the Straits Settlements, where official attention was focused, was over

257

250 per 1 000 births; by 1911, it had risen to over 290 per thousand, with nearly two-thirds of the deaths occurring neonatally and post-neonatally.[4] In Singapore, the rates were especially high, from 319.9 in 1902 to 324.9 in 1911, with a range during this period from 306.2 (1906) to 347.8 (1908) and with some 54–60% of these deaths occurring before the infant was three months old. These infant mortality statistics were estimates, claimed by some to be inflated both as a consequence of the under-reporting of births and as a result of the inclusion of the deaths of infants born outside the Straits Settlements. But against this, it was argued that at least some neonatal deaths were probably also suppressed. Adjustments to the figures to exclude immigrant infant deaths reduced the rate, but by only around 20 per thousand.[5]

Most infant deaths were registered at the local police post without certification by a medical practitioner. However, even where there was a certificate, the stated cause of death was at times questionable, with the practitioner dependent upon the parents' own assessment of their infant's illness. A number of infants were recorded as having died of *Tetanus neonatorum* (tetanus, usually due to umbilical infection), caused, it was argued, by the unhygienic conditions of village midwifery. A number again died of 'prematurity'. However, most died of unspecified 'fever' or 'convulsions', disguising a variety of infant illnesses and disabilities. The major contributing factors to the infant mortality rate were to remain the subject of debate for some decades ahead.

The infant mortality rate varied significantly from one settlement to another and between ethnic communities. The infant mortality rate in Singapore was generally higher than elsewhere in the Settlements, always over 300 and typically nearer 350 per 1 000 live births. Only Malacca's rate approached this. It increased relatively steadily from a registered low rate of 215 in 1902 to a rate of 369.1 in 1911, exceeding even that of Singapore, and was suggestive, like the Singapore rate, of the impact of urbanization on infant health. The Penang rate peaked in 1907 at 306.5 but had declined by 1911 to a low 234.1. In the rural areas of Province Wellesley and the Dindings, in contrast, the infant mortality rate was usually around 150, although this figure was possibly low due to the under-reporting of neonatal mortality and was distorted by a relatively small population (especially in the Dindings) from which the rates were derived. The infant mortality rate for Europeans

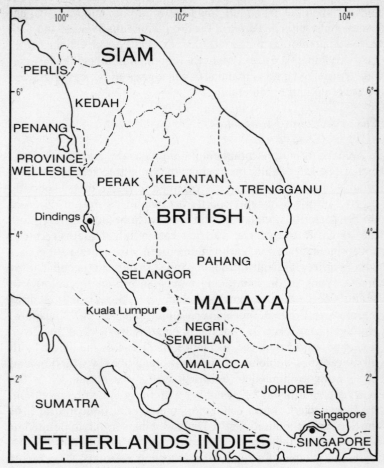

Map 4 British Malaya

was comparatively low, but was based upon only a few births and deaths per annum. The rates for Eurasians and 'others' were unpredictable and again usually referred to very small numbers, although they were at least three times greater than those of Europeans. The Indian infant mortality rate, although still relating to a relatively small population, was fairly constant at around 250 per 1 000. Chinese and Malay rates averaged for the settlements, for the years 1905–11, 288 and 244 respectively. However at times the rates of both Malays and Chinese soared to over 400 per 1 000, most often in the urban settlements of Singapore and Malacca, but occasionally also in Penang. Further, whilst on average the Chinese infant mortality rate was higher, Malay and Chinese rates vied for top place from year to year in unpredictable fashion, reflecting the complex manner in which various factors interacted to make early life vulnerable.

The Conditions of Urban Life

Analytic attention to the infant mortality rate, and the development of a public health programme that sought to reduce the rate, occurred initially in Singapore, partly in response to its especially high infant mortality rate, partly because of its concentration of the Settlements' population, and partly also because of its role as the administrative centre. The high rate of infant deaths received government attention early in the twentieth century, together with a variety of health problems other than those peculiar to or most striking in the estate and mining sectors of the colony. In June 1905, the then Colonial Secretary, E.L. Brockman, first drew attention to the high morbidity and mortality rates of Singapore. He noted that some 20% of the population was sick at any given time and associated the incidence of sickness and death with urbanization. Problems of overcrowding, poor ventilation and insanitation continued to be discussed for the remainder of the year, culminating on 22 December with the passing of a motion in the Legislative Council, calling for an inquiry into the mortality of the Settlement. Subsequently, Dr W. J. Simpson was appointed to undertake the inquiry; he visited Singapore in July and August 1906 and produced a report the following February. The report drew attention to the over-development of land with buildings, the overcrowding of these buildings, the absence of light and air in housing, and the lack of drainage and sewage removal so that 'the smell of faecal matter and urine was very strong in Singapore, not only in a large number of houses but also in the morning in the streets'.[6] People lived in 'rabbit warrens, consisting of scores of cubicles where daylight never penetrates, and air is always foul and germ laden'.[7] The report, and subsequent commentators, argued that in light of the appalling conditions of the urban dwellers—largely Chinese artisans and labourers—a high infant mortality rate and a high adult morbidity and mortality rate were to be expected: 'When one considers what life must be like for a small child or a sick person in a cubicle in one of these houses, the wonder is, not that they die, but that they live.'[8]

Conditions remained poor. In 1910, the infant mortality rate in Singapore had increased over previous years to 343 per 1 000, a rate that the *Straits Times*, at least, associated with 'foul wells, impure milk, and homes that are saturated with filth and robbed of all purification by air and sunlight, [making] it almost impossible to rear children'.[9] These problems persisted. In 1918, a Commission of Inquiry into urban conditions in Singapore again drew attention to the relationship between overcrowding and infant mortality. It argued that there was little difference at birth in the health status of infants born in rural or urban areas and to poor or wealthy parents, and that the major factor in their differential survival rates was subsequent environmental conditions.[10] The Commission drew attention to the disproportionate age structure in certain urban areas, suggesting that there were far fewer children than might normally be expected given the number of adults, and that this was explicable by the high infant mortality rate.[11] Later reports continually returned to the impoverished conditions of urban dwellers. The 1927 Annual Report of the Medical Department, for example, noted that 80% of almost 10 000 women (8 037 of 9 981) visited in their homes after the birth of their child were living in single rooms or cubicles where the worst type of overcrowding and insanitation prevailed.[12] The 1933 Report similarly noted that 'with so many of the wage earners living in such ill ventilated and insanitary dwellings, it is not surprising that tuberculosis in urban areas is so prevalent and that the infantile death rate is high'.[13]

Poor living conditions occurred elsewhere in the colony also. In Penang overcrowding, lack of sanitary facilities and polluted water supplies were again a feature of urban life early in the century,[14] and later commentators constantly referred to the 'evils of overcrowding, ignorance of hygiene and bad housing' and the fact that in areas immediately outside the town, health was prejudiced by a 'growing tendency for people to crowd into ill constructed village shanties'.[15] The lower infant mortality rates recorded in the least urbanized parts of the colony, although possibly too low due to under-reporting, nevertheless provided further evidence of the significance of relatively healthy living conditions to infant health, even in areas with poor medical services.[16] But in rural areas, too, there were problems of overcrowding and insanitation. As late as

1935 it was estimated that only half the dwellings provided for plantation labour on rural estates in the Straits Settlements conformed to a minimum standard, and constant inspection by the Department of Labour was necessary.[17]

Maternal Health, Labour and the Economy

The poor health and nutritional status of women prior to and during pregnancy and during confinement after childbirth was also used sporadically to World War II to explain the high infant mortality rate. Venereal disease amongst indigenous and other 'native' (non-European) women, congenital syphilis, and anaemia due both to the demands of pregnancy and malaria, were all factors that affected foetal development and the subsequent survival chances of the infant.[18] Beri-beri was believed both to affect the women's ability to lactate, and to be transferred to the infant through breast-milk.[19] Dietary restrictions during pregnancy and confinement were considered to cause vitamin and mineral deficiencies that disadvantaged mother and child, so that both were debilitated,[20] although there is little evidence to support this contention. In addition, it was argued, particularly in the 1930s, that general economic conditions affected women's nutritional intake and thus their own and their infants' health. The Government of the Federated Malay States in 1933 noted that 'economic stress of the past two years . . . now appears to be manifesting itself in a lowered vitality of mothers and infants',[21] and a health report of Kedah published in 1936 suggested that unfavourable climatic conditions, resulting in a poor rice crop, had led to general sub-nutrition that was at least as important as the absence of adequate health services in explaining the high infant and child mortality rates.[22] For residents of the Straits Settlements, the monetization of the economy was itself considered detrimental to maternal and infant nutrition, particularly where wages were insufficient to cover the cost of a varied diet, but also because of an increasing tendency for rural and to a lesser extent urban dwellers to sell various home-grown foodstuffs to purchase 'a more sophisticated but less nourishing diet'.[23]

While downturns in the economy were used to explain in part the equivocal health status of women and its effect on infant health, economic growth was also considered to influence the infant mortality rate, albeit indirectly. Here, the argument was simply that working women neglected their infants. During periods of high demand for labour, it was claimed, women were more likely to seek paid employment soon after delivery, and thus leave their small infants in the care of others to be fed artificially. The rise in the infant mortality rate in the Straits Settlements in 1934, from 168 to 172, was considered to be the result of 'an abnormal demand for labourers [whereby] women were employed in industry to a greater extent than is usual. It is generally recognised that during periods of unemployment which do not lead to actual starvation, infantile mortality is low. The return of prosperity usually causes an increase in infantile deaths in countries that have a high birth rate'.[24] In the Federated Malay States, the same argument was advanced: 'the increased employment of mothers and the increased purchasing power which leads to artificial instead of breastfeeding may be a possible explanation' of the increased infant mortality rate of 163 in 1934 compared to the 1933 rate of 146.[25] The subsequent year the improved infant mortality rate of 144 (and 162 in the Settlements) was related partly to a reduced demand for labour and a decline in the employment of women.[26] The authors of medical reports in the 1920s and 1930s appeared uncritically willing to allocate the blame for high infant mortality rates away from the government and government sources, and in so doing, overlooked the contradictions and paradoxes of their arguments: women were responsible for high infant mortality rates during both periods of economic constraint and growth, because of their economic and employment status as well as because of patterns of childcare and mothering (see below).

Later reports again argued that women's participation in paid employment negatively affected infant health, although the conditions of their employment appear to be significant. A 1940 study of infant mortality and child welfare in Kedah, for example, maintained that low wages paid to labour forced families to depend on two incomes, and this led to the early return after childbirth of women to work; delay in return to work and hence failure to contribute to family income created sufficient worry to interfere with the women's ability to lactate in any case. In addition maternity leave provisions placed considerable stress on the women throughout pregnancy (which arguably affected foetal development and thus infant health). For example, on the estates examined in the report, maternity leave payments were provided for one month before and one month after delivery. These were

calculated on the amount earned by the women during the preceding six months, thus placing pressure on the women to work
hard and long hours during a period when considerable rest was
required.[27]

Midwifery Practice and Neonatal Mortality

Whilst mothers were explicitly blamed in the above explanations
of the high infant mortality rate, for the most part their actions and
behaviour were related to the general processes of economic
development in the colony. There appeared to be little opportunity here for direct intervention by the medical departments.
However, other factors, associated with infant death, allowed for
immediate intervention. Traditional midwifery practices were
among the first to be addressed. Medical officers were concerned
with the failure of village midwives (*bidan*) to use aseptic instruments to cut the umbilicus, although they also believed that the
delayed cutting of the cord until the cessation of pulsation caused
maternal haemorrhage and that, additionally, the midwives lacked
the skill to identify problems of late pregnancy and complications
of labour or to handle such complications with competence.

Any dirty old woman could practice midwifery. The majority of them
were illiterate, superstitious, filthy and unintentionally cruel. Filthy scissors, dirty pocket knives, pieces of bamboo, broken crockery and at times
even finger nails were used for cutting the baby's cord. Black powder and
ashes were applied to the cord which was then covered with a leaf. The
bodies were then bound firmly like mummies from head to foot in yards of
cloth. They were given black coffee, rice and bananas to eat from birth
and were bathed in cold water straight from the well.[28]

Again, in even more vitriolic terms:

These women thrive on superstition, and the dreadful consequences of
their revolting habits were everywhere encountered. These relics of
mediaeval times are moreover in a strong position, because their craft is
generally a family accomplishment handed down from mother to
daughter. The Malay *bidans* still have a virtual monopoly in most of the
rural villages, and though most of them are filthy, illiterate and obstinate,
it is well worth the attempt to try to teach them the rudiments of simple
midwifery practice.[29]

Concern with the high incidence of *Tetanus neonatorum* led to
moves to bring midwifery practice under government control.

Legislative measures to control midwifery in the Straits Settlements were foreshadowed in 1905, when the Honorary Visiting Surgeon, Dr P. Fowlie, noted that 'the time will come in Singapore when the practice of midwifery and its regulation must be a subject for legislation and in anticipation of that time it would seem desirable that the training of Natives in the art should be begun forthwith—and the sooner the better'.[30] In 1906 the Administrative Report for Penang called for special instruction to be provided to native women in midwifery and hygiene,[31] and in 1908 notice was given of a Midwives Bill to be introduced 'at an early date' to prohibit the practice of midwifery by women other than those holding a certificate of competence following training by the colonial medical service. Midwives were to receive as part of their training instruction in child rearing and infant feeding, as a means of reaching indirectly the mothers themselves.[32] Legislation in fact was not introduced until 1917. Its provisions for the registration of midwives were extended in 1923 with a new ordinance which constituted a Central Midwives Board. This legislation made registration compulsory only within the municipal limits of Singapore, Penang and Malacca. It was not extended to rural areas of the Settlements until 1 January 1930, and similar provisions for compulsory registration in the Federated and Unfederated Malay States were not introduced until 1954.[33]

The training of midwives and health workers commenced much earlier. In October 1910, the first European nurse was appointed in Singapore to the Straits Settlements Medical Department to gather information on early infant life and to instruct women in child care; a year later the Singapore Municipality appointed female inspectors within its Health Department to make home visits in urban areas to advise women on the care of their newborn.[34] From 1910, too, a training scheme was implemented whereby the Government covered the cost of tuition and the Singapore Municipality the cost of uniforms and subsistence, to train four local women at a time 'to help indigenous women care for their infants'.[35] A graded training scheme for midwives was also introduced, offering from six months' to three years' instruction; by 1914, fifteen women had qualified.

In Malacca, a Lady Inspector was appointed from 1908. From 1912 lectures were offered in Malay to midwives, covering topics such as the antiseptic care of patients and the dressing of the umbilicus. All midwives in whose practice there had been known incidence of tetanus were interviewed, and all were issued with a free supply of antiseptic, cotton wool and lint.[36] The Lady Inspector also instructed newly confined mothers on the care of the cord and on general principles of hygiene.

Training in Penang was rather slower. By January 1930 there were still only fourteen trained midwives for a population of 190 000. Unqualified midwives were gradually replaced by women who had received training at government expense in a six-month residential course; in the interim, practising midwives were encouraged to attend at least one class a week for some months, at the end of which they received a certificate with a warning to each 'that if her work did not improve she would not be allowed to practice, and that her certificate would be taken away from her and that she would "lose face"'.[37] Government-trained midwives were issued with free obstetrics baskets that included an enamel bowl, forceps and surgical scissors; private midwives could purchase the baskets for $8.[38] Contemporary reports suggest some resistance by midwives to training and registration, although the reports are themselves rather antipathetic to the midwives;

> The bidans were so ignorant that they had to be taught again and again the names of the contents of their baskets, such as lotions for baby's eyes, cord dressings, etc., and how to use them . . . even after several years of intensive training some of them still need the most careful watching—being prone to slip back into dirty habits and superstitious practices.[39]

By 1935, however, all practising midwives were registered, and according to the Penang Health Sister, 'the bona fide midwives [untrained registered *bidan*] have improved so much that many of them . . . are as competent and conscientious as the qualified ones'.[40]

By the 1920s, some degree of training was also being offered to midwives in the Federated Malay States,[41] and later also in the Unfederated States, although for the most part it remained necessary to permit the supervised practice of village midwives, with brief instruction in antisepsis and the recognition of complications of pregnancy and parturition.[42] In addition, in rural areas particularly, there was some suggestion of resistance to Western ways by mothers as well as by the midwives, and a reluctance by both to report complications to the colonial authorities.[43]

Parallel with the training and registration of midwives, positive efforts were also made to encourage women to seek Western medical advice and to discourage their use of village midwives. Museums that operated as propaganda against village midwives were set up in Infant Welfare Centres in the 1920s with various confiscated equipment, including old midwifery baskets 'full of appalling exhibits that must have caused many deaths'[44] and including long-tube feeders, comforters, unsuitable clothing and dressing material as 'a warning lesson to mothers'.[45] Beyond this, staff in the Infant Welfare Centres sought to establish regular contact with pregnant women and to encourage them to present themselves to hospital at the onset of labour.[46] The main function of the Centres, however, was to educate the women, not only with regard to ante-natal care, but especially in care in infancy and early childhood.

Infant Feeding Practice and the Ways of Mothering

While many commentators argued that midwifery practice was an important component in the high infant mortality rate, others argued that the major cause of early death was a complex of preventable factors, defined as 'domestic' and including 'racial habits and customs, ignorance of elementary hygiene and nutrition, and the artificial feeding of infants'.[47]

In defining this domestic problem, indigenous and other native women were described as ignorant of the general concepts of hygiene and basic cleanliness, of acceptable methods of child care and child rearing, and of 'correct infant feeding and weaning practice'. Early reports maintained that the 'want of knowledge on the part of Mothers or Guardians have [sic] a great deal to do with the high mortality'[48]; this want, it was to be argued, derived from 'simple ignorance with only conservatism behind it rather than a system of superstitions which would be a still more tedious obstacle'.[49] In addition, however, many colonial officers explained such 'ignorance' in explicitly racist terms. Mrs Hamblin, a health worker in Negri Sembilan before World War II, characterized Malay women as 'distinguished by their lethargy and apathy in health matters' and although the 'Chinese took advice more readily than the other elements of the Asiatic population; the Tamils often tried to act on the advice given them but were often handicapped by lack of intelligence'.[50] Miss E. Darville, Health Sister in Penang from 1927 to 1941, again characterized Malay women as fatalists. 'They are inclined to be lazy, and those dwelling in rural

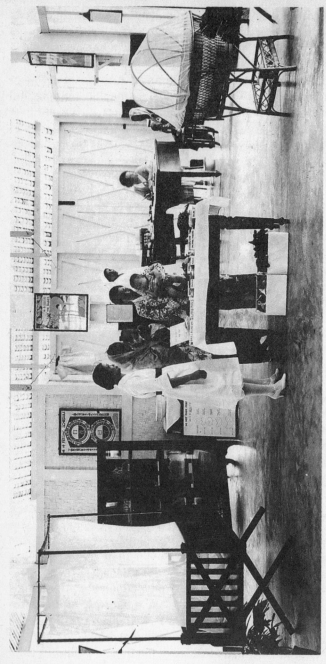

Fig. 12.1. Infant Welfare Centre, Balik Pulau, Penang, c.1933. Cot on far left and cradle on far right were both made by fathers attending the clinic; the mosquito nets in both cases were made by local mothers. The cupboard near the cot constitutes the Centre's 'museum', and includes feeding bottles, midwifery baskets, and wax models of 'good' food. From Bodleian Library (Rhodes House Library, Colonial Records Project, Mss Indian Ocean S134).

districts are ignorant and superstitious, but good mannered and charming . . . the majority of the Malay women in the rural districts of Penang are ignorant, and many of them appear to have only the mentality of a child of ten.'[51] Chinese women, by contrast, were 'industrious and intelligent', but 'they have large families and this causes a great deal of poverty'; Indian women were 'illiterate and superstitious with many very unhygienic habits . . . [but were] good mothers according to their lights in spite of being ignorant'.[52]

These and other health workers provided details of the extent of maternal 'ignorance', particularly in infant feeding practice but also more generally in child care. Miss Darville described Malay and Chinese feeding practices thus:

[Malay] babies a few weeks old were brought to the [Infant Welfare] centre sucking black coffee from a long tube feeder or dirty tin. They were bathed in cold water straight from the well, and bound round like mummies with yards of material until they were six or seven months old. A thick shawl was suspended from a hook in the ceiling to form a cradle, the child being almost suffocated when placed inside . . .
A large number of [Chinese] babies were artificially fed from birth, and were also given pork to eat. The mother worked in the fields and left the child in the care of the grandmother . . . It was the usual thing for the mother to give her newborn baby daughter a bottle, while the older baby, if a son, continued with the fresh supply of breastmilk which should have been given to the sister.[53]

Annual Medical Department reports provided further instances of maternal ignorance and error:

Errors of feeding [are] usually due to ignorance, or national habits rather than poverty. Artificial feeding, starchy foods such as flour, rice and potatoes being fed to a few days old infants [sic]. In Yeo Chu Keng Road, a rachitic infant of 5 months, weighing 7 lbs., was found to be sharing his fare from a clean long tube feeding bottle with a little suckling pig—there seemed nothing wrong with the pig.[54]

Artificial feeding and weaning practices had been identified from the earliest discussions as major contributory factors to the high infant mortality rate. In 1907 it was estimated that over 94% of infant deaths were due to conditions largely removable, and that nearly 37% of all deaths were the result of 'improper feeding' including the use of adulterated and polluted fresh and imported cows' milk.[55] The Annual Report of the Straits Settlements for

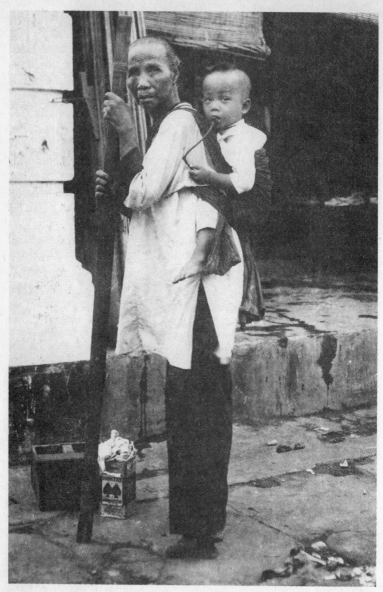

Fig. 12.2. Chinese Grandmother and Toddler, Singapore, c.1910. Note child is sucking on teat with feeding tube, of the type confiscated by health workers. From Royal Commonwealth Society, London, Files of the British Association of Malaya, BAM/1–Singapore; reproduced courtesy of Royal Commonwealth Society.

1910 suggested that most infantile convulsions, the major stated cause of infant death, were due to the 'faulty feeding of infants, [with] boiled rice and starchy food entering the dietery [*sic*] even from the first month of life'.[56]

The extent to which infants received a mixed regime from birth, and the incidence of artificial feeding in addition to or instead of breastfeeding is unknown. However, bottle feeding appears to have occurred early and was widespread in urban areas, certainly by the turn of the century. Condensed milk was available in Singapore from the 1880s, and infant food preparations were marketed, increasingly aggressively, from 1896.[57] Chinese infants 'adopted' and imported from China through Hong Kong to Singapore for sale to brothel keepers were fed diluted condensed milk on the ships, with a reported high mortality rate in consequence,[58] and bottle feeding was widespread in urban Malaya. In 1926, for instance, of 8 539 infants seen on home visits by Singapore municipal health workers, 21% were bottle fed exclusively and 4% were on a mixed regime; in Malacca the same year, 29% of 1 121 newborn infants were bottle fed.[60] The following year, of 9 507 infants in Singapore for whom the method of feeding is known, 18% received artificial milk only and an additional 2% received both breast and bottled milk. In Malacca, the figures provided imply that only 33.5% were breastfed, and even presuming an error of transposition, the proportion of infants receiving sweetened condensed milk as their major source of nutrition was extremely high.[61]

The argument put forward with respect to expatriate women,[62] that the tropical climate of Malaya mitigated against lactation, appears not to have been applied to non-European women. However, it was argued seriously that 'many of the poor were unable from bad health or debility to nurse their own infants', whilst lacking the resources to purchase milk[63] or to purchase sufficient milk to provide the infant with the necessary nutrients. As a result, Health Department workers and later the Infant Welfare Centres supplied condensed milk to women deemed needy. In 1914, the Malacca Municipality provided 804 tins of condensed milk to various poor women on the advice of the Lady Inspector.[64] Infant health centres, including those run by the Government, the Municipalities, and by voluntary associations such as the Singapore Children's Welfare Society, all maintained supplies of tinned milk, bottles and teats,[65] and offered advice on artificial feeding in addition to seeking to encourage prolonged breastfeeding. Thus, despite various statements by medical officers and institutions regarding the preferability of breast milk, children's services, including the infant health centres, effectively promoted bottle feeding.

Maternal Education: Home Visiting and Infant Welfare Centres

Government medical officers argued that a direct approach to native women would be resisted, and that the most effective way of educating them to be 'better mothers' was first to instruct the midwives in elementary child care: 'The only way of teaching native mothers to feed their children properly and the necessity of cleanliness etc., is by first teaching the women that attend them in childbirth and through them educating the mothers.'[66] However, direct approaches to women also occurred early. I have noted above that home visiting commenced in Singapore in 1910, and a year later the Singapore Municipal Health Department appointed women as inspectors to visit newly confined women, using a list of births provided daily from the office of the Registrar of Births and Deaths. Malacca and Penang also had limited home visiting by Lady Inspectors within urban areas. Extension work in the rural areas occurred later. In Malacca, Miss I. M. Simmons and Miss A. McNeill began to visit villages (*kampung*) from May 1927, calling on newly delivered women and offering advice on health matters.[67] The same year Miss Darville was appointed as Health Sister in Penang and commenced home visiting 'to give advice to the mother on the care and feeding of the child and herself . . . A few words of praise, sometimes a scolding, is all that is needed in some houses'.[68]

Home visiting continued as the most effective means of first contact between health workers and indigenous women, given the high proportion of home births and the low utilization of Western medical services. At the same time, medical centres operated to provide public health education as well as to treat illness. The Women and Children's Dispensary at the Kandang Kerbau Maternity Hospital in Singapore opened in June 1921, for example, and reportedly 'a very great proportion of the time . . . [was spent] with outpatients . . . directed to giving information concerning the diet suitable for children and the avoidance of causes of unnecessary bad health'.[69] But education was the special task of the Infant Welfare Centres, established by the Government Medical Departments throughout the Straits Settlements and Federated Malay States by the late 1920s and in the Unfederated States by the late 1930s. Singapore and Malacca also had clinics run by the Municipalities, and in Singapore, too, the voluntary Children's Welfare Society ran two centres and made home visits for a ten-year period from 1923, and also provided crèche facilities for locally employed women from 1930. Often the centres began in a very small way. The first clinic in Penang, for example, opened in 1927 in a rented shop house. Women were encouraged to attend at preliminary home visits made by the Health Sister and a Chinese nurse/interpreter. The initial session attracted nine women only, five Chinese and four Malays. None of the latter returned, apparently because they were distressed by having their babies weighed. By the end of the first month, only forty women had presented themselves, but after five months, the clinic had had 2 500 attendances.[70] By 1936, there were seventy centres and nine sub-centres in the Settlements and Federated Malay States, each of which was staffed at least by a health nurse, a midwife and an attendant.

At clinic sessions held at the Infant Welfare Centres, medical attention was provided for minor ailments, with more serious cases of illness being referred to the nearest government dispensary. Ante-natal check-ups were provided; village midwives were supervised and provided with dressings and disinfectant. Infants were weighed and had their temperatures checked; at this time advice on infant feeding and care would be imparted to the mothers. Cecily Williams describes the operation of Trengganu centres in the later 1930s thus:

> The present method is for the Health Nurse to go to the centre at 7 in the morning with about 4 helpers, generally a dresser, a nurse and two bidans. Two go visiting in the district with her, looking up new-born babies particularly. The other two helpers prepare the centre, food display and so forth. They begin weighing babies, taking temperatures and writing up cards. At about 9 o'clock the visiting team returns, and the Health Nurse then sees the mothers and babies for as long as is necessary.[71]

While in operational terms effort was concentrated upon practical activities, official sources stressed the educational role of the centres—the 'proper preventive work of educating mothers':[72]

Their chief functions are educational and advisory. Efforts are directed towards teaching mothers how properly to feed, clothe and care for their infants and many visits are paid to the homes of mothers for this purpose. By these means it has been found possible to overcome many of the ignorant prejudices which in the past have been so inimical to infant welfare . . . An attempt is also made by the staff of the centres to educate the unskilled women and restrain them from some of their more objectionable and injurious practices.[73]

Such 'education' and 'restraint' was not always subtle:

If a mother has been careless or lazy in giving the treatment suggested, then she is scolded . . . Malays are obstinate almost to the point of stupidity when told to go to the hospital for advanced illnesses, and much time is often wasted trying to tell them they will be cared for or cured if only they will trust themselves to the district nurses in charge.[74]

But advice was not enough to encourage or increase clinic attendance, and hence centres sought methods of 'more obvious appeal',[75] such as the issue of milk rations and holding regular baby shows with monetary prizes for the winners. The Chief Health Officer of Singapore in 1927, Dr Brooker, noted that 'year by year' the baby shows were 'getting a larger hold on the popular imagination—a fact which should have useful public health results',[76] and shows became an early feature of newly opened centres. The Klang Infant Welfare Centre, for example, opened in 1928 and 'after being in operation for only six months, its influence had extended so widely that 470 competitors were entered for the first Baby Show'.[77] The Singapore Children's Welfare Society conducted a monthly as well as an annual show, with cash prizes for the healthiest, fattest and cleanest babies; and government and municipal centres both saw the shows as a first step in carrying 'the knowledge of public health into the very life of the family'.[78]

Other methods, too, were utilized to publicize the work of the centres and increase clinic attendance. Direct appeal was made to government servants in Kuala Lumpur to encourage their wives to attend ante-natal sessions at the clinics and to take their infants along for advice and treatment if indicated.[79] Exhibitions were mounted at horticultural/agricultural shows, often with a particular emphasis: the 1927 health exhibition at the Penang Show focused largely on the prevention of hookworm, although the display also included posters advocating breast feeding and bottles for artificial feeding.[80] In Penang, an annual tea party was also held from 1929 until the outbreak of war, to which parents were invited with invitations printed in English, Chinese, Tamil and *jawi* (Malay in Arabic script); fathers were especially encouraged to attend.[81]

Conclusion: The Decline of Early Death

Although published data from year to year are not directly comparable, the statistics that are available indicate an impressive increase in home visiting by nursing staff and in clinic attendance by the women and infants with whom they made contact. In 1926, 64 432 home visits and clinic consultations of infants were made in Singapore; an additional 23 138 home visits to newborn infants were made in Malacca. In 1930, the total number of home visits in the Straits Settlements combined had risen to 274 219, and clinic consultations to 99 450. Six years later, the number of home visits had increased by over 50% to 428 179 and clinic attendance had increased over 250% to 244 068. In the Federated Malay States, there are few published figures on home visits, but Infant Welfare Clinic attendance increased over three-fold, from 56 916 in 1925 to 195 144 in 1938.

Official reports took considerable satisfaction from the fact that clinic attendance increased dramatically over the years, and that there was therefore a demonstrably changed attitude by the population towards European medicine and the colonial medical institutions. The Federated Malay States triumphantly reported in 1926:

> It is interesting to note the change that has taken place in the attitude of the parents towards the aim and object of the centres. They were originally full of fears and prejudices and attended only after much persuasion and in a very hesitating manner; they vouchsafed no signs of approval or otherwise at the instructions given them and appeared completely mystified and far from happy. Today on visiting the centre one can see for oneself that these same people are now thoroughly at home and have lost their fears, their attendance weekly is regular and they bring not only their own babies but persuade their neighbours to do the same.[82]

Increased clinic attendance throughout the colony allowed this kind of romantic and optimistic interpretation of the role of the centres. However, as contemporary analysts recognized, the factors that influenced infant morbidity and mortality were complex. Changes in the infant mortality rate overall showed a downward trend. In the Straits Settlements the corrected infant mortality rate (i.e., excluding infants born outside the colonies) fell from 255.02 in 1906, to 179.23 in 1921 to 168.3 in 1936. In the Federated Malay States, the infant mortality rate dropped from 203.11 as late as 1927, to 142 in 1936. But changes to the infant mortality rates did not always correlate with the activities of the Medical Department. Moreover, the infant mortality rates were sufficiently variable within administrative regions and within ethnic groups to prevent any confident statements regarding the role of the state in effecting reductions, whether by controlling midwifery practice or by bringing women under the supervision and guidance of Infant Welfare Centre staff.

State and settlement trends were rather more consistent than those for ethnic groups. By the mid to late 1930s, the infant mortality rate had declined in all states and settlements (excepting Labuan) to around 165 per 1 000; the proportional decline in the rate from earlier years depended largely on the original marked disparity between regions. This disparity in itself defies too broad generalization, since both the administrative regions which were least economically developed and most peripheral to the colonial economy, and those most highly developed and best served by government, had higher infant mortality rates than those that prevailed in the Federated Malay States and Settlements of the mid and northwest coast of the peninsula (Perak, Selangor, Province Wellesley, Dindings). Each state holds a rather different pattern of decline. Sporadic reversals in the rate of decline occurred both because of the improved reliability of statistics, which tend to increase the number of reported deaths and thence the apparent rate, and as a result of epidemics. Influenza, for example, hit the population badly in 1918 especially, and in 1926 the incidence of malaria was extremely high, affecting infant as well as adult morbidity and mortality rates. However, other rises and falls are less easily explained and suggest the need for a more detailed inquiry into local conditions.

The variation between ethnic groups is rather more confusing. Certain inclines in the rate correspond, as they do for geographic area, to broader health crises such as the influenza pandemic and the high incidence of malaria. In general the infant mortality rate declined for all ethnic groups. But amongst the Malay population in the Straits Settlements the decline over the period 1906–36 was very slight (from 242.3 to 221.8), representing a decline of just

8.5%. This is less than 20% of that recorded for the other major ethnic groups, the Chinese and the Indians, for whom the respective declines over the period are 45.4% and 44.3%. This suggests the possible concentration of effort and services in urban centres to the disadvantage or disregard of the rural, predominantly Malay, population. In the Federated Malay States, in the 1930s the infant mortality rate amongst the Malay community actually rose by over 13%; here, it had in 1931 in fact been lower than that recorded for the Chinese and Indians (135, compared with 148 and 154 respectively). Yet state-by-state data suggest greater variability again. Thus, whilst the overall Malay rate in 1931 was lower than that for the Chinese and Indians, the highest of all rates in that year was the Malay rate in Pahang (169), reflecting perhaps the fact that this population was least well served by infant welfare services or any other medical services. In 1936, the Chinese rate for the Federated Malay States combined fell between the higher Malay rate and the lower Indian rate (139, 149 and 136 respectively), but the highest rates recorded were for Chinese in Pahang and Negri Sembilan (166 and 162). And in this year the total rate, and most breakdowns of the rate both by ethnicity and by administrative area, were higher in the Straits Settlements than in the Federated Malay States, even though the former settlements were far better served by Infant Welfare Centres and were, proportionate to the population, also considerably better off in terms of hospitals and dispensaries (see Table 12.1).

It was in light of these confusing statistics that socio-economic explanations, originally proffered around the turn of the century, regained currency among colonial officials. Fluctuations in the infant mortality rate, always regarded as a 'sensitive indicator' of the health status of the community, became a cost of economic development and were seen as an inevitable short-term result of increased urbanization and industrialization.

Even so, there was an appreciable downturn in infant mortality rates. This continued following the Pacific War. Under the continued efforts of the colonial medical officers, then under the auspices of the state departments of health of independent Malaya, further infant welfare centres were built, supplementary feeding programmes were introduced, and ante- and post-natal care was promoted and extended. For the period under discussion in this paper, these factors, together with the increased surveillance by health workers of mothers and their infants, which assisted the

TABLE 12.1

MEDICAL FACILITIES, STRAITS SETTLEMENTS AND FEDERATED MALAY STATES, 1936

Settlement/ State	Population	Hospital Beds	Dispensaries Outdoor	Travelling	River	Infant Welfare Centres	Infant Welfare Sub-Centres	Infant Mortality Rate (per 1000 births)
STRAITS SETTLEMENTS								
Singapore	603 163	1 753	5	1	—	5	6	169
Penang	205 994	680	3	1	—	6	2	152
Province Wellesley	148 406	400	3	1	—	6	1	150
Malacca	202 828	500	5	2	—	10	—	189
Total	1 160 390	3 333	16	5	—	27	9	168[a]
FEDERATED MALAY STATES								
Perak	830 093	2 312	12	8	2	3	—	142
Selangor	575 775	1 475	12	4	—	9	—	137
Negri Sembilan	249 853	966	4	5	1	1	—	144
Pahang	192 230	1 980	8	4	1	2	—	153
Total	1 847 951	6 733	43	21	3	16	—	142
GRAND TOTAL	3 008 341	10 066	59	26	3	43	9	162

(a) Includes Dindings and Labuan.
Sources: Straits Settlements, *Annual Departmental Report 1936* (Singapore, Government Printing Office, 1938), 1:909; Federated Malay States, *Annual Reports on the Social and Economic Progress of the People of the Federated Malay States* (Kuala Lumpur, Government Printing Office, 1938).

early diagnosis and treatment of a number of illness of early childhood, probably did contribute to the decline in infant deaths. Yet it is possible that the infant mortality rate would have declined without the development of these services. Crude death rates also fell at this time: in the Straits Settlements from 37.82 in 1906 to 31.81 in 1926 to 19.20 in 1936. Anti-malarial measures, sanitation and hygiene programmes (including the provision of latrines), the increased administrative of vaccination and medical treatment to control and treat various infectious diseases, and other public health programmes all reduced the incidence of life-threatening illness and disease, and these measures were reflected in the demographic statistics of all age groups for the period. The health and medical services oriented towards mothers and infants provided a back-up to other broader-based public health programmes and served a useful role in the dispensation of medicine and medical advice where illness occurred. The significance of the 'educational' role of the infant welfare clinics remains in doubt however. This appears to be the manifest product of colonial ideology, and specifically the view that women—mothers and midwives—caused infant deaths, a view informed by racism and sexism rather than empirical reality. To re-evoke a metaphor from the introduction of this chapter: the battle to reduce the infant mortality rate was waged against women, with nursing staff in infant welfare centres in the front-line. The real war against death and disease, however, appears to have been fought elsewhere.

1. This paper focuses especially on the Straits Settlements (Malacca, Penang and Singapore) and to a lesser extent on the Federated Malay States of Perak, Negri Sembilan, Selangor and Pahang. The Unfederated Malay States of the Malay Peninsula are referred to occasionally only.

2. Among the unofficial European records that address loss and grief, see F. A. Swettenham, *Malay Sketches* (London, John Lane–the Bodley Head, 1913), chapter 14; and H. Clifford, *Malayan Monochromes* (London, John Murray, 1913), chapter 4. Of indigenous nineteenth century sources, the Tuhfat al-Nafis provides perhaps the most detailed depictions; see Raja Ali Haji bin Ahmad, *The Precious Gift (Tuhfat al-Nafis)*, An annotated translation by V. Matheson and B. Watson Andaya (Kuala Lumpur, Oxford University Press, 1982), 259–61, 288–9, 300–1. For Abdullah's account of his daughter's death, including his advocation of submission to Allah's will and thus the privatization of grief that follows this faith, see Abdullah bin Abdul Kadir, *The Hikayat Abdullah*, An annotated translation by A. H. Hill (Kuala Lumpur, Oxford University Press, 1970), 286–7.

3. *Straits Times*, 2 May 1907, 7.

4. Neonatal refers to the first four weeks after birth; post-neonatal is used here for the subsequent two months.

5. Government of Straits Settlements, *Annual Departmental Reports 1905* (hereafter *SSAR 1905*) (Singapore, Government Printing Office, 1906), 189, 628.

6. Government of Straits Settlements, Commission Appointed to Inquire into the Causes of the Present Housing Difficulties in Singapore, and the Steps which should be Taken to Remedy such Difficulties (hereafter Housing Commission), *Proceedings and Report. Vol. 1: Instruments of Appointment and Report* (Singapore, Government Printing Office, 1918), A63.

7. *Straits Times*, 26 June 1907, 7.

8. Housing Commission, op. cit., A63.

9. *Straits Times*, 7 July 1910, 6.

10. Housing Commission, op. cit., A4.

11. Ibid.

12. *SSAR 1927* (Singapore, Government Printing Office, 1928), 781.

13. *SSAR 1933* (Singapore, Government Printing Office, 1934), 400.

14. *Straits Times*, 26 June 1907, 7.

15. J. W. Scharff, *A Note on Public Health Administration in the Northern Settlement (Penang)* (Penang, The Criterion Press, n.d. [c.1932]).

16. *SSAR 1936* (Singapore, Government Printing Office, 1938), 1:922–3.

17. *SSAR 1935* (Singapore, Government Printing Office, 1927), 2:162.

18. See for example *SSAR 1905*, 681; *SSAR 1935*, 2:815; Files of the Institute of Medical Research, IMR 54/1931, 23.

19. *SSAR 1910* (Singapore: Government Printing Office, 1911), 581. J. Albert, 'Studies on Infantile Beri-beri Based on Five Hundred Fourteen Cases', *The Philippines Journal of Science* 45, 2 (1931), 297–318, argued that infants nursed by women with beri-beri were also infected, and that this accounted for over 28% of all infant deaths. The incidence of maternal and infantile beri-beri need not coincide for this to occur. In an autobiographical account, Hobbs argued that Chinese women in Malacca fed a red rice porridge called *chobee* produced large quantities of milk and were able to breast-feed with ease; in an experiment, women fed with dehusked but not pounded rice produced a 'copious milk supply and thriving babies, instead of the miserable starved infants, whose mothers were without breast milk, presumably because they had lived on pounded rice'. See H. M. Hobbs, 'Welfare Clinics in Malaya', Rhodes House Library, Colonial Records Project 1962, *Mss Indian Ocean S38*, 1–2.

20. *SSAR 1936*, 1:900–1.

21. Government of Federated Malay States, *Colonial Reports. Annual Reports on the Social and Economic Progress of the People of the Federated Malay States, 1933* (hereafter *FMSAR 1933*) (Kuala Lumpur, Government Printing Office, 1934), 9.

22. W. J. Vickers and J. H. Strahan, *A Health Survey of the State of Kedah with Special Reference to Rice Field Malaria, Nutrition, and Water Supply, 1935–1936* (Kuala Lumpur, Kyle, Palmer and Co., 1936), 2.

23. *SSAR 1936*, 1:922.

24. *SSAR 1935*, 2:815.

25. *FMSAR 1934* (London, His Majesty's Stationery Office, 1936), 9.

26. *FMSAR 1935* (London, His Majesty's Stationery Office, 1936), 9.

27. Files of the Colonial Office, Social Services Department, CO859/53/12257 (1941), 2.

28. E. W. Darville, 'Maternity and child welfare work in Penang, 1927–35, 1935–41. Lectures given at the London School of Hygiene and Tropical Medicine, 1935; Account of the work done by E. W. Darville in the Government Welfare Clinics, Penang, by Mrs Crane-Williams, 1933 (Typescript)', Rhodes House Library, Colonial Records Project, *Mss Indian Ocean S134*, 17.

29. Scharff, 26.

30. *SSAR 1905*, op. cit., 715

31. *SSAR 1906* (Singapore, Government Printing Office, 1907), 237.

32. *SSAR 1908* (Singapore, Government Printing Office, 1910), 499.

33. L. Manderson, 'Bottle Feeding and Ideology in Colonial Malaya: The Production of Change', *International Journal of Health Services* 12, 4 (1982), 612.

34. *SSAR 1911* (Singapore, Government Printing Office, 1912), 519.

35. *SSAR 1910*, 507.

36. *SSAR 1914* (Singapore, Government Printing Office, 1915), 482.

37. Darville, op. cit., 19.

38. Ibid.

39. Ibid.

40. Ibid., 22.

41. Files of the Institute of Medical Research, IMR 59/1923, 'Annual Report for 1922', 2.

42. Files of the Colonial Office, Social Services Department, CO859/46/12101/4A, 1943, 9.

43. G. I. H. Braine, 'State of Kelantan, Annual Report of the Medical Department 1948', Rhodes House Library, Colonial Records Project, *Mss Indian Ocean S37*, 31.

44. Mrs Crane-Williams, in Darville, op. cit., 52.

45. *SSAR 1934*, 1014.

46. Ibid., 1010

47. Files of the Colonial Office, Social Services Department, CO859/14/3550/18 (1939), Annex 1: Miss I. Simmons to Haynes, 29 June 1939.

48. *SSAR 1905*, 681.

49. *SSAR 1922* (Singapore, Government Printing Office, 1924), 572–3.

50. Files of the Colonial Office, Social Services Department, CO859/46/12101/317, Medical Education Committee on Training of Nurses for Colonial Territories. Papers circulated to Committee Members: CNC (A) 12, Statements in Sub-Committee A of the C.N.C., 4th Meeting, 11 March 1944, 6.

51. Darville, op. cit., 7–8

52. Ibid., 11

53. Ibid., 10.

54. *SSAR 1927* (Singapore, Government Printing Office, 1928), 902.

55. *Straits Times*, 2 May 1907, 7. Published and unpublished records indicate that milk supplies were indeed polluted and diluted. Dixon refers to locally supplied milk as an 'appalling liquid . . . flavoured with cow dung and usually speckled with dead flies'; A. Dixon, 'Milk production in Singapore', Royal Commonwealth Society, London, *Files of the British Association of Malaya*, BAM IV/7. Imported milk was often also of poor quality, at times light on fats and solids; see Files of the Institute of Medical Research, IMR 164/1925, 'Analysis of Milk Supplied by the Cold Storage–N. Z. Dairy Co., Anchor Brand.' See also Manderson, op. cit. 600.

56. *SSAR 1910*, 581, *SSAR 1914*, 482; Files of the Colonial Office, Social Services Department, CO859/14/3550, 1939, 39.

57. Manderson, op. cit., 598–605.

58. Files of the Colonial Office, C0237/265/22834, 1900, 838.

59. Manderson, op. cit., 610.

60. *SSAR 1926* (Singapore, Government Printing Office, 1928), 423–4.

61. *SSAR 1927*, 781–2.

62. A. Castellani, 'The Adaption of European Women and Children to Tropical Climates', *Proceedings of the Royal Society of Medicine* 24 (1931), 95–8. Castellani argued that lactation was difficult for European women: 'the secretion of the mammary glands becoming scanty after a short time; very few women can nurse their babies for more than a few weeks' (96).

63. *SSAR 1914*, 482.

64. Ibid.

65. Nestles donated weighing machines, milk, feeding bottles, teats and valves to government clinics and the Singapore Children's Welfare Society in Singapore (*SSAR 1927*, 902) and to the government clinics in Malacca (ibid., 730), and also supplied milk bottles to the Penang clinics (Darville, op. cit., 10). Private individuals also donated milk to the Penang clinics (ibid., 55).

66. *SSAR 1908*, 6.

67. *SSAR 1927*, 730.

68. Darville, op. cit., 23.

69. *SSAR 1922*, 572–3.

70. Darville, op. cit., 11–12.

71. Files of the Colonial Office, Social Services Department, CO859/153/12402/ 8, 1948, C. D. Williams and J. W. Scharff, 'Preventive Paediatrics. An Experiment in Health Work in Trengganu in 1940–41', 25.

72. *FMSAR 1930* (Kuala Lumpur, Government Printing Office, 1931), 56.

73. *FMSAR 1934*, 20.

74. Mrs. Crane-Williams, in Darville, op. cit., 49.

75. *SSAR 1927*, 734.

76. Ibid.

77. *FMSAR 1928* (Kuala Lumpur, Government Printing Office, 1929), 49.

78. *SSAR 1936*, 2:952.

79. Files of the Institute of Medical Research, IMR 72/1923; for Malacca, see *SSAR 1926*, 420.

80. Darville, op. cit., 43.

81. Ibid, 41–2; on p. 27 she notes that a number of men did in fact attend the clinics with their infants and small children.

82. *FMSAR 1926* (London, His Majesty's Stationery Office. 1927), 38.

INDEX

ACEH: and war captives, 42, 43
Acupuncture, 168–9, 173
Agriculture: and fertility, 11, 39–40,
    43; impact of new crops, 13–15; and
    influenza pandemic, 249–50;
    rice shortages, 49, 59–60. *See also*
    Cultivation System; Famine
Agung, Sultan of Mataram, 39, 42–3
Ambon, 246
Anatomy, 178, 180–1
Animism: and low birth rates, 39–40
Astrology, 173–4
Ayutthaya, 37; founding linked to
    cholera, 144; smallpox in, 147

BALI: *baris* dance, 134–5, 141 n56;
    and Islam, 127–32, 139 n18;
    population trends in, 34, 36, 47;
    ritual and welfare, 117–18, 136.
    See also Cholera; Leprosy; Plague;
    Rangda; Siwa-Buddhism; Smallpox;
    Tantrism
Balian (healer), 119, 135
Bangka, 242
Bangkok: cholera in, 148–56
Banten, 34, 37, 39, 72, 86; population,
    34
Batavia, 37, 43, 76, 82, 83, 84, 88 n14;
    artesian wells, 196–7; canals, 192,
    196, 208 n26; Chinese in, 190, 191,
    192, 204; Chinese Hospital, 197,
    198, 202; Ciliwung River, 192, 207
    n9; death rate in, 206; Europeans in
    189, 191–3; Indonesians in, 191,
    193–5; populations trends, 189–90,
    206–7 n3; public health
    programmes, 195–9; Tanjung
    Priok harbour, 208 n26; Western
    medicine in, 198–202. *See also*
    Cholera; Dysentery; Malaria;
    Medical training; Water supply
Beri-beri, 74, 81, 108, 200, 262, 280
    n19
Bikol region (Philippines): cholera in,

92, 104, 106, 110 n4 & 5, 112 n27
    & 30, 113, n33 & 38; famine in, 92,
    107, 108, 112 n30, 113 n37;
    mortality rates in, 92, 97–107
Birth control, 5, 11, 26 n29, 27 n39,
    41, 45 n29
Birth rates, 40
Bleeker, P., 192, 193, 201, 207 n16
Borneo: birth rate, 40; population 36,
    47
Bosch, Dr Willem, 59, 62
Brockman, E. L., 260
Bronchitis, 82
Brunei: birth rate, 40; population, 47;
    stature, 38
Buddhism: demographic impact of,
    41, 42; sutra chanting to ward off
    pestilence, 148–9, 150–1, 154–5, 175
Burg, Dr C. L. van der, 52, 55,
    199–200
Burial, 176, 196, 225, 247. *See also*
    Cremation
Burma: population, 36; 'roasting' after
    childbirth, 39; and war captives, 42
Buton, 247

CALON ARANG (Widow-Witch),
    121–5, 137 n1
Cambodia: population, 35, 36
Carey, P. B. R., 61
Celibacy, 11
Census: Burma, 39; Indonesia, 36–7,
    40, 254; Java, 34, 72–3; Philippines,
    26 n33, 93. *See also* Parish records;
    Tributos; Village registration
Champa: population, 36
Childbearing age at, 39
Children: and parental attitudes, 13,
    23 n5, 27 n39, 38. *See also* Infant
    feeding; Infant mortality
Chinese: in Batavia, 190–2, 204; in
    Malaya, 259–60, 269–71, 273, 277;
    riots against, 247–8
Chinese medical traditions, 164–6,

170, 171–2. *See also* 'Humours'; *Yin and yang*
Cholera (*Cholera asiatica*), 12, 14, 16, 19, 53–4, 142–3, 205, 206; associated with wet season, 110 n5, 135; in Bali, 132–6, 137; in Batavia, 78, 190, 192–3, 194, 195, 199–200, 203, 204, 207 n6; distinguished from *Cholera nostras*, 49, 52–3; in Java, 49, 50, 51, 52–5, 60, 64, 74, 75–8, 83; 'mixtures', 18, 55, 200; in Philippines, 20, 92, 104, 106, 108, 110 n4, 112 n27 & 30, 113 n33 & 38; in Siam, 22, 143–61; Siamese terminology for, 156–8; vaccine, 76, 82, 88; in Vietnam, 154, 161 n57, 176, 179, 183
Christianity: and fertility, 40–2
Comets, 145
Concubinage: demographic impact of, 39
Crawfurd, John, 61–2, 153–4
Cremation, 119, 130, 140 n38, 148, 149
Cultivation System: impact of on health, 50, 85

DAENDELS, Governor-General, 56, 67 n18, 192
Damrong Ratchanuphap, Prince: historical writing of, 144–5, 150, 154, 156
Dance: to exorcise disease, 134–5, 154
Darville, Miss E., 267, 269, 272
Đặng Văn Ngừ, Dr, 182
Daum, P. A., 203–4
Demographic equilibrium: 16th to 19th centuries, 8–9
Dengue fever, 56
Despiau, J. M., 178
Dewa Majapahit, 125, 126, 127, 131
Diarrhoea: infantile, 12, 14; in Java, 51, 52
Diphtheria, 74, 82
Dissection, 180–1
Đỗ Phong Thuần, 181
Dokter-djawa, 58, 74, 87 n9, 197–8
Doumer, Governor General Paul, 178
Drainage: of fish ponds, 88 n28; of swamps, 58, 65, 79–80, 84, 89 n45, 196. *See also* Swamps
Drug use, 23 n2, 65. *See also Sirih*
Dukun (local healer, Java), 51, 200–3, 243, 244

Durand, Maurice, 172
Durga (Balinese Goddess of Death), 121–4
Dysentery, 12, 181; in Batavia, 82, 191, 192, 201; in Java, 49, 51, 52, 74, 81, 83

EDUCATION, health: in Java, 222–3, 243; in Malaya, 260, 272–5, 279; in Vietnam, 179
Erlangga (r. 1010–42, Java), 121–3
Europe: comparisons with, 18, 37–8; impact of, 9. *See also* Medical intervention; Plague; Western medicine

FAMINE, 10, 108, 114 n49; in Bengal, 49; in Bikol region, 92, 107, 108, 112 n30, 113 n37; in India, 85, 86; in Semarang, 52, 60; in Siam, 147; in Vietnam, 15
Fertility: patterns of, 11, 25, 39–43, 65
'Fever', 12, 51, 52, 55–60, 72, 74, 76, 89 n35, 258; in Batavia, 190, 194, 207 n6
Fleas: Bacot and Martin research on, 221–2; and plague, 213, 214, 219, 220–2
Flight: as factor in spreading disease, 149, 155, 158, 248
Flu, Dr P. C., 216, 220
Folklore: disease in, 253
Food consumption: and health, 65
Fromm, Dr, 59

GIA LONG: and medicine, 177, 178
Gianti Peace (1755), 9, 35, 42
Goitre, 138
Gonorrhoea, 51
Gorkom, Dr W. J. van, 206, 216–18, 219, 223, 228

HAFFKINE'S VACCINE, 220, 230 n18
Hải Thượng Lãn Ông, 171–2, 177, 181
Hamblin, Mrs, 267
Haw Par medical compendium, 179
Health inspectors (*inspecteurs*), 72, 74, 88 n12. *See also* Plague Service
Helminthic diseases, 15
Hồ Chi Minh, 183
Hồ Đắc An, 181
Hồ Đắc Di, Dr, 180
Hogendorp, W. van, 61
Horoscopy, 173–4

Housing: destruction of in epidemic control, 76, 212; improvements to combat plague, 212, 214, 215, 222, 223, 225, 227, 228, 230 n30, 233–4
Huard, Pierre, 172
'Humours', 18, 168, 201; 'hot' and 'cold', 18; 172, 183
Hydrick, J. L., 223
Hygiene: improvements in, 13, 19, 65, 83–4, 222–3. *See also* Education

INDONESIA. *See* Aceh; Bali; Batavia; Influenza; Java; Lombok; Madura; Sulawesi; Sumatra; Sumba; Surabaya
Infant feeding: artificial, 263, 269–72, 282 n65; breast, 11, 26 n27, 271, 272, 280 n19, 281 n62
Infant mortality, 5, 14, 62, 83, 228; in Batavia, 83, 195; in Malaya, 257–82
Infant Welfare Centres: in Malaya, 267, 268, 269, 272–5, 277, 279
Influenza, 12, 82; complications of, 236; demographic impact of, Indonesia, 238–9, 254; groups at risk, 240–2, 250; impact on agriculture, 249–52; in Indonesia, 235–56; 1918 pandemic, 21, 72–3, 79, 235–6, 276; and weather conditions, 245–6
Injections: popular attitudes towards, 21, 30 n69, 183, 219, 230 n19
Insecticides, 89 n45, 227
Islam: demographic impact of, 41, 42; penetration of Java, and smallpox, 126–32, 140 n39

JACOBS, Julius, 133–4, 137 n1, 140 n43
Java: mortality patterns in, 49–52, 70–90; population trends, 36, 43, 46, 84, 207 n4. *See also* Cholera; *Dukun*; Dysentery; Education; Housing; Leprosy; Malaria; Pharmacopoeia; Plague; Plague Service; Semarang; Smallpox; Surabaya; Tuberculosis; Typhoid; Yaws
Java War (1825–30), 49, 50, 62
Jayakusunu (ruler of Bali), 118
Johor: population, 36

KEDAH (Saiburi): and cholera, 148, 150, 151, 156; population, 34, 36
Koch, Robert, 159 n3

LAMPHUN (Haripunjaya), 143
Langlois, Fr., 178
Legislation: emergency regulations, Java (1919), 243; Epidemic Diseases Ordinance, Java (1911), 252; Indies Health Act (1882), 206; Influenza Ordinance, Java (1921), 252; midwifery, 265
Lesser Sunda Islands: population, 36, 47
Leprosy, 179; in Bali, 119–20, 137; in Java, 49, 51, 66 n7
Lice: and plague, 215, 221–2
Life expectancy, 5
Lombok, 130, 131, 132, 240
Luzon: population, 34, 36

McNEIL, Miss A., 272
Macaling, Ratu Gege (Balinese protective deity), 132–6
Madura, 42, 43, 76, 215, 247
Magic: in Bali, 117–41; in Java, 246; in Vietnam, 174
Majapahit: fall of and smallpox, 125–7, 131, 132, 140 n48; and Islam, 126–32
Makassar: plague in, 229 n5; stature, 38; and war captives, 42
Malaria (*Plasmodium* parasite), 12, 19, 108, 179, 205, 276; in Batavia, 191, 192, 200; and 'fever', 56, 74, 78; in Java, 49, 50, 51, 55–9, 74, 78–80, 83, 84; and public works, 56, 57, 67 n18; and rinderpest, 57; and spread of *sawah* cultivation, 56–7, 64, 88 n23. *See also* Drainage; Mosquitoes; Quinine
Malaya: medical facilities in, 278; population, 36, 43. *See also* Education; Infant feeding; Infant mortality; Infant Welfare Centres; Midwives, Penang
Malnutrition, 6, 15, 19, 67 n22. *See also* Nutrition
Maluku: influenza in, 240; population, 36, 47
Mantra: used against disease, 127–9, 132, 133, 139 n32
Mantri (health workers), 218–19, 222–3
Marriage: age at, 11, 25–6 n26, 38
Mataram, 42–3; population, 34
Mayadanawa (ruler of Bali), 119, 138 n6

Measles, 82
Medical intervention: efficacy of, 10,
  13, 14, 15, 20–1, 64–5, 82–4, 87, 89
  n41 & 44, 200, 243, 279. *See also*
  Cholera vaccine; Plague vaccine;
  Quinine; Smallpox vaccine
Medical profession, status of:
  Vietnam, 177–9
Medical training: in Batavia, 197–8; in
  Java, 228; in Vietnam, 178–9,
  180–1. *See also* Midwives
Mekong Delta: population, 36
Meningitis, epidemic cerebrospinal,
  74–5
Mentawei Island, 40
Meteorite showers, 149
Midwives, training of: in Batavia, 198;
  in Malaya, 264–7
Migration: to frontier areas, 11; in
  Java, 50, 57
Mindanao: population, 36
Morbidity, 15–16, 28 n49, 65, 117–41,
  189–209
Mortality: 'background' and 'crisis',
  12–13, 49–51; decline in, 10–15, 21,
  65; in Philippines, 91–114. *See also*
  Infant mortality
Mosquitoes (*Anopheles*), 55, 192, 194,
  203, 221
Moxabustion, 168–9, 173
Muruts (North Borneo): and
  gonorrhea, 41
Music: and epidemics, 141 n56

NAKHON SITHAMMARAT, 146, 156
Neo-Confucian ideology: and
  medicine, 178
Nguyễn Đinh Chiểu, 169, 170, 174
Nias, South: birth rates in, 40
Nutrition: and children, 89 n48;
  improvements in, 6, 11, 13, 14–15;
  and pregnancy, 262. *See also* Food
  Consumption; Infant feeding;
  Malnutrition

OTTEN, Dr L., 216, 218, 220, 221,
  222; and plague vaccine, 225–6
Ouwehand, C. D., 192, 193, 206

PAHANG: population, 36
Parasitic infestation, 6, 14, 181
Paratyphoid A, 74
Parish records: as data source, 7, 22,
  91–2, 93–5, 102–7

Patani, 146; population, 36
Pax imperica, 10–11, 43
Pegu: stature in, 38
Penang: and cholera, 148, 149, 150,
  151
Penicillin, 182
Pharmaceuticals: in Vietnam, 168,
  173, 176
Pharmacopoeia, indigenous, 17; in
  Java, 201, 203, 209 n58, 245; in
  Vietnam, 169–71, 181–2
Philippines. *See* Bikol region;
  Cholera; Luzon; Mindanao;
  Mortality; Parish records; *Tributos*;
  Tuberculosis; Visayas
Plague: bacillus (*Pasteurella pestis*),
  178, 210; in Bali, 120–5, 137;
  combattive measures, 212, 214, 215,
  216, 218–19, 220, 222, 223, 227; in
  Europe, 6, 14, 122; in India, 219,
  220–1; in Java, 20–1, 22, 74, 76, 81,
  89 n33, 210–34; in Siam, 143–4, 146;
  and spleen puncture, 212, 218, 225,
  229 n7; vaccine, 211, 213, 219, 220,
  226–7. *See also* Housing
Plague Service, Java, 212, 216, 218,
  219, 220, 222–3, 225
Pneumonia, 82
Poliomyelitis, 75
Polygamy: royal, 38–9
Population growth: pre-colonial,
  33–47; 19th century, 8, 9–13, 65,
  189–90; world comparisons, 13, 25
  n19
Post-mortem examination, 192. *See
  also* Dissection
Print media: and medicine, 179; and
  public health, 213
Professionalization, of physicians,
  29 n60, 177
Purwokerto Demonstration Health
  Unit, 89 n41
Pulse taking, 166–7

QUARANTINE, 76–7
Quinine, 58–9, 64, 79, 80, 88 n14 &
  25 & 26, 89 n31, 182, 186 n57, 200

RAADT, Dr O. L. E. de, 215, 222, 227
Rabies, 179
Rangda (widow-witch), 121–4, 138–9
  n17
Rats: field rat as plague host, 227–8;
  and plague, 138 n14, 210–34

Religion: and disease, 17–21. *See also*
Buddhism; Christianity; Islam;
Siwa-Buddhism; Tantrism
Raffles, Sir Thomas Stamford, 62; and
1815 census, 37 n(g)
Riau, 242
Rinderpest, 57, 108
Ritual: as response to disease, 117–18,
123, 133, 136, 175, 204, 245.
See also Buddhism; Dance
Rivai, Dr Abdul, 243–4
Roorda van Eysinga, P. P., 203
Rosier, H. J., 225

SA'DAN TORAJA: birth rate, 40
Sanitation: improvements in, 14, 83,
89 n44, 279; lack of, 196, 260–1
Scabies: in Java, 51, 64
Secularization, 6, 13, 21
Semarang, 76, 78, 79, 88 n14
Semmelink, Dr J., 53
Siam: population, 34–6; stature in, 38;
and war captives, 42. *See also*
Cholera; Plague; Smallpox; Typhoid
Simmons, Miss I. M., 272
Simpson, Dr W. J., 260
Sirih chewing, 201, 208 n49. *See also*
Drug use
Siwa-Buddhism, 131–2, 139 n20
Slaves, 40, 42, 139
Smallpox, 12, 14, 23, 108, 139 n20; in
Bali, 64, 68 n53, 125–32, 137; in
Bengal, 68 n53; inoculation, 131,
153, 197; in Java, 49–52, 60–4, 74,
76, 78, 80–1, 83, 197, 208 n31;
linked with commerce, 131, 139
n30; 7-year cycle of, 64; in Siam,
146–8, 157; vaccination, 10, 19, 27
n28, 60–4, 68 n49, 82, 83, 88 n14,
89 n31, 131, 178; variolation, 62–3,
68 n44; in Vietnam, 178. *See also*
Islam
Sources, problems of: crisis mentality,
6, 12; early texts, 4, 8, 9, 16;
statistics, 73–5. *See also* Parish
records
Spirits: propitiation of, 117–41, 154–5,
172–6, 245
Songkhla, 146, 156, 160 n39
Stature, 38
Streptomycin, 182
Sulawesi, 240; population, 36, 47
Sulfonamide, 182, 183
Sulu: population, 36

Sumatra: population, 36, 47
Sumba: gonorrhea in, 41
Sumba, East: birth rate, 40
Sumbawa, 247
Supernatural: and disease, 16–21.
See also Magic; Spirits
Surabaya, 42–3, 76–8, 88 n14, 205,
213–14
Swamps: and sickness, 144, 160 n39,
192, 194
Swellengrebel, N. H., 214, 215, 221,
222
Syncretism: in approaches to healing,
17–18, 20–1, 183–4, 202–3
Syphilis, 51, 74, 179, 183, 262

TANA TORAJA: influenza in, 240
Tantrism, 122, 138
Temples: building of as protection
against disease, 118; of medicine
(*Y Miếu*), 177
Tetanus neonatorum, 258, 264
Thiel, P. H. van, 214
Thiphākọrawong, Chaophrayā:
historical writings, 149–53, 156–7
Tidore: and concubines, 39
Timor, 240
Toba Batak: and birth rates, 40
Tôn Thất Tùng, Dr, 180, 181, 182
Torajans: and birth rates, 40
Trachoma, 75, 82
Trade: and disease, 11, 55, 76–8,
124–5, 210, 213
Traditional medicine, 16–21, *See also*
Dukun; Pharmacopoeia; Vietnam
Tributọs: records of, 92–3
Tụ Đức, King (r. 1847–88), 178
Tuberculosis, 15; in Java, 75, 82, 192;
in Philippines, 6, 12; in Vietnam,
179
Tuệ Tĩnh, 170–1, 177
Typhoid (*Typhus abdominalis*), 12,
14; in Java, 49, 50, 51, 59–60; 74,
81, 83, 89 n35, 192; in Siam, 147,
157

USANA BALI, 117, 119, 137 n1

VACCINATION. *See* Cholera; Plague;
Smallpox
Venereal disease, 41–2, 262; in Java,
51, 74, 81. *See also* Syphilis
Vietnam, *See* Cholera; Education;
Medical training; Pharmaceuticals;

Pharmacopoeia; Smallpox,
Vietnamese
Vietnamese medical traditions:
Northern (*Thuốc Bắc*), 164–9, 173,
174, 176, 179; Southern (*Thuốc
Nam*) 169–72, 173, 179, 181–2;
spirit, 172–3, 174–5, 176; Western
(*Tây Y*), 178–9, 180–4; Eastern
(*Đông Y*), 180, 182–3
Village registration: Java, 70–3
Visayas: population, 34, 36

WALES, H. G. Q., 145
Warfare: and pestilence, 123, 134,
147; and population trends, 42–3
Water supply: improvements to, 14,
76, 83; pollution of, in Batavia, 192,
193, 195, 196, in Europe, 205, 209
n70, in Malaya, 261
Western medicine, 19; in Indonesia,
199–202, 244–5; in Malaya, 267,
272–3, 275; in Siam, 153, 158; in
Vietnam, 178–9, 180–4
Women: medical examination of, 166;
as medical practitioners, 202, 209
n53; work and childcare, 263–4;
workloads of and fertility, 39–40.
See also Marriage; Midwives;
Nutrition

YAWS (*framboesia*): in Java, 49, 51
Yersin, Dr, 178, 186 n48
Yin and *yang*, 17, 164, 173